Current Topics in Anaesthesia

General Editors: Stanley A. Feldman
Cyril F. Scurr

5 Neonatal Anaesthesia and Perioperative Care
Second Edition

Neonatal Anaesthesia and Perioperative Care

Second Edition

David J. Hatch
MB, BS, FFARCS
Consultant in Anaesthesia and Respiratory Function
The Hospital for Sick Children, Great Ormond Street, London;
Formerly, Sub-Dean, Institute of Child Health, University of
London

and

Edward Sumner
MA, BM, BCh, FFARCS
Consultant in Paediatric Anaesthesia and Intensive Care
The Hospital for Sick Children, Great Ormond Street, London

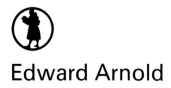

Edward Arnold

First published in Great Britain 1981 by
Edward Arnold (Publishers) Ltd,
41 Bedford Square,
London WC1B 3DQ

Edward Arnold (Australia) Pty Ltd,
80 Waverley Road,
Caulfield East,
Victoria 3145,
Australia

Edward Arnold,
3 East Read Street,
Baltimore,
Maryland 21202,
USA

Second edition 1986

British Library Cataloguing in Publication Data
Hatch, David J.
  Neonatal anaesthesia and perioperative care.——
  2nd ed.——(Current topics in anaesthesia; v. 5)
  1. Pediatric anaesthesia   2. Infants (Newborn)——
  Surgery
  I. Title   II. Sumner, Edward   III. Series
  617'.96798   RD139

ISBN 0 7131 4494 7

Text set in 10 on 11 pt Monotype Times
by Butler & Tanner Ltd
printed in Great Britain by Butler & Tanner Ltd
Frome and London

General preface to series

The current rate of increase of scientific knowledge is such that it is recognized that '... ninety per cent of all the existing knowledge which can be drawn upon for the practice of medicine is less than 10 years old'.*

In an acute specialty, such as anaesthesia, failure to keep abreast of advances can seriously affect the standard of patient care. The need for continuing education is widely recognized and indeed it is mandatory in some countries.

However, due to the flood of new knowledge which grows in an exponential fashion greatly multiplying the pool of information every decade, the difficulty which presents itself is that of selecting and retrieving the information of immediate value and clinical relevance. This series has been produced in an effort to overcome this dilemma.

By producing a number of authoritative reviews the Current Topics Series has allowed the General Editors to select those in which it is felt there is a particular need for a digest of the large amount of literature, or for a clear statement of the relevance of new information.

By presenting these books in a concise form it should be possible to publish these reviews quickly. Careful selection of authors allows the presentation of mature clinical judgement on the relative importance of this new information.

The information will be clearly presented and, by emphasizing only key references and by avoiding an excess of specialist jargon, the books will, it is hoped, prove to be useful and succinct.

It has been our intention to avoid the difficulties of the large textbooks, with their inevitable prolonged gestation period, and to produce books with a wider appeal than the comprehensive, detailed, and highly specialized monographs. By this means we hope that the Current Topics in Anaesthesia Series will make a valuable contribution by meeting the demands of continuing education in anaesthesia.

Westminster Hospital London

Stanley A. Feldman
Cyril F. Scurr

*Education and Training for the Professions.
  Sir Frank Hartley, Wilkinson Lecture
  Delivered at Institute of Dental Surgery, 30.1.78
  University of London Bulletin, May 1978, No. 45, p. 3

Preface

For this second edition we again follow the general philosophy of the series by concentrating on those aspects of neonatal care which are of immediate clinical relevance to the anaesthetist, whether in the operating theatre or in the intensive care unit. We include essential new information on drugs and techniques and incorporate the new and greater understandings which are emerging from the increasing survival of babies with gestational ages as low as 26 weeks.

As before, the first chapter is devoted to perinatal physiology, because the differences between the anaesthetic needs for the newborn and the older child depend largely on differences in physiology. The chapter has been expanded to include new information in this field but we have continued to link anatomy, physiology, pharmacology and neonatal medicine with intensive care and anaesthetic practice. The title of this second edition has been extended to include perioperative care: this reflects our expansion of Chapters 2 and 4 to contain material which we hope will be of interest to non-anaesthetic medical colleagues, including surgeons and neonatologists, who are also involved in the care of small babies.

The contents of those chapters which deal with clinical matters are, as before, almost entirely based on our own experience at the Hospitals for Sick Children, Great Ormond Street, London, where more than 500 anaesthetics are administered annually to neonatal patients for all types of surgery. The clinical approach is based on concepts and techniques which have proved safe over many years of use. The references have again been limited to a brief list at the end of each chapter and contain only those we consider to be important or those which will provide an easy guide to further study of the subject.

Neonatal intensive care for medical problems has traditionally been the province of neonatal paediatricians and this volume does not attempt to cover all aspects of this subject which include, for example, detailed care of the very preterm baby and infant feeding. We have, however, mentioned those aspects of perioperative care which we believe are essential to the safe practice of neonatal anaesthesia. Because of the increasing survival of babies of low gestational age, the application of the term 'neonatal' has broadened and much of the information in this volume is now relevant to many babies beyond the first month of extrauterine life.

1986

D.J.H.
E.S.

Acknowledgements

This edition could not have been completed without advice from many medical colleagues. We are particularly grateful to Mr Marc de Leval, Dr Michael Dillon, Dr Peter Helms, Mr Harold Nixon and Mr Jaroslav Stark of Great Ormond Street for helping with various sections.

We also thank Dorothy Duranti, Rita Hatch and Diana Newlands for help with preparation of the manuscript, the Department of Diagnostic Imaging, Great Ormond Street, for providing x-rays, and Ray Lunnon and Carol Reeves of the Department of Illustration, Great Ormond Street, for producing many beautiful photographs. We are grateful also to the authors and publishers who have kindly allowed us to use certain Figures and Tables.

D.J.H.
E.S.

Contents

Perinatal physiology

Introduction and definitions

Prior to birth the fetus lives in a protected environment and, although most organs are capable of function even weeks before full term, it is not until after delivery that the functions of the placenta are at once replaced by the lungs, kidneys and gastrointestinal tract. After birth, itself a great physiological stress, the baby faces a harsh environment. The delivery may have been traumatic, and drugs and anaesthesia given to the mother may still be affecting the baby. After birth, organs and physiological systems develop at different rates; for example, the liver reaches maturity long before the kidneys or the central nervous system. The development of the neuromuscular junction is related to the length of extrauterine life rather than to gestational age. During the early days of life, adaptations occur in all systems, sometimes even with a transitional stage, to fit the baby eventually for adult life. The degree of maturity at birth and the rate at which these adaptations occur depend largely on the gestational or postconceptual age—the age at birth expressed in weeks after conception.

The neonatal period is generally regarded as the first 28 days of extra-uterine life. By the end of this period most physiological systems have matured reasonably well in healthy infants born at term, but those of low postconceptual age may take considerably longer to mature. No magical change occurs on the 28th day, and many of the problems discussed in this book have relevance in older infants. The differences between the baby and the adult, however, are clearly greatest in the newborn neonate, especially if birth occurs before term.

Preterm infants can themselves be classified according to their weight as well as their gestational age (Fig. 1.1). Significant physiological differences occur, particularly with regard to metabolism, between preterm infants who are small for gestational age (SGA), appropriate size for gestational age (AGA) or large for gestational age (LGA). Both SGA and LGA babies have a higher mortality rate than AGA babies at all gestational ages, and an accurate assessment of postconceptual age is therefore essential when assessing the risks of anaesthesia. In the absence of a reliable menstrual history from the mother, postconceptual age can be approximated by careful examination of the baby (see p. 57), but accurate assessment may require estimation of the lecithin/sphingomyelin ratio of the amniotic fluid. This is discussed in more detail on p. 3.

1

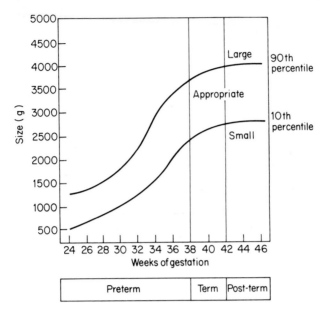

Fig. 1.1   Percentile chart of weight in relation to gestational age. (Reproduced, with permission, from Lubchenco, 1976)

Respiration

The lungs during fetal life

Before birth all gas exchange and acid–base balance is performed by the placenta, but the development of the lungs must prepare them to be able to take over full respiratory function by weeks 24–28 of gestation. The bronchial tree is fully developed by week 16, as are the preacinar blood vessels, whose development follows that of the airways. Respiration is not possible at this stage, however, because the airways are blind-ending tubules completely lined by non-respiratory cuboidal epithelium. During the fourth to sixth months the respiratory portion of the lung becomes delineated as blood vessels grow beneath this cuboidal epithelium, thinning it, whilst new branches, all with thin-walled epithelium, also develop. By week 28 the preacinar pattern of airways, arteries and veins is complete, the blood/gas barrier is thin and capillary vessels are present within the alveolar wall. Muscularization of the intra-acinar arteries does not however, keep pace with the appearance of new vessels.

Specialized type II pneumocytes of the alveolar epithelial lining become discernible by electron microscopy during the sixth month of gestation; these contain the osmophilic inclusion bodies widely thought to be the site of production of surfactant. This lipoprotein complex lowers surface tension in the fluid lining of the alveoli once a fluid/air interface has developed.

Without surfactant, the lungs would be unable to retain gas within them and would be unstable because the pressure within them required to prevent collapse due to surface tension is inversely proportional to their radius (Laplace formula). As areas of lung collapse, the collapsing forces increase and thus a state of unstable equilibrium exists. Although surfactant can be detected in lung extracts from human fetuses from week 23 onwards, the quantity which can be detected increases greatly towards term and this is one of the main reasons why the older fetus has a greater chance of surviving in air than those delivered very prematurely. Surfactant can be detected in fetal tracheal fluid by week 28 and clearly the potential for normal extrauterine life exists by this stage of development.

Recent work shows that it is possible to make accurate assessments of fetal maturity from measurements of biochemical substances in the amniotic fluid. The concentration of sphingomyelin in the amniotic fluid remains fairly constant throughout pregnancy whilst surfactant production is accompanied by the appearance of lecithin. A lecithin/sphingomyelin (L/S) ratio of more than 2.0 is normally present by weeks 35–36, and is 98 per cent accurate in predicting that an infant will not develop idiopathic respiratory distress syndrome of the newborn (RDS). The 2 per cent of infants with L/S ratios of 2.0 or more who do develop RDS usually have a history of asphyxia *in utero*, are born to diabetic mothers or have rhesus

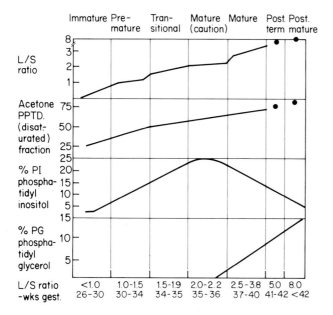

Fig. 1.2 Lecithin/sphingomyelin ratio and amniotic fluid phospholipids in relation to gestational age and lung maturity. (Reproduced, with permission, from Kulovich, Hallman and Gluck, 1979)

incompatibility and hydrops fetalis. Low L/S ratios (<1.5) are less reliable predictors of lung development, as are intermediate values, and measurements of the acid phospholipids phosphatidyl inositol (PI) and phosphatidyl glycerol (PG) have been found to be more accurate. PI levels in amniotic fluid reach their peak by weeks 35–36, whilst PG appears by week 35 and peaks at birth (Fig. 1.2). The presence of PG indicates a definite degree of lung maturity and is not affected by diabetes or asphyxia.

During the last 3 months of gestation there is further differentiation of the respiratory region of the lung, with additional respiratory bronchioles developing whose terminal saccules are capable of acting as gas-exchanging areas. New alveoli continue to grow, however, until 8 years of age, and their size increases until adult life.

During fetal life the lungs are filled with fluid, and although the respiratory muscles contract vigorously from time to time from an early stage of development, they cannot move much fluid in and out because of the large frictional forces involved. Ultrasound studies in humans have clearly demonstrated that these breathing movements are a normal feature of fetal life, and they may well be essential for normal lung development. This view is supported by the fact that infants with spinal muscular atrophy which begins *in utero* have small lungs whilst those whose disease begins after birth do not.

A chance observation in fetal lambs (Liggins and Howie, 1972) showed that steroids infused into lambs born prematurely caused unexpected survival. It has since been confirmed that steroids injected into the mother accelerate lung maturation in human fetuses, and this is now widely performed in obstetric practice. Careful evaluation is still required, however, with respect to any harmful long-term effects.

Gas transport in fetal life

The oxygen tension of fetal blood of 4 kPa (30 mmHg) is considerably lower than that of the mother, although levels of fetal Po_2 remain stable even with wide variations in maternal Pao_2. Raising the maternal Po_2 by 20 kPa (150 mmHg) increases fetal Po_2 by only 1.1 kPa (8mmHg), and falls in maternal Po_2 will also have relatively less effect on the fetus. Fetal blood has a greater affinity for oxygen than adult blood, which enables it to carry more oxygen in the presence of a relatively low Po_2; the oxygen/haemoglobin dissociation curve is shifted to the left (Fig. 1.3). This is due to the fact that fetal haemoglobin (HbF) is relatively insensitive to 2,3-diphosphoglycerate (2,3-DPG), which in itself lowers the oxygen affinity of the haemoglobin molecule. A decrease in pH (Fig. 1.4) and a rise in body temperature will move the dissociation curve to the right; conversely, a rise in pH or fall in body temperature will have the reverse effect. It might be thought that the increased affinity of fetal blood for oxygen would hinder the release of oxygen at the tissues, but the simultaneous uptake of carbon dioxide shifts the dissociation curve to the right. Because the tissue oxygen tension is so low—about 2 kPa (15mmHg)—and because the dissociation curve is so steep, adequate oxygen delivery to the tissues is ensured.

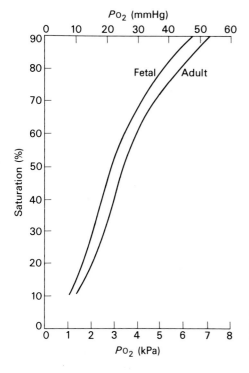

Fig. 1.3 Oxygen dissociation curves for fetal and adult blood. (Reproduced, with permission, from Darling *et al.*, 1941)

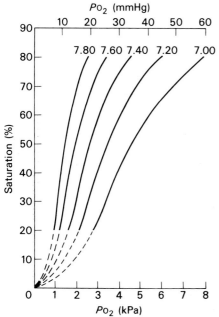

Fig. 1.4 Oxygen/haemoglobin dissociation curves for fetal blood at various pH levels. (Reproduced, with permission, from Hellegers and Schrueffer, 1961)

One method of expressing the position of the dissociation curve is to measure the oxygen tension at which the blood is 50 per cent saturated. This is known as the P_{50}. For adult blood the P_{50} is about 3.6 kPa (27 mmHg) whilst at birth it is around 2.7 kPa (20 mmHg). It rises slowly, reaching the adult value by 6 months of age. At birth approximately 70 per cent of the haemoglobin is HbF, and total replacement of this by HbA does not occur until about 3 months after birth. The steepness and position of the fetal oxygen/haemoglobin dissociation curve are advantageous for normal fetal gas exchange. After birth, however, severe tissue hypoxia can occur if arterial oxygen tension is allowed to fall substantially, since the AV oxygen content or 'unloading capacity' of HbF is considerably less than that of HbA (Fig. 1.5). In neonatal pulmonary disease with hypoxaemia this factor has led some workers to advocate exchange transfusion, replacing fetal blood with adult blood with its lower oxygen affinity.

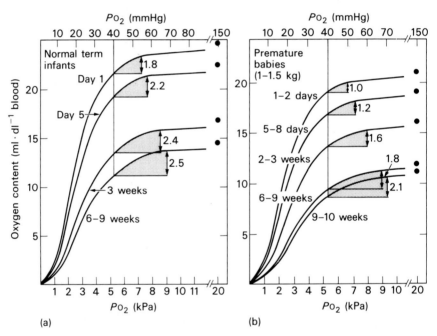

Fig. 1.5 The blood oxygen-releasing capacity at various ages from birth. (a) Term infants. (b) Preterm infants. The shaded areas represent AV oxygen content in ml $O_2 \cdot dl^{-1}$ blood. (Reproduced, with permission, from Delivoria-Papadopoulos, Roncevic and Oski, 1971)

Adaptation to extrauterine life

During vaginal delivery the baby's thorax is squeezed as it passes through the birth canal and up to 35 ml of fluid drains out of the mouth. As the thoracic cage re-expands at birth, this volume of fluid is replaced by the entry of an equivalent volume of air into the trachea and main air passages. At birth the type II pneumocytes rapidly discharge their surface active phospholipids into the alveolar space, and are then seen to be vacuolated rather than containing dense inclusion bodies.

Many factors stimulate the newborn infant to take its first breath, including non-specific stimuli such as sound, touch, temperature and the effect of gravity, but one of the main factors appears to be a sudden resetting of the chemoreceptors. The sudden increase in sensory activity arising at the moment of birth activates the reticular system and causes a resetting of the respiratory centres, so that levels of oxygen and carbon dioxide tension which previously did not stimulate respiration now do so. The arterial oxygen tension falls during the birth process from its fetal level of about 4 kPa (30 mmHg); levels as low as 2 kPa (15 mmHg) have been reported. Increased glycogen stores protect the newborn infant to some extent from hypoxic tissue damage; CO_2 tension rises from about 6.7 kPa (50 mmHg) with a consequent fall in pH from its fetal level of 7.2. The reduction in blood flow through the umbilical vessels is also an important factor in initiating the onset of respiration, possibly by causing a sudden change in blood flow through the carotid bodies. The chemoreceptors are certainly not essential since, in experimental animals, respiration will start

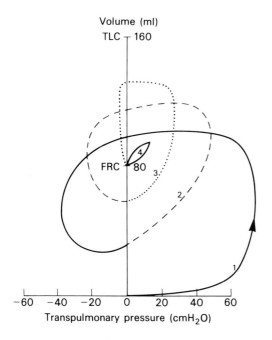

Fig. 1.6 The first four breaths. Each successive breath requires less pressure and adds increasing volume to the lungs. (Based on data from Karlberg and Koch, 1962)

if they are denervated. Chemoreceptor responses become sensitive to small changes in arterial blood gas tensions early in postnatal life.

After the onset of the first breath, which may require inspiratory pressures of $70\,cmH_2O$ or more, a functional residual capacity (FRC) of 30–35 $ml\cdot kg^{-1}$ is rapidly established (Fig. 1.6). Remaining lung fluid is removed by the pulmonary lymphatics and lung capillaries which open up with lung expansion. A normal FRC is usually established within 60 minutes of birth. The rapid rise in arterial oxygen tension which follows the onset of respiration leads to a dramatic fall in pulmonary vascular resistance and an uptake of up to 100 ml of blood into the pulmonary circulation. The fall in pulmonary vascular resistance with increased pulmonary blood flow, together with a reduction in inferior vena caval return due to clamping of the umbilical cord, cause left atrial pressure to exceed right atrial pressure with closure of the foramen ovale. As the arterial oxygen tension rises, the smooth muscle in the ductus arteriosus constricts and closure is usually physiologically complete within 10–15 hours. These cardiac and pulmonary changes are obviously interrelated; ventilation improves both pulmonary perfusion and surfactant release, which in turn help further improve ventilation. Surfactant synthesis is dependent upon satisfactory oxygenation and acid–base state. The chain of events in newborns who fail to breathe immediately after birth is described in Chapter 6.

Respiratory function in the newborn

Over the first few hours of life the newborn infant establishes a tidal volume of approximately $6\,ml\cdot kg^{-1}$ and breathes at between 30 and 40 breaths per minute. Many healthy infants weighing less than 1.5 kg have respiratory rates of 50-60 per minute for the first 2 months of life. The dead space/ tidal volume ratio is about 0.3, which is similar to the adult, but alveolar ventilation is approximately twice that of the adult at $150\,ml\cdot kg^{-1}\cdot min^{-1}$ due to the high neonatal metabolic rate. Consequently, changes in inspired oxygen concentration will rapidly affect arterial oxygen tension. The FRC of around $30\,ml\cdot kg^{-1}$ established in the first few minutes of birth changes very little throughout the newborn period. Although this appears little different from the adult value (Table 1.1), this expression is probably misleading because lung volume correlates more closely with height than with weight. FRC in the neonate expressed in relation to crown–rump length is significantly smaller than in the adult.

The lungs are relatively stiff at birth, and calculations of the surface forces involved, together with experiments on excised lungs, have suggested that a force of some 3 kPa ($30\,cmH_2O$) would be required for the first breath. Recent work has shown, however, that such opening pressures are not required in practice, and this may have important implications in resuscitation. The compliance of the lungs (volume change per unit pressure change) increases over the first few hours from about $1.5\,ml\cdot cmH_2O^{-1}$ to about $6\,ml\cdot cmH_2O^{-1}$ (Fig. 1.7). By the end of the first week of life, however, the specific compliance (compliance/lung volume) is similar in value

Table 1.1 Normal values in full-term infants compared with adults

	Infant	Adult
Weight (kg)	3.0	70
Surface area (m²)	0.19	1.8
Surface area/weight (m²·kg⁻¹)	0.06	0.03
Respiratory frequency (breaths·min⁻¹)	30–40	12–16
Tidal volume (V_T) (ml·kg⁻¹)	6–8	7
Dead space (V_D) (ml·kg⁻¹)	2–2.5	2.2
V_D/V_T	0.3	0.3
Vital capacity (VC) (ml·kg⁻¹)	35–40	50–60
Thoracic gas volume (TGV) (ml·kg⁻¹)	35–40	30
Functional residual capacity (FRC) (ml·kg⁻¹)	27–30	30
Lung compliance (C_L) (ml·cmH₂O⁻¹)	5–6	200
Specific compliance (C_L/FRC) (ml·cmH₂O⁻¹·ml⁻¹)	0.04–0.06	0.04–0.07
Airways resistance (R_{aw}) (cmH₂O·l⁻¹·s⁻¹)	25–30	1.6
Work of breathing (g·cm⁻¹·l⁻¹)	2000–4000	2000–7000
Diffusion capacity ($D_{L_{CO}}$) (mlCO·kPa⁻¹·min⁻¹)	6–22.5	112.5–187.5
Resting alveolar ventilation (V_A) (ml·kg⁻¹·min⁻¹)	100–150	60
Resting oxygen consumption (V_{O_2}) (ml·kg⁻¹·min⁻¹)	6.8	3.3
Arterial oxygen tension (Pa_{O_2}) (kPa)	9–10.6	10.6–12.6
(mmHg)	(65–80)	(80–95)
Arterial carbon dioxide tension (Pa_{CO_2}) (kPa)	4.7	4.7–6.0
(mmHg)	(35)	(35–45)

to the adult. The neonatal chest wall is very compliant, so total compliance and lung compliance are approximately equal.

The striking changes in the mechanical properties of the lungs during the first few hours of life could be due to changes in resting lung volume or, more probably, to true alterations in the elastic properties of the lung tissue, compatible with the removal of fluid from the lungs. Serial measurements of lung volume over the first few hours of life show little change. Attempts to measure total lung capacity in the newborn by adding crying vital capa-

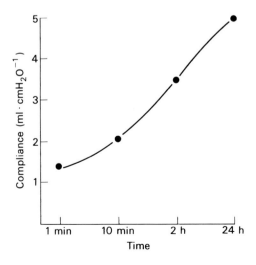

Fig. 1.7 Changes in compliance in full-term infants during the first 24 hours after birth. (Reproduced, with permission, from Godfrey, 1981)

city to FRC suggest that it is about 60 ml·kg^{-1}, indicating a relatively small inspiratory reserve capacity. For this reason, increases in alveolar ventilation are mainly achieved by increase in frequency of respiration.

Calculations of chest wall compliance in the neonate have shown it to be about five times as great as lung compliance. This compares with the adult, where lung and chest wall compliance are approximately equal. The very compliant nature of the chest wall in the newborn undoubtedly enables it to change shape dramatically during passage through the birth canal, and means that very little of the work of breathing is required to move the chest after birth, but it does have some disadvantages. The relatively low outward recoil force of the chest wall available to oppose the inward recoil force of the lung is probably the main reason why resting FRC is relatively low in the newborn, predisposing it to hypoxia. In addition, absolute pleural pressure is less negative with respect to atmosphere than in the healthy young adult, causing an increased tendency to closure of small airways. This again will lead to an increase in intrapulmonary shunting and hypoxia. FRC measurements in neonates obtained by gas dilution methods give lower results than thoracic gas volume (TGV) estimations obtained plethysmographically, particularly in the first 10 days of life (Fig. 1.8). This tendency to gas trapping behind closed airways in neonates forms the basic rationale for the use of continuous distending pressures at this age. There is clear evidence that perfusion is high relative to ventilation throughout the neonatal lung, with a threefold increase in venous admixture compared to the adult.

The resistance to the flow of gases through the airways decreases from

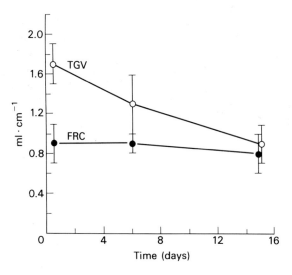

Fig. 1.8 Serial studies of FRC (black circles) and TGV (white circles) in small premature infants, showing evidence of gas trapping. (Reproduced, with permission, from Auld, 1967)

about $90 \, cmH_2O \cdot l^{-1} \cdot s^{-1}$ in the first minute to about $25 \, cm \, H_2O \cdot l^{-1} \cdot s^{-1}$ by the end of the first day, by which time an intrathoracic pressure change of only $5 \, cmH_2O$ is needed for normal tidal breathing. The resistance of the nasal passages in the newborn is approximately 50 per cent of the total resistance for caucasians and 30 per cent of the total for negroes. These values are lower than the figure of 63 per cent commonly quoted for adults, which is important as neonates are obligatory nose breathers. Nasal resistance can be significantly increased by the presence of an indwelling nasogastric tube, particularly if placed in the larger nostril. Since the absolute size of the peripheral airways is small in infants, they are particularly prone to develop small airways obstruction, and airways resistance forms a larger fraction of total resistance than in the older child or adult. Because of this, neonates with retarded maturation of the lungs and reduction in the number of peripheral airways, as may be seen with congenital diaphragmatic hernia or following oligohydramnios, tend to have reduced total airways resistance.

The diffusing capacity of the newborn infant is similar to the adult when expressed in relation to surface area, although it may be slightly lower in prematurity. The dead space/tidal volume ratio is also approximately the same as in the adult, but there is a higher dead space ventilation per minute because of the rapid rate of respiration (see Table 1.1).

Gas exchange in the newborn

Oxygen consumption in the newborn at neutral environmental temperature is approximately $7 \, ml \cdot kg^{-1} \cdot min^{-1}$, which is about twice that of the adult on a weight basis. Measurements made at below neutral environmental temperature will be misleadingly high because of the increase in metabolic rate in response to cold. The respiratory quotient is low in the immediate postnatal period at about 0.7, increasing to 0.8 by the end of the first week.

Studies of arterial blood gas tensions in the newborn show that the relative hypoxia of the fetus is largely corrected by 5 minutes after birth, the hypercapnia by 20 minutes and the acidosis by 24 hours. The arterial oxygen tension in the neonate remains lower than the adult value, at about 10–10.7 kPa (75–80 mmHg) and the arterial carbon dioxide tension is also a little low at about 4.7 kPa (35 mmHg). This reduced oxygen tension is thought to be due to persistent amounts of right-to-left shunting through remaining fetal channels, or to intrapulmonary shunting through poorly ventilated or unventilated areas of lung, or to the draining of small amounts of systemic blood into the left side of the heart from the bronchial circulation. It should be remembered that umbilical arterial blood is distal to the ductus arteriosus, and will be contaminated by any blood that has been shunted from right to left through this. Radial to umbilical arterial oxygen tension differences of up to 1.3 kPa (10 mmHg) have been demonstrated. Oxygen tension rises rapidly in the first months of life (Fig. 1.9). Although the newborn appears somewhat hypoxic by adult standards, it must be remembered that his oxygen dissociation curve is shifted to the left and therefore his arterial oxygen saturation is probably over 95 per cent; more-

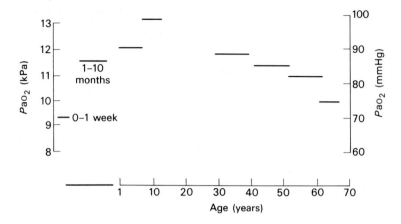

Fig. 1.9 Oxygen tensions in the newborn and at various subsequent ages. (Data from Sorbini, Grassi and Solinas, 1968, and Mansell, Bryan and Levison, 1972)

over, because of the higher haemoglobin level in the newborn period the actual volume of oxygen transported in the arterial blood is proportionately higher than in the adult.

Control of breathing in the newborn

Chemoreceptor responses to Po_2, Pco_2 and pH are present at birth, and the resetting of their sensitivity at the moment of birth has already been described. Cutting the sinus nerve in the newborn lamb abolishes the response to oxygen but does not affect the response to carbon dioxide, suggesting that, as in the adult, Po_2 acts mainly through the peripheral chemoreceptors in the carotid and aortic bodies, whilst Pco_2 and pH act mainly on the central chemoreceptors in the medulla.

Response to carbon dioxide

The mature newborn infant increases his ventilation in response to an increase in inspired carbon dioxide concentration. The slope of the carbon dioxide response curve when corrected for the smaller ventilatory capacity of the newborn is similar to that of the adult, at a value of approximately 40 per cent of resting minute ventilation per mmHg (0.133 kPa). At birth, however, the chemoreceptors are functioning at a lower arterial carbon dioxide tension and thus the carbon dioxide response curve is shifted to the left when compared with the adult, so that the increase in ventilation with increasing carbon dioxide tension begins at a lower level of carbon dioxide (Fig. 1.10). The ventilatory response in neonates is mainly achieved by an increase in tidal volume, whilst in adults increase in both tidal volume and frequency occurs.

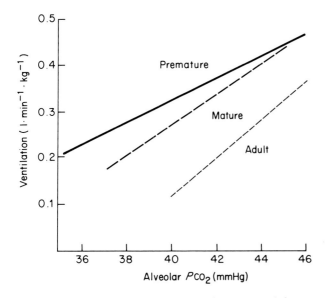

Fig. 1.10 Different CO₂ response curves for premature infants, term infants and adults. (Reproduced, with permission, from Godfrey, 1981)

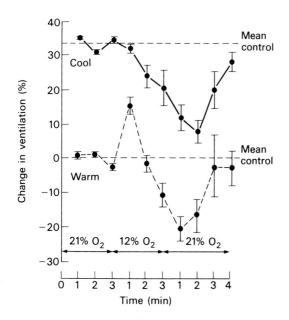

Fig. 1.11 Percentage change in ventilation while breathing air and 12% oxygen in normal full-term infants in cool and in warm environments. (Reproduced, with permission, from Ceruti, 1966)

Response to oxygen

Increasing the concentration of oxygen in the inspired gas depresses respiration, and giving low concentrations of oxygen stimulates it. Unlike the effects of carbon dioxide, however, change in inspired oxygen concentration has only a transient effect on ventilation in the immediate postnatal period, passing off after about 2 minutes. This transient response develops into a fully sustained adult response by the 10th day of life. In a cool environment the newborn infant does not respond to hypoxia by an increase in ventilation, and respiratory depression is seen as the only response (Fig. 1.11). After the first week of life, however, hypoxia invariably increases ventilation.

Hypercapnia potentiates the ventilatory response to hypoxia in the neonate as in the adult, although the converse effect is less certain.

Pulmonary reflexes

There are two pulmonary reflexes which may be important in the control of respiration in the newborn.

1. Head's paradoxical inflation reflex.   When the lungs are inflated the infant makes an extra inspiratory effort before exhaling. This reflex can be demonstrated even during deep anaesthesia. Although it has been suggested that it is important in the initiation of respiration, the newborn rabbit has been shown to be capable of initiating respiration after all the pulmonary reflexes have been abolished by vagotomy.

2. Hering–Breuer reflex.   This reflex is evoked by a more gradual inflation of the lungs than Head's reflex and consists of transient apnoea following inflation. Weakness of this reflex may lead to apnoeic spells.

Besides the classic chemical and mechanical influences on breathing in the newborn there is now much more understanding of the influence of sleep state and chest wall reflexes. Paradoxical rib cage movement occurs during rapid eye movement (REM) sleep due to inhibition of the intercostal muscles whilst the diaphragm remains active. Compression or vibration of the rib cage shortens the duration of inspiration during REM, not non-REM, sleep. The significance of this in preterm infants is discussed later.

Periodic respiration

Pauses of up to 5 seconds occurring five or six times an hour in infants at sea level, and more frequently at high altitudes, are normal. They also occur more often in premature infants, especially during REM sleep. These episodes of periodic breathing may develop into frank spells of apnoea, and the peak incidence of these occurs between days 3 and 10 of life. Periodically breathing babies have a lower arterial oxygen tension than those breathing normally, although still within the normal range. They do not have an altered sensitivity to carbon dioxide, although they do not display the lowered carbon dioxide threshold described above. Periodic breathing may be abolished by increasing lung volume (e.g. constant distending pressure) or by increasing the inspired oxygen or carbon dioxide concentrations.

No constant changes in heart rate occur during periodic breathing, which appears to have no serious consequences and usually ceases by 4–6 weeks of age.

The work of breathing

The work of breathing can be calculated from the area of a pressure/volume loop for an individual breath and may be subdivided into elastic work and flow-resistive work, as illustrated in Fig. 1.12. Work can also be calculated

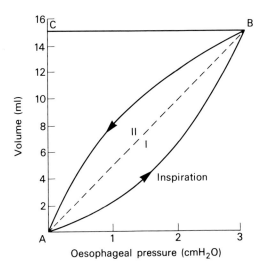

Fig. 1.12 A pressure/volume respiratory loop. Elastic work = the area of triangle ABC. Inspiratory and expiratory flow-resistive work are represented by areas I and II, respectively. Total pulmonary work = area ABC + area I. (From data of Cook *et al.*, 1957)

from formulae based on the measured compliance and resistance or from the oesophageal pressure required to produce a given tidal volume.

Calculations of the work of breathing in the newborn suggest that its value is about 0.004J (40 g·cm) per breath or 0.14J (1400 g·cm) per minute. About 75 per cent of this work is elastic work and the rest is flow resistive. Quiet breathing in healthy babies requires little work, and calculations based on the time constant obtained from normal data for compliance and resistance suggest that a respiratory rate of 35–40 per minute is the most efficient with regard to energy consumption for the healthy neonate. In respiratory disease, increased pulmonary stiffness (reduced compliance) or increased airway resistance may lead to a significant increase in work, and this in turn will lead to an increase in oxygen consumption by the respiratory muscles. The work of breathing may then represent a substantial proportion of metabolic rate.

Respiratory function in the preterm infant

The preterm infant is particularly prone to develop respiratory difficulties. The distinction has already been drawn in the introduction to this chapter between preterm infants who are small for gestational age (SGA), appropriate size for gestational age (AGA) and large for gestational age (LGA). It will be clear from the preceding description of lung development during fetal life that an accurate assessment of postconceptual age is essential, particularly in view of the relationship between the low lecithin/sphingomyelin ratios of prematurity and the subsequent development of RDS. In addition, the preterm infant suffers from the following disturbances of respiratory function.

1. Arterial oxygen tension is reduced as a result of increased maldistribution of blood and gas within the lungs. This may result either from increased compliance of the chest wall or from reduction in inspiratory muscle activity, both of which will lead to reduction in lung volume and increase in small airway closure.

2. For a given oxygen tension the oxygen content of the blood of preterm infants is lower than at term because the oxygen/haemoglobin dissociation curve is shifted to the right. The capacity of blood to release oxygen to the tissues is also reduced (see Fig. 1.5).

3. Reduced glycogen stores compared to the mature neonate result in less protection against hypoxic tissue damage.

4. The slope of the ventilatory response curve to carbon dioxide is flatter in the preterm than in the mature neonate, leading to a less effective response at higher levels of CO_2. The response to oxygen is similar in preterm and term neonates, although the ability to sustain ventilation when hypoxic takes 2–3 weeks to develop. The preterm neonate is thus less well defended against hypercapnia and hypoxia.

5. The premature infant attempts to inspire for longer against an obstruction than a mature infant or adult, suggesting that inflation of the lung is necessary to inhibit inspiration. Pulmonary reflexes may thus be more important in the control of respiration in the preterm neonate.

6. Respiratory work uses about 1 per cent of the full term neonate's energy consumption, but this may be considerably increased in prematurity.

7. Since the preterm neonate may spend 60–70 per cent of its time in REM sleep (the amount of time decreasing with increasing maturity), the inhibition of nerve impulses to the inspiratory muscles known to occur in REM sleep, leading to a fall in FRC, together with the relative chemoinsensitivity of the preterm, may contribute significantly to the irregular respiration and frequent apnoeic pauses seen in these neonates. Treatment with methylxanthines and doxapram has been effective and the stabilizing effect of a continuous distending pressure is well recognized.

Anatomy of the airway

The neonate has a relatively large head because of the advanced development of the brain, but the neck is short and the shoulders and chest are narrow.

Various anatomical differences can make the neonate difficult to intubate. The tongue is large in relation to the size of the oropharynx and this may interfere with visibility and the easy positioning of a laryngoscope blade.

The vocal cords lie opposite the lower border of the C4 vertebra, and at about the fourth year of life are found at the adult level of C5 or C6. Thus, the infant glottis lies higher and more anteriorly than in the older child and is behind a soft and often 'folded' epiglottis. The infant epiglottis inclines to the posterior pharyngeal wall at an angle of 45 degrees, and the vocal cords are angled more forwards and downwards than in the adult. During growth the epiglottis reaches the adult position closely approximated to the base of the tongue.

The anatomical differences mean that specialized equipment and techniques are required for intubation in this age group.

The trachea is approximately 4 cm in length and between 6 and 8 mm in diameter in a term baby, and bronchial intubation is more likely than in older children. The right main bronchus is intubated more easily than the left, as the latter crosses the midline from the right side at a sharper angle than the right. The right main bronchus is also wider than the left, corresponding to the difference in volume between the lungs, and this ratio is unchanged from birth to adult life.

The narrowest part of a child's airway is at the level of the cricoid ring, which is easily damaged by the inadvertent use of a tracheal tube which is too large but which may have passed through the glottis. Because there is a complete ring of cartilage at this level, any oedema will narrow the airway: 1 mm of mucosal oedema at the cricoid level may reduce the area of the airway by as much as 60 per cent in a newborn infant.

Heart and circulation

Fetal circulation

Because the fetal ductus arteriosus is relatively very large it allows equal pressures in the aorta and pulmonary artery, so that the flow to the lungs depends on the relative resistance of the lungs and the placenta.

The fetal circulation has a very low pulmonary blood flow (10 per cent of the right ventricular output) because the pulmonary vascular resistance is high. Placental blood flow is high because the vascular bed has a very low resistance and carries at least 50 per cent of the output of both ventricles, and fetal blood is oxygenated from the maternal blood. Blood with the highest oxygen content passes as quickly as possible to the coronaries and the developing brain. The ductus venosus takes umbilical oxygenated blood through the liver into the very short inferior vena cava with only minimal mixing of desaturated blood from the gut. The crista terminalis (the superior margin of the foramen ovale) directs the blood from the right to the left atrium and thence to the aorta via the left ventricle. Most of the pulmonary flow bypasses the lungs by right-to-left shunting through the patent ductus arteriosus (PDA) because the pulmonary vascular resistance is higher than the systemic (Fig. 1.13).

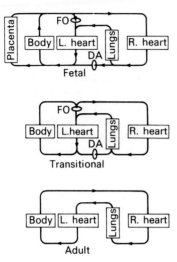

Fig. 1.13 Changes in the circulation after birth. (Reproduced, with permission, from Dawes, 1968, and Born *et al.*, 1954)

DA, ductus arteriosus
FO, foramen ovale

About 70 per cent of the cardiac output returns via the inferior vena cava and 20 per cent via the superior vena cava; the remaining 10 per cent comes from the lungs and coronary sinus.

Adaptation to extrauterine life

With the first breath and clamping of the umbilical cord, cessation of umbilical blood flow causes a reduction in right atrial pressure. At the same time, increasing pulmonary blood flow causes the left atrial pressure to rise and this rise is sustained with the onset of regular respiration. This reversal of the pressure difference between right and left atria results in the closure of the foramen ovale. Although potentially patent in 30 per cent of normal adults, it is held closed by the difference in pressure between the atria, and eventually seals in most cases. Pulmonary vascular resistance (PVR) gradually falls under the influence of increasing arterial oxygen tension (Pao_2), decreasing carbon dioxide tension ($Paco_2$) and rising pH. This leads to a further reduction in right atrial pressure, making closure of the foramen ovale more secure. Bradykinin release from inactive precursors into the pulmonary circulation also contributes to the fall in PVR. The fall in temperature and pH of umbilical venous blood at birth may trigger this release.

The above represents the transitional circulation between the true fetal circulation and that of the adult where left and right are completely separated.

The media of the ductus arteriosus, unlike other vessels, has spirally arranged dense smooth muscle. Closure of the PDA by contraction of this smooth muscle begins at the pulmonary artery end under the stimulation of increasing Pao_2 after the first breath and closure of the foramen ovale.

This physiological closure is completed in 10-15 hours, but permanent closure needs 2-3 weeks during which fibrosis occurs. Isolated ductus tissue from the fetal lamb is relaxed by prostaglandins E_1 and E_2, which may ensure patency of this vital channel during fetal life. The ductus is capable of producing thromboxanes locally, which may also be important in maintaining its patency. The exact role of substances which constrict the fetal ductus such as catecholamines, prostaglandin $F_{2\alpha}$, bradykinin and angiotensin is unknown. During fetal life increases in PaO_2 cause the ductus to narrow, and as gestational age increases towards term more constriction is seen for a smaller rise in PaO_2. The lack of response to PaO_2 which may cause the PDA to remain open may be due to action of prostaglandins E_1 and E_2.

After closure of the ductus arteriosus, normal 'adult' separation of pulmonary and systemic circulations is complete. Persistent patency beyond the age of 4 months may be caused by a defect in the media of the PDA.

In the normal infant, pulmonary artery pressure falls to adult levels in about 2 weeks, with most of the change occurring in the first 3 days.

Until the duct is firmly closed by fibrosis after 2-3 weeks, it may become patent with exposure to hypoxia as may occur in babies with congenital heart disease or respiratory distress syndrome (RDS). In infants of less than 1.5 kg who survive RDS the incidence of PDA may be 20 per cent. The premature ductus is much less sensitive to the factors which cause closure; many more remain open in these babies. This is caused not only by exposure to low PaO_2 but also by other factors such as fluid overload at a time when the oxygen mechanism for closure of the duct may not be fully developed. If the PVR is less than systemic there will be a left-to-right shunt through the duct, causing heart failure, pulmonary oedema and increased work of breathing to the extent that the duct may need urgent medical or surgical attention. The presence of a PDA in a baby dependent on mechanical ventilation may contribute to the development of bronchopulmonary dysplasia—an indication to close the ductus (p. 63).

Attempts are often made to close the duct using small doses of a prostaglandin synthetase inhibitor such as a salicylate or indomethacin. Indomethacin may be given orally for three doses, 6-hourly, of $0.2\,mg\cdot kg^{-1}$. It is contraindicated if the baby is jaundiced or has necrotizing enterocolitis, as it may cause gastrointestinal damage, a bleeding tendency and oliguria. It is possible to monitor the effects of a closing ductus using echocardiography, as the size of the left atrium will decrease with reduction of the left-to-right shunt. However, indomethacin also increases pulmonary vascular resistance, an effect intensified by hypoxia and more marked in the preterm than the mature baby. This resultant rise in PVR in the preterm baby may outweigh the advantage of using this technique to reduce blood flow through the PDA. Conversely, the E prostaglandins, low calcium, low glucose and a high pulmonary artery pressure all tend to maintain patency of the duct. Prostaglandin E_1 or E_2 may be used therapeutically in doses of $0.05-0.1\,\mu g\cdot kg^{-1}\cdot min^{-1}$ by intravenous infusion (or orally each hour) to maintain ductal patency in babies with cardiac lesions where ductal blood flow is essential to maintain life. Such lesions include severe tetralogy of

Fallot, tricuspid atresia, pulmonary artery atresia, hypoplastic right ventricle and preductal coarctation of the aorta. It is especially useful in severely cyanosed infants with pulmonary atresia until a systemic–pulmonary shunt of the Blalock–Taussig type can be created surgically. Any tendency to apnoea may be exacerbated after the start of the infusion and facilities for respiratory support must be immediately available.

Cardiovascular system at birth

At birth, the heart rate is rapid—averaging between 130 and 160 per minute—and this gradually falls to around 100 by 5 years of age.

Neonates have a lower blood pressure than older children or adults.

The mean systolic blood pressure is 10.7 ± 2.1 kPa (80 ± 16 mmHg) and the mean diastolic blood pressure is 6.1 ± 2.1 kPa (46 ± 16 mmHg) (Fig. 1.14). In the 2 hours after delivery the blood pressure falls slightly from an initial higher level, partly caused by compensation for the placental transfusion and partly because of the mechanisms operating during birth asphyxia which tend to induce hypertension. Maintenance of normal blood pressure is mainly due to baroreceptors in the carotid sinus and aortic arch. Afferent impulses pass through the vagus to nuclei in the brain stem. The efferent pathway passes through the sympathetic adrenergic nerves and the cardiac vagus nerve. All these reflexes function even in the premature infant.

The aortic chemoreceptors seem to be important for cardiovascular control in the newborn; hypoxia alone causes hypotension, vasoconstriction and variable heart rate changes, although bradycardia is the usual response.

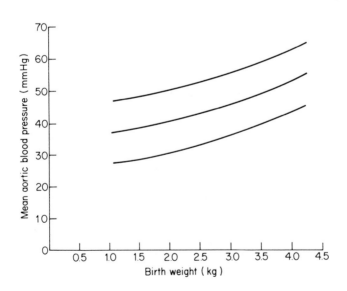

Fig. 1.14   Mean aortic blood pressure related to birth weight over the first few days of life. (Reproduced, with permission, from Kitterman, Phibbs and Tooley, 1969)

These responses differ from those to hypoxia and acidosis which cause hypertension. The aortic chemoreceptors are important in the fetus to respond to hypoxia by constriction in peripheral vascular beds and to maintain the placental blood flow at all costs. Blood flow is diverted to the brain and myocardium.

The fetus has little capacity to increase the cardiac stroke volume and so bradycardia causes a fall in cardiac output, an effect which lasts well into the neonatal period. Similarly, to increase cardiac output the infant depends on increasing the cardiac rate. Thus hypoxia causes bradycardia followed by heart block and asystole. Ventricular fibrillation is very uncommon in the newborn so there is very little need for an electrical defibrillator in a special care baby unit.

The neonatal response to posture is less efficient, and marked hypotension is seen with the baby tilted into a head-up position. If 25 per cent of the blood volume is removed at exchange transfusion there is a marked tachycardia mediated by carotid sinus baroreceptors, which does not compensate for a fall in blood pressure and which takes up to 15 minutes to recover. Peripheral vasoconstriction occurs most severely in the skin, muscles, liver, intestines and kidney. These inadequate responses suggest that the mechanisms associated with circulating catecholamines are immature at birth and the renin–angiotensin system may be more important in the neonate for the maintenance of the circulation in stressful situations such as birth asphyxia. Renin activity is high in the fetus, and fetal tissues respond to angiotensin II. In experimental animals nephrectomy abolishes the response to haemorrhage in the newborn. Angiotensin II is a more powerful vasoconstrictor than adrenaline or noradrenaline. Although very high levels of angiotensin II are found after severe birth asphyxia, it may not be as important in maintaining resting blood pressure and cardiac output as it is in the stressful situation.

Stimulation of the sympathetic nerves to the heart in newborn experimental animals produces myocardial contractility comparable to that of the adult, although there is some evidence that, in the human, innervation of the fetal and neonatal myocardium may be incomplete. Thus responses elicited, although similar in sensitivity to the adult, may be of shorter duration. From 20 weeks' gestation the adrenergic tone on the heart is two to three times the cholinergic, but by term the two influences are balanced. After the second week of life, cardiac tone is dependent on dominance of the parasympathetic nervous system—that prevailing in the adult. The response to exogenous catecholamines increases with increasing gestational age so that even in the term baby the response to a dopamine infusion, for example, may not be as full as with the older child.

Cardiac output falls during the neonatal period, with an average initial value of 400–$500 \, \mathrm{ml \cdot kg^{-1} \cdot min^{-1}}$ for the output of both ventricles. Initially the left ventricular output is greater because of shunts through the ductus arteriosus and foramen ovale. By the end of the first week of life the output of the two ventricles becomes the same as fetal channels close, and reaches 150–$200 \, \mathrm{ml \cdot kg^{-1} \cdot min^{-1}}$. As the cardiac output falls, peripheral vasoconstriction must occur to produce the gradual rise in blood pressure seen in postnatal life. A fall in peripheral temperature relative to the core temperature from the normal difference of 2°C is a very sensitive guide to the adequacy of cardiac output in the newborn.

Premature infants have a relatively higher cardiac output than term babies. The cardiac index of a normal preterm baby is 5.5 $l\cdot min^{-1}\cdot m^{-2}$ surface area (term baby 3.3 $l\cdot min^{-1}\cdot m^{-2}$).

Animal work shows that strips of fetal myocardium develop much less active tension during isometric contraction than do those from an adult. This is likely to be due to the smaller proportion of sarcomeres and to the fact that these are randomly arranged rather than in parallel sequences as in the adult. Moreover, in the adult, 60 per cent of cardiac muscle is contractile mass, whereas in the newborn the figure may be as low as 30 per cent, resulting in less myocardial contractile ability. However, neonatal cardiac muscle is much less susceptible to hypoxia than is mature muscle if the pH is normal, thus reflecting a greater ability for anaerobic metabolism. In studies on fetal and neonatal animals, falls in cardiac output of up to 25 per cent occur in response to hypoxia ($Pao_2 < 2.7\,kPa$ (20 mmHg)) in association with severe metabolic acidosis (pH < 7.15).

Transitional circulation (persistent fetal circulation)

The circulation of the neonate is labile and may revert to the fetal pattern with blood flowing from the right side of the heart to the left through the ductus arteriosus from pulmonary artery to aorta and/or through the foramen ovale, if subjected to conditions which promote pulmonary vasoconstriction.

The lability of the pulmonary vasculature is a particular feature of neonatal physiology and is caused by abundant arteriolar smooth muscle, extending more peripherally than later in life. The pulmonary vasculature constricts in response to hypoxaemia, hypercapnia, acidaemia and to a low Fio_2 via an adrenergic mechanism since it is abolished after sympathectomy.

Some infants, cyanosed after birth but without lung disease, are found at cardiac cathetization to have a high pulmonary artery pressure and a right-to-left shunt through a PDA or patent foramen ovale. This is termed 'persistent fetal circulation' or, more correctly, 'transitional circulation' since the lungs are perfused. This state is particularly important in some babies with RDS, congenital diaphragmatic hernia, meconium aspiration syndrome and in babies with persistent transitional circulation of unknown aetiology, who may die in a vicious circle of cyanosis, acidaemia and falling cardiac output unless steps are taken to reverse the high pulmonary vascular resistance. At post-mortem examination all alveolar duct and wall arterioles, normally non-muscular, are found to be fully muscularized, and where muscle is normally found in the intra-acinar arteries the width of muscle is doubled. It is possible that this abnormality is a failure of the normal post-natal regression of muscle followed by a rapid differentiation of pericytes and intermediate cells into mature smooth muscle cells. The overgrowth may be triggered by vasoactive substances released from endothelial cells in the presence of hypoxia.

The pulmonary vascular resistance (PVR) may fall with ventilator-induced respiratory alkalosis and high Fio_2 if the lungs are compliant. The histamine-releasing drug tolazoline may be used but there may be lack of response, probably because of depletion of lung histamine after the use of curare, morphine or contrast medium. Dopamine may increase PVR and it may be more logical to use dobutamine for inotropic support in these babies. Sodium nitroprusside and prostaglandin D_2 have also been used to reverse pulmonary hypertension both in man and in experimental animals.

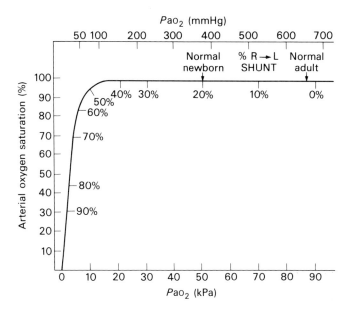

Fig. 1.15 Oxygen saturation/tension curve, showing effects of various volumes of venous admixture. Down to arterial oxygen tension of 17.3 kPa (130 mmHg), each 1 per cent of venous admixture reduces arterial tension by 2 kPa (15 mmHg). Below 17.3 kPa, the rough rule does not apply. (Reproduced, with permission, from Swyer, 1975)

In the newborn there is a physiological right-to-left shunt of the order of 20 per cent (adult 7 per cent). In states of persistent fetal circulation this may increase to 70–80 per cent, in which case the infant will be cyanosed even when breathing increased inspired oxygen concentrations (Fig. 1.15).

Cerebral circulation

In normal adults the process of autoregulation of cerebral blood flow tends to allow a constant flow with changes of mean systemic blood pressure between 60 and 130 mmHg. There is no reason to believe that this process is not present in the normal newborn, although in preterm babies the reflex is likely to be immature—slower in onset and less complete. Autoregulation is readily disturbed by hypercapnia and hypoxia and after severe hypotension, but in the newborn is regained by a period of mild hyperventilation of 30 minutes or so. Total cerebral blood flow may be lower in the preterm than the term baby, which in turn is less than in an older child on the basis of body weight.

A major cause of neonatal death is intraventricular haemorrhage (IVH), but for those of low birth weight this is the commonest cause of death or neurodevelopmental handicap. Although the pathogenesis of IVH is uncertain, the blood probably dissects into the adjacent ventricular system from ruptured veins in the subependymal germinal matrix of the immature brain. After 28 weeks' gestation this germinal matrix regresses, leaving a loose latticework of connective tissue giving little support to arteries and veins. Thus the anatomy of the circulation over the basal ganglia is unusual, with short, thin-walled, poorly supported capillaries opening at right angles into the branches of the internal cerebral vein which in turn flows into the vein of Galen at a right angle. There is a potential for venous obstruction, and surges of arterial or venous pressure may cause rupture of the capillaries. IVH is associated with prematurity, respiratory distress of all types, mechanical ventilation, metabolic acidosis, hypoxia and hypercapnia. Immediately after an IVH there is severe reactive cerebral oedema, but there is also a very high incidence of late hydrocephalus following such a haemorrhage.

Surges of arterial pressure may occur if autoregulation has been disturbed by hypoxia followed by stressful manoeuvres such as intubation or venepuncture. Hypoxia also causes venous congestion and endothelial damage. Surges of venous pressure are caused by constant distending pressure, especially CPAP using a Gregory-type headbox. Intubated babies have the smallest rise in venous pressure during crying or seizures. The osmotic effects of large bolus injections of 8.4% sodium bicarbonate or hypertonic dextrose are also incriminated. In asphyxiated babies all attempts should be made to keep systemic blood pressure within the normal limits of 40–70 mmHg systolic.

Ultrasound investigation at the bedside is used to detect IVH and allows prediction of the outcome according to the size of the haemorrhage. This investigation may be used until the age of 9 months, when the anterior fontanelle is too small to provide an adequate window for full ultrasonography.

Temperature control

There are several reasons why heat balance in a newborn neonate can be seriously affected by environmental temperature. The surface area/weight ratio is large—approximately three times that of the adult. The insulating capacity of the subcutaneous tissue is less than one-half that of the adult even for a full-term infant, and for premature infants it is even less. The ability to shiver in response to cold is poorly developed even at term and in premature infants this mechanism again is even less well developed.

Vasoconstriction and vasodilatation of skin blood vessels does occur, together with behavioural movements such as adoption of nestling or huddling positions, but these physical thermoregulatory processes can compensate for only a limited range of changes in environmental temperature.

The main thermoregulatory mechanism in the newborn is chemical. Cold exposure releases noradrenaline at sympathetic nerve endings, depolarizes the cell membrane and, by activating adenylcyclase, increases the circulating level of 3'5'-cyclic AMP. This in turn activates protein kinases which enhance the action of hormone-sensitive lipase, causing hydrolysis of triglyceride stores to free fatty acid and glycerol. About 11 per cent of total body fat in the full-term neonate is located in the brown fat stores principally found at the base of the neck, in the axillae, between the scapulae and in the mediastinum. The extra calories produced by oxidation of triglycerides from brown fat stores have been shown to be capable of maintaining the cold-induced increase in heat production evoked by an environmental temperature of 25°C for about 3 days in the full-term baby.

Additional sites of heat production are the brain and liver, hepatic glucose production occurring by glycogenolysis and providing the main source of energy in these sites. Full-term newborns are capable of a threefold increase in metabolic rate over basal levels, but in spite of this excellent metabolic response the neonate is unable to maintain body temperature outside a narrow range of environmental temperatures because of the rapid rate of heat transfer. The ideal thermal environment will be that in which oxygen consumption is minimal. This is known as the neutral thermal environment or neutral temperature range. This temperature range is fairly

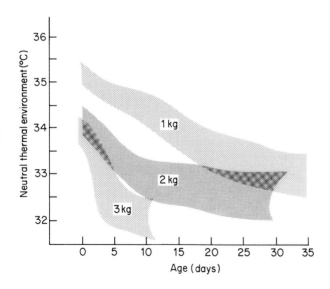

Fig. 1.16   Neutral thermal environment for babies of varying birth weight in the first few days of life. (Reproduced, with permission, from Hey and Katz, 1970)

narrow for the naked newborn baby, and its mean on the first day of life increases from approximately 33°C in full-term babies to almost 36°C in babies of very low birth weight (Fig. 1.16). The neutral temperature range is widened and lowered by covering the baby with a layer of clothing (Fig. 1.17). The limits of thermoneutrality are defined by upper and lower critical temperatures. Rise in environmental temperature above the upper critical temperature leads to recruitment of thermoregulating processes such as sweating and to an increase in body temperature, whilst an environment cooler than the lower critical temperature causes an increase in the thermogenic processes described above. Metabolism of brown fat increases metabolic rate and oxygen consumption, and any existing hypoxia is likely to be worsened. It was shown many years ago that the mortality rate of premature infants was markedly reduced by increasing the environmental temperature. The metabolic response to cold is inhibited by hypoxia, general anaesthesia, hypoglycaemia, intracranial haemorrhage and prematurity. Because it is sympathetically mediated, it can also be prevented by beta blockade. The metabolic response to cold continues throughout the neo-

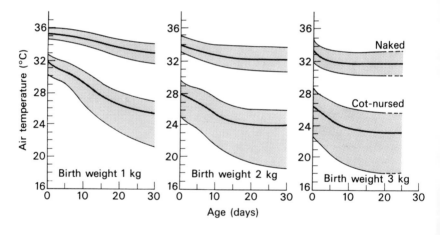

Fig. 1.17 Summary of the changes in optimum environmental temperature which occur with age in babies weighing 1, 2 or 3 kg at birth. The dark line indicates the 'optimum' temperature (at the lower limit of the neutral environmental temperature range), and the shaded area the range of temperature within which a baby can be expected to maintain a normal body temperature without increasing either heat production or evaporative water loss more than 25 per cent. The higher temperatures are appropriate for a baby being nursed naked in a draught-free environment of moderate humidity (50 per cent saturation), and the lower temperatures are appropriate for a baby clothed and well wrapped up in a cot in a similar environment. It must be remembered that the environmental temperature inside a single-walled incubator is *less* than the internal air temperature recorded by the thermometer; the effective environmental temperature provided by the incubator can, however, be estimated by subtracting 1°C from the air temperature for each 7°C by which the incubator air temperature exceeds room temperature. (Reproduced, with permission, from Hey, 1971)

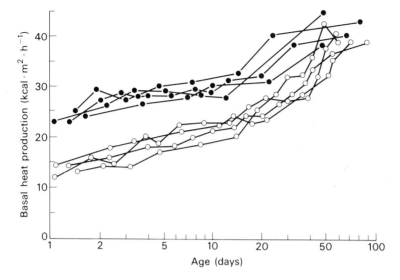

Fig. 1.18 The rise in heat production in a neutral thermal environment (standard or basal metabolism) which occurred with increasing age in four babies of 28–30 weeks' gestation (white circles) and four babies of 38–40 weeks' gestation (black circles). Heat production per unit surface area usually reaches a level comparable to that found in adults by the third month of life. (Reproduced, with permission, from Hey, 1971)

natal period although oxygen consumption is increasing rapidly, especially in the first few days of life (Fig. 1.18).

Heat transfer

The newborn baby loses heat in a cold environment in any of the following four ways.

Conduction

Conductive losses are generally small since it is unusual for an infant to be laid in contact with a cold surface. Such losses will depend on the baby's skin temperature, the area of contact and the conductive properties of the surface on which the baby is laid.

Convection

Convective heat loss depends on skin/air temperature gradients and air velocity. Even within an incubator the air circulation may be considerable, and small neonates may only maintain their body temperature if they are covered or if other attempts are made to reduce air currents.

Radiation

As with convection, radiant heat loss decreases as environmental temperature rises (Fig. 1.19). When the infant is in a protected enclosure, radiant
loss probably becomes the most significant form of heat exchange. Radiant

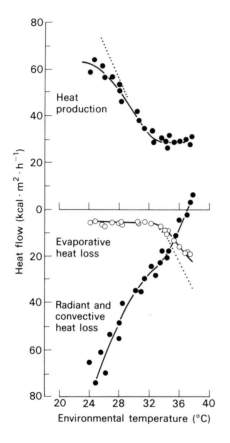

Fig. 1.19 The effect of environmental temperature on heat balance in a naked baby, weight 2.1 kg, gestation 36 weeks, when 3–7 days old, in surroundings of uniform temperature and moderate humidity. Conductive heat loss was small enough to be neglected. Heat loss by radiation and convection is large in a draught-free environment of 26°C, and falls to nothing when the environmental temperature equals body temperature (37°C). Heat production rises in a cold environment and evaporative water loss increases in a warm environment, but these changes are not enough to keep deep body temperature completely constant (the dotted lines indicate the changes that would be necessary for body temperature to remain constant). Neutral conditions are provided by an environment of 33°C. (Reproduced, with permission, from Hey, 1971)

loss in an incubator occurs between the infant and the wall of the incubator,
and between the wall of the incubator and the surrounding environment.
The effective temperature in the incubator is thus affected by environmental
temperature. Every 7°C difference between the inside and the outside of the
incubator lowers the effective temperature in the incubator by 1°C. Radiant
heat loss can be minimized by using double-walled incubators or a small
Perspex shield placed over the baby inside the incubator, or by clothing the
baby.

Evaporation

Evaporative heat loss occurs both from the respiratory tract and from the body surface. Evaporative heat loss from the skin surface is considerable at birth when the neonate is covered with liquor amnii, as in a cold labour ward, but skin evaporative loss is not considered of great importance in normal circumstances. Evaporative loss from the lungs is increased with hyperventilation but again is not of great significance in normal circumstances.

About 70 per cent of normal heat loss is dry loss by radiation, convection and conduction, whilst 25 per cent occurs by evaporation from skin and lungs, 3 per cent in warming the inspired air and 1–2 per cent in excreta. Since evaporative heat loss is practically unchanged over a wide range of ambient temperatures, dry heat losses account for more than 90 per cent of total heat loss in response to cold.

Effects of hypothermia

The main danger of hypothermia in the neonate is the increase in oxygen consumption, diverting valuable oxygen supplies from the tissues and increasing the mortality from hypoxia, particularly in RDS. Hypothermia also decreases surfactant synthesis and is associated with coagulation abnormalities. The action of many drugs, particularly muscle relaxants and anaesthetic agents, is prolonged in hypothermic neonates.

Effects of hyperthermia

Although less common than reductions in temperature, raised environmental temperature can also be harmful to neonates. Increase in rectal temperature above 37°C can lead to a threefold increase in water loss by evaporation, although efficient sweating does not develop until 36–37 weeks of gestation. Neonates, including prematures, also vasodilate when their rectal temperature rises, enabling them to increase their heat losses fourfold. Oxygen consumption increases if the infant becomes restless or if his body temperature rises. Low birth weight infants exposed to raised environmental temperature or suffering from pyrexia may have an increased number of apnoeic attacks. It is known that a rise in temperature, as well as hypothermia, increases the mortality in premature infants but it is not known whether this is due to apnoeic attacks, to hypernatraemia from increased fluid loss or to cardiovascular strain from increased cardiac output. These harmful effects of a raised environmental temperature, however, occur below the temperature at which oxygen consumption increases and within the neutral temperature range (see Fig. 1.18).

Special problems of prematurity

The thermoregulatory responses to cold stress, both physical and chemical, are found to be more and more well developed with increasing maturity. The newborn neonate of less than 30–32 weeks' gestation appears virtually unable to increase heat production in response to cold. SGA babies cannot maintain their body temperature as well as AGA babies because of their larger surface area/weight ratio, diminished subcutaneous tissue insulation and a possible deficiency of essential nutrients.

The respiratory quotients both of full-term neonates and of those suffering from intrauterine malnourishment are around 0.7 both in thermoneutral and cold environments, indicating predominantly endogenous fat oxidation. More glucose utilization tends to occur in dysmature infants, however, probably largely by gluconeogenesis. Administration of intralipid infusions has been advocated in order to supply adequate nutrients for chemical thermoregulation.

Haematology

Haematopoietic activity is detectable by 14 days' gestation in the human embryo, starting in the yolk sac from aggregates of primitive mesenchymal cells. Subsequently the liver becomes the principal organ for blood formation and, although haematopoiesis begins in the bone marrow in the fifth month, the liver continues this role until the first week of postnatal life. Early erythrocytes are larger than those at birth. Platelets are present by 11 weeks of gestation, but the normal adult platelet count is achieved by 30 weeks of gestation. White cells are present only in very small numbers up to 20 weeks, but at birth the count is $20\,000 \cdot mm^{-3}$ with a wide normal range; 70 per cent are neutrophils, possibly with less phagocytic activity than later in life.

The mean cord haemoglobin of premature infants is $17.5 \pm 1.6\,g \cdot dl^{-1}$ and for full-term babies $17.1 \pm 1.8\,g \cdot dl^{-1}$. Babies who are small for gestational age may be rendered relatively polycythaemic by placental insufficiency. The concentration of haemoglobin may rise by $1–2\,g \cdot dl^{-1}$ in the first days of life as a result of placental transfusion and low oral fluid intake, with a decrease in extracellular fluid volume. Hb values taken from heel or finger prick may be $1–2\,g \cdot dl^{-1}$ higher than those from central venous blood because of the sluggish peripheral circulation of the newborn. By 1 week, the value of Hb compares with that of cord blood, but thereafter declines progressively. This phenomenon is known as physiological anaemia of infancy (Fig. 1.20). Premature babies have an even greater fall in Hb levels— the average level being $8\,g \cdot dl^{-1}$ at 4–8 weeks of life in the 1.5 kg group relative to $11.4\,g \cdot dl^{-1}$ in the full-term baby (see Table 1.2). The reason for this earlier and greater fall in the premature baby is not entirely clear, although it may be related to an even shorter red cell survival time than in the term baby.

The haemoglobin fall mainly results from a decrease in red cell mass (as shown using ^{51}Cr-labelled red cells) rather than from a dilutional effect of

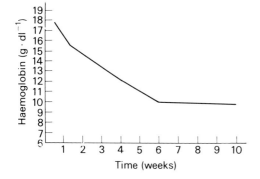

Fig. 1.20 The relation between haemoglobin concentration and age from birth in a group of infants weighing less than 1.5 kg. (Reproduced, with permission, from Stockman and Oski, 1978)

increasing plasma volume. Red cell survival is lower in the neonate (60–70 days at term; 30–40 days in premature infants) and there is less red cell production.

The reason for lower red cell survival is not known, although metabolic differences such as increased glucose consumption exist and increased glycolytic enzymes seem to confer greater susceptibility to injury and earlier destruction. The fetal red cell, with its relatively larger size and greater degree of wall rigidity, is less compliant and possibly more likely to be damaged in small vessels. The increased permeability of the cell membrane to Na^+ and K^+ predisposes erythrocytes of the newborn to damage by an adverse osmotic environment.

The changes in erythropoiesis which occur in the first weeks of life are caused by the improved oxygenation of the newborn. The reticulocytosis, which may be as high as 80 per cent in early fetal life, falls to 4 per cent at birth and decreases rapidly to less than 1 per cent at 5 days of age. Red cell production is mediated through the effect of tissue oxygen tension on the output of the hormone erythropoietin, which is made in the liver in the fetus (kidney in the adult). The hormone is detectable in the fetal blood at

Table 1.2 Normal haematological values during the first week of life in the term infant

Value	Cord blood	Day 1	Day 3	Day 7
Hb (g·dl⁻¹)	16.8	18.4	17.8	17.0
Haematocrit (%)	53.0	58.0	55.0	54.0
Red cells (mm³ × 10⁶)	5.25	5.8	5.6	5.2
MCV (μm³)	107	108	99.0	98.0
MCH (γγ)	34	35	33	32.5
MCHC (%)	31.7	32.5	33	33
Reticulocytes (%)	3–7	3–7	1–3	0–1
Nuc. RBC (mm⁻³)	500	200	0–5	0

MCV, mean corpuscular volume; MCH, mean corpuscular haemoglobin; MCHC, mean corpuscular haemoglobin concentration.

(From Lubin, 1978)

birth, but thereafter levels fall rapidly until between 8 and 12 weeks when erythroid activity recommences. The return to full active erythropoiesis occurs at similar minimum Hb levels even in infants with widely differing values at birth. In the preterm infant, resumption of active erythropoiesis begins earlier in postnatal life than in the full-term infant. The anaemia of prematurity is not seen in babies with cyanotic congenital heart disease or respiratory insufficiency. These infants continue to produce erythropoietin during the first weeks after birth and thus show no decline in marrow activity. In the healthy infant, the lower limit of normal Hb falls by about $1 \, g \cdot dl^{-1}$ per week. Values of less than $8 \, g \cdot dl^{-1}$ at any age require explanation, but not necessarily correction.

Factors which influence the magnitude of physiological anaemia include the nutritional status of the infant, and supplies of vitamin E, folic acid and iron may be inadequate in the face of a rapid increase in growth later in the first year of life. The use of oral iron supplements does not prevent the early anaemia of prematurity, and indeed the anaemia is not associated with a low serum iron. However, late anaemia will occur without supplemental dietary iron after the first 5-6 months of life. Iron supplementation of $1 \, mg \cdot kg^{-1} \cdot day^{-1}$ is always necessary for preterm babies as rapid growth outstrips the iron available from normal stores or dietary sources.

The commonest situations associated with anaemia in the neonatal period are haemorrhage (including multiple sampling for haematology or blood gases), haemolytic disease of the newborn caused by rhesus incompatibility and anaemia of prematurity. The neonatal haematocrit ranges from 52 to 58 per cent (Table 1.2). Haematocrit up to 70 per cent is reported but this causes a reduction in blood flow to vital organs, particularly the kidneys.

Fetal haemoglobin

Before birth, fetal haemoglobin (HbF; α_2, γ_2 globin chains) accounts for 90-95 per cent of all Hb production and is the major haemoglobin of fetal life. The maximum rate of synthesis declines after 35 weeks' gestation and at term accounts for 50-60 per cent of haemoglobin production. The replacement of fetal by adult haemoglobin is a function of maturity of the fetus and is uninfluenced by the timing of the birth. The rate continues to decrease and at 3 months only 5 per cent of synthesis is HbF. Adult haemoglobin (HbA; α_2, β_2) synthesis increases to 35-50 per cent of new Hb at birth so that at this stage the relative concentration of HbF is 80 per cent to HbA 20 per cent. Adult Hb has the ability to combine with low molecular weight phosphorylated compounds such as 2,3-diphosphoglycerate (2,3-DPG), causing a marked reduction in oxygen affinity. HbF does not appear to react in this way. The consequence of the high HbF level and the relatively low concentration of red cell 2,3-DPG is a shift in the oxygen dissociation curve to the left (equivalent to adult blood of pH 7.6), thus favouring transport of oxygen from the maternal to the fetal circulation (see Fig. 1.4). Neonatal blood has an oxygen-carrying capacity at least 1.25 times that of adult blood. These two factors afford some protection for the baby under the conditions of relative hypoxia experienced during the birth process. The oxygen dissociation curve gradually shifts to the right as the concentrations of HbA and 2,3-DPG increase, so oxygen delivery to the tissues may actually increase in spite of a falling Hb.

Blood volume

The blood volume of an infant with a normal haemoglobin is estimated to be 80–85 ml·kg^{-1} body weight. For the premature baby a higher figure, perhaps as much as 100 ml·kg^{-1} may be the case. The blood volume of the newborn is more variable than that of an older infant, depending on the magnitude of the placental transfusion. Because of this wide variation, difficulties are created if blood replacement intraoperatively or otherwise is to be based on a percentage of blood volume.

Because the placental vessels contain approximately 100 ml of blood at term, the blood volume of the infant can be increased by up to 60 per cent under conditions such as delayed clamping of the cord or placing the infant below the level of the placenta which favour blood flow from the placenta to the baby. The volume of blood in the placenta is unchanged during the last 10 weeks of gestation, so the preterm baby may receive a relatively larger percentage increase in his blood volume. Although the haematocrit is the same in all babies whenever clamping of the cord takes place, in those in which clamping is delayed, haematocrit values are as high as 65 per cent after 48 hours, compared with the normal of 45–48 per cent.

It has been suggested that an alternative method of calculation based on the more constant plasma volume may be more precise. The plasma volume is generally accepted as 5 per cent of body weight (50 ml·kg^{-1}) and so total blood volume can be regarded as 50 + haematocrit, as ml·kg^{-1}.

Coagulation

Several aspects of the coagulation mechanism are defective in the neonate as compared with the adult. The infant is at risk from bleeding, not only because of reduced platelet function or reduced plasma coagulation factors but also because of the susceptibility to acute infections or metabolic disorders associated with disseminated intravascular coagulopathy.

It is widely stated that premature infants have increased vascular fragility—perhaps caused by inadequate connective tissue support of capillaries, although there is no firm evidence to support this.

Platelet counts even in the premature baby are in the same range as for normal adults, but there is evidence that all newborns have a mild transient defect in platelet function. This is without a great deal of clinical significance. Primary platelet aggregation is followed by release of serotonin and adenosine diphosphate, after which secondary aggregation occurs and this is irreversible. Neonatal platelets have lower than normal levels of serotonin and may also be mildly deficient in adenine nucleotides. The platelet defect is accentuated by high levels of unconjugated bilirubin, by phototherapy or by maternal ingestion of aspirin.

The levels of plasma proteins may be normal at birth, although there may be a deficiency of certain plasma proteins involved in the coagulation system. Synthesis of the vitamin K-dependent factors (II, VII, IX and X) by the liver is suboptimal until adult levels are attained after the age of 2 months. Newborns have grossly deficient stores of vitamin K at birth and deficiency will ensue, especially in breast-fed babies. By the second or third day of life, levels may drop to as low as 5–20 per cent of the adult level before rising later in the first week of life secondary to production of vitamin K by the microflora of the colon. Minimal levels of clotting factors are seen on the second or third day of life, at which time the prothrombin time may be very prolonged.

This fall after birth and the risk of spontaneous bleeding (haemorrhagic disease of the newborn) or increased surgical bleeding may be partly prevented by the administration of 1 mg vitamin K parenterally. Nowadays this is given routinely. Vitamin K does not fully correct the clotting deficiencies in the neonate, as defective synthetic capacity of the production of coagulation factors by the liver continues for the first weeks of life. Preterm babies continue to have poor prothrombin activity even after vitamin K, because of their greater hepatic immaturity than term infants. The prothrombin time (PT) and partial thromboplastin time (PTT) are prolonged in preterm infants. The thrombin time (TT) is also prolonged, possibly because of the presence of breakdown products of fibrin which may have heparin-like activity. Severe deficiency in vitamin K-dependent factors may also occur in infants of mothers taking antiepileptic drugs such as phenytoin during pregnancy. Proteins produced by the liver, but which are not vitamin K-dependent such as factor V and fibrinogen, are in the normal range at birth. There is no transplacental passage of clotting factors so a deficiency of any one of them is detectable from cord blood taken at birth.

The fibrinolytic enzyme system is also relatively underdeveloped in the neonate. The plasminogen level is low at term and is even lower in the preterm baby.

Nervous system

Development of the nervous system

At birth the brain is relatively large, being 10 per cent of the total body weight; by 6 months of age it has doubled in size and by 1 year has trebled. About 25 per cent of the adult number of brain cells is present at birth. The cells of the cortex and brain stem are complete in number after 1 year of life. The cerebellum has less of its total complement at birth but reaches its final number before other areas.

The rapid growth in the first year of life is also the result of myelination and elaboration of the dendritic processes necessary for the full complex behaviour of the older child and adult.

Nutritional deprivation during the period of the postnatal growth 'spurt' of the infant brain may give rise to impairment of cerebral development and may explain the vulnerability of the brain in inborn errors of metabolism. Certainly, infants who have suffered both prenatal and postnatal undernutrition have reduced quantities of brain cells, lipids and protein and decreased dendritic connections.

There is now good evidence that newborn motor behaviour is not, as has previously been thought, entirely at subcortical levels. Cortical potentials are elicited during neonatal seizures which are manifest clinically, corresponding with the extent of dendritic growth in the motor cortex before birth. However, at birth, myelination of the nerve fibres is incomplete, and reflex responses not seen later (such as the Moro reflex) may be elicited. These reflexes depend on cutaneous stimulation and the resultant action is more widespread in immature babies. Such differences may be used to assess the gestational age of a baby.

Incomplete myelination in the CNS also explains the increased sensitivity to opiates and general anaesthesia.

In the very young, functional and anatomical immaturity give rise to low pain sensitivity and limited conscious behaviour, but even small preterm babies move away from noxious stimuli and the cardiovascular signs of autonomic stimulation and stress hormone release in response to pain are similar to the adult. Babies react to painful stimuli in a non-specific fashion and do not appear to differentiate the origins of the pain. Newborns have a higher circulating level of beta-endorphins than have adults, and the immature blood-brain barrier may allow these to cross and affect the central nervous system. This may explain the reduced need for analgesics in this age group.

The sleep pattern depends on the degree of development of the CNS. Whether *in utero* or after premature delivery, the amount of slow-wave sleep increases during the third trimester of gestation when about half of sleep is non-REM. Slow-wave sleep is necessary for functional development of the respiratory control area of the brain. At the 36th week, the baby develops a biological rhythm with a definite pattern of slow-wave, REM and transitional sleep.

The high incidence of convulsions in the first months of life is not fully understood, but can be attributed to a number of factors, including poor myelination, immaturity of central inhibitory mechanisms, increased water content of the brain and a higher metabolic rate. Because dendritic connections are poorly developed at birth, fits do not spread throughout the cortex as they would in an older child and thus the clinical manifestation is often fragmentary.

By 12 weeks of gestational life, motor nerve fibres reach the extremities of the limbs, but by 28 weeks the neuromuscular junctions are more highly differentiated in the tongue and the diaphragm than in the hand. Gamma-efferent activity is less sustained than in the adult and this may contribute to the relative hypotonia of the newborn. At this stage the muscles are functionally a uniform group, having the characteristics of adult 'slow' fibres. Early in neonatal life the 'slow' and 'fast' groups develop at the same time that fibres lose their overall sensitivity to acetylcholine and the subneural apparatus of the neuromuscular junction appears. Together with this, an adult pattern of sensitivity develops restricted to the motor endplate. Indirect tetanic stimulation is poorly sustained and there is some evidence of early tetanic fade. Because of the anatomical and physiological differences, a different response to the muscle relaxants is elicited (described on p. 105).

Immunology

Immunity is the ability of an organism to respond to foreign matter by using a variety of mechanisms involving different types of cells and cellular products to destroy or inactivate the foreign substances.

During its development the fetus is normally protected by its environment from infection, so the immune system is only called upon after birth to respond to outside agents. Bacterial colonization occurs rapidly after birth not only from the mother but also from a hospital environment, and the baby may become infected by pathological organisms to which he has impaired resistance. Physical, humoral and cellular mechanisms of immunity have reduced efficiency in the newborn, so every effort should be made to prevent bacterial infection—especially in the preterm baby.

Neonatal anaesthesia and intensive care involve invasive manoeuvres such as intubation and venepuncture which provide a route for organisms; also the skin of a neonate is very delicate and easily becomes infected.

The primary immune response consisting of the inflammatory response and phagocytosis is impaired in the fetus and newborn. The chemotactic response of polymorphonuclear leucocytes is reduced, as is opsonization due to lower levels of complement—especially C_3—and low immunoglobulin levels. The febrile response which implies increased metabolic activity and the release of pyrogens from leucocytes is not well developed and the phagocytosis of ingested pathogens may be further reduced in disease states of the newborn such as RDS or septicaemia.

Immunoglobulin IgG passes from the maternal circulation to the fetus by passive and active transport mainly during the third trimester of pregnancy. The levels usually exceed the maternal level $(0.02\,\mathrm{g\cdot l^{-1}})$ and are higher in the full term baby than the preterm. There is no transport of IgA or IgM, so these are absent at birth unless the immune system has been challenged *in utero* by an infection such as congenital rubella. After birth the level of IgG falls with a half-life of between 20 and 30 days, so there is a relative hypogammaglobulinaemia, lowest between the second and fourth months. This is rarely of clinical importance except in preterm babies if IgG levels fall to less than 10 per cent of normal.

The number of T cells is reduced at birth by about 50 per cent, but their function is relatively normal and there is very little reduction in the ability to reject skin grafts. The number of B cells is similar to an adult's, but there is a reduction in antibody production in response to exogenous antigen.

About 80 per cent of serious neonatal infections are caused by *Escherichia coli* or group B haemolytic streptococcus.

Kidney

Fetal kidney

The kidneys produce dilute urine from as early as the third month of intrauterine life, although the excretory and regulatory requirements of the fetus are satisfactorily carried out by the placenta. The only known function of the fetal kidney is the maintenance of amniotic fluid volume; renal agenesis my lead to oligohydramnios and compression deformities. It is important to consider the possibility of absent kidneys in newborn babies with pneumothorax and pulmonary hypoplasia where amniotic fluid deficit may prevent proper maturation of the lungs. The contribution the kidneys make to fetal homoeostasis must, however, be small, as infants born with absent kidneys may have normal plasma elecytrolytes, urea and creatinine. It is only at birth that the kidney must take up its role of excretion of the nitrogenous end-products of metabolism, and plays its part in stabilizing the volume, osmotic pressure and chemical composition of extracellular fluid.

The neonatal kidney has often been regarded as immature, but comparison with the adult kidney assumes that these neonatal and adult organs have similar tasks to perform. This is clearly not so, if only because of the effect of growth. Approximately 50 per cent of dietary nitrogen in the newborn is incorporated into new tissue, thus relieving the kidney of half of its excretory load. As will be seen below, the neonatal kidney appears to be well able to cope with the work it is normally required to perform, although it is less well equipped to counter the effects of severe dehydration, excessive water or solute load, trauma and acidosis.

At birth, the glomeruli are smaller than in the adult, but their filtration surface in relation to body weight is similar. The tubules are not fully grown and may not extend into the medulla.

Glomerular filtration rate and renal plasma flow

It is difficult to decide how to compare these aspects of renal function in neonates and adults. Whatever basis is used is largely a matter of convention and less important than an understanding that glomerular filtration rate (GFR) and renal plasma flow (RPF) increase with growth in a predictable way. For many years comparisons were made per unit of surface area, as this was thought to relate most closely to basal metabolism. On this basis, GFR is low and does not reach adult values until the second year of life (Table 1.3). RPF rises even more slowly from the neonatal value of $150 \, ml \cdot 1.73 \, m^{-2} \cdot min^{-1}$ to adult values ($600 \, ml \cdot 1.73 \, m^{-2} \cdot min^{-1}$) by 24 months. It is extremely unlikely that neonatal renal function is as inefficient as these figures would suggest; since the surface area/weight ratio is three times greater in the neonate than in the adult, it seems probable that surface area is not the most appropriate basis on which to make the comparison.

It has been suggested that renal function should be related to some measure of body fluid volume, but no single volume is appropriate for all situations and, as with surface area, fluid volumes can only be estimated.

Weight, which can be measured directly, has the advantage of being the only routinely used measure in clinical practice. There is now evidence that, in early infancy, age- and weight-related variations are best minimized by expressing the GFR per kilogram rather than per surface area.

Irrespective of the basis of comparison, the GFR, RPF and tubular reabsorption mechanisms are poorly developed in the neonate, particularly in the first week of life. Renal cortical perfusion is particularly poor, and peripheral vascular resistance is increased. In the piglet, RPF does not

Table 1.3   Changes in glomerular filtration rate in early infancy

| Age | GFR ($ml \cdot 1.73\,m^{-2} \cdot min^{-1}$) | |
	Mean	Range
2–3 hours	24	3– 38
2– 8 days	38	17– 60
10–22 days	50	32– 69
37–95 days	58	30– 86
Adult	120	105–150

(From data of Edelman, 1979)

become normal until the end of the first month of extrauterine life, and it seems likely that it follows a similar pattern in the human. This may account for the fact that neonates suffering from birth asphyxia or severe dehydration are particulary vulnerable to renal vascular insults such as venous thrombosis. Tubular reabsorption of glucose has been shown to be similar in relation to GFR in neonates and older children. There is, however, poor reabsorption of filtered amino acids and the renal bicarbonate threshold is low. The restrained GFR probably prevents overperfusion of the poorly developed tubules, and limits the loss of sodium and water, especially in response to water loading.

Concentration and dilution

The ability of the neonatal kidney to concentrate urine in response to water deprivation is less than in the adult. In the first week of life the neonate cannot concentrate his urine much above $600\,mmol \cdot l^{-1}$; even when no water has been given for 3 days following birth, concentrations above $500\,mmol \cdot l^{-1}$ are seldom reached. This is, however, largely due to solutes such as urea being excreted at too low a rate to be concentrated rather than to impairment of tubular reabsorption alone, and the apparent defect is less on a high protein diet. Concentrations of non-urea solutes are similar in neonates and in adults.

The neonate has virtually no diuretic response to a water load for the first 48 hours after birth. By the end of the first week dilute urine can be produced, but output tails off before the full water load has been excreted.

Sodium

The neonatal kidney is poor at retaining sodium, especially during prematurity. The premature kidney leaks three times more sodium than at term, and hyponatraemia is therefore common.

Excretion of a sodium load is also poor, rising from approximately $1.5 \, \text{mmol} \cdot 1.73 \, \text{m}^{-2} \cdot \text{h}^{-1}$ at birth to reach the normal adult value of 15–$16 \, \text{mmol} \cdot 1.73 \, \text{m}^{-2} \cdot \text{h}^{-1}$ by 1 year.

Sodium loss may be considerable during the diuretic phase which follows relief of urinary obstruction.

Potassium

Potassium levels are high at birth, and well tolerated. Even values as high as $10 \, \text{mmol} \cdot 1^{-1}$ can occur without changes in the ECG and without treatment necessarily being required. Such high levels would of course give rise to concern, and levels above $5 \, \text{mmol} \cdot 1^{-1}$ demand investigation. Serum potassium levels fall gradually in the first 48 hours of life, but mainly because of a shift into the cells with correction of acidosis rather than by renal excretion.

Acid–base changes

The pH of cord blood immediately after birth is lower than that of the mother, due to intrapartum asphyxia. In the premature infant a metabolic acidosis may persist for several days (see p. 46), but in the full-term infant the pH usually rises to the normal adult level within 12 hours of birth. Metabolism of milk produces hydrogen ion in excess of bicarbonate. This is excreted in the urine as titratable acidity and ammonium ion, and is substantially greater on a diet of cow's milk than on breast milk. After the first few days of life the ability to acidify the urine is normal, but the excretion of titratable acidity is low due to low phosphate excretion, and ammonium excretion is reduced in proportion to GFR. During acidosis only a modest increase in acid excretion is possible, resulting in the rapid development of acidaemia in response to only a small increase in hydrogen ion.

Extrarenal factors affecting neonatal metabolism

Growth

By the end of the first week of life, the normal full-term neonate on a diet of breast milk may be consuming $2 \, \text{g} \, \text{protein} \cdot \text{kg}^{-1}$ body weight $\cdot \text{day}^{-1}$. The growing infant, however, incorporates about 50 per cent of this protein into body tissues, together with water, phosphate, potassium and other substances. The phenomenon of growth thus relieves the kidney of some of its excretory load: growth has been described as 'the third kidney'. It has been shown, however, that an adequate calorie intake is essential to protect nephrectomized puppies from the development of uraemia, hyperkalaemia or hyperphosphataemia by this anabolic mechanism.

Diet

An adequate intake of carbohydrate, fat, protein, sodium, potassium, calcium, chloride and other solutes is essential for growth. Although fat and carbohydrate are completely metabolized to carbon dioxide and water, an excessive intake of other solutes (e.g. by intravenous administration) will increase the solute load for excretion, which can be approximately estimated by the equation:

$$\text{Solute load (mmol)} = 4 \times \text{dietary protein (g)} + \text{dietary Na (mmol)} + \text{dietary K (mmol)} + \text{dietary Cl (mmol)}$$

Table 1.4 Representative dietary intakes and urinary excretion of infants receiving cow's milk and human breast milk, and of adults, expressed per kg body weight per day

| Per kg body weight per day | Infants | | Adults |
	Cow's milk	Human breast milk	
Water (ml)	150	150	30
Sodium (mmol)	4	1	1
Potassium (mmol)	5	2	1
Chloride (mmol)	4	2	1
Calcium (mg)	200	50	15
Phosphorus (mg)	150	23	20
Magnesium (mg)	18	6	4
Protein (g)	5	2	1
Calories (J)	420	420	168
Renal solute load (m)*	33	13	7
Urine osmolality $(m \cdot l^{-1})$†	330	130	280

* Calculated from the formula of Ziegler and Fomon (1971).
† Assuming a urine volume of 100 ml·kg^{-1} body weight per day in the infant and 25 ml·kg^{-1} body weight per day in the adult.

(From Barratt, 1974)

Table 1.4 shows that although the calorific value of equivalent volumes of cow's milk and breast milk is similar, the renal solute load of cow's milk is nearly three times as high. An infant who is unable to concentrate his urine above $300\,\text{mmol·l}^{-1}$ will be in negative water balance on a daily intake of cow's milk of $150\,\text{ml·kg}^{-1}$, and, because he is unable to complain of thirst, could become seriously dehydrated even on this apparently adequate fluid intake. Barratt (1974) commented that cow's milk for such an infant is as sea-water for a shipwrecked sailor, causing dangerously hyperosmolar states.

Surgery

In adults there is a well-defined metabolic response to surgery and trauma, including rapid utilization of glycogen stores, protein breakdown, and the release of antidiuretic and adrenocortical hormones, causing water and salt retention. This is also seen in the newborn, particularly after fetal distress or birth trauma. The trauma of surgery in the neonatal period does not seem to produce this metabolic response unless the surgery is major or the baby's general state poor. In these babies there is a severe shift of fluid from the intravascular compartment to the third space. In acute renal damage the kidneys tend to retain salt and water because of the reduced GFR, although in chronic renal disease such as renal dysplasia, where salt and water retention is diminished, the antiduiretic response to surgery is not seen.

Normal water and electrolyte metabolism

The total body water content of the newborn neonate is proportionately higher than the adult, due principally to a relative excess of extracellular fluid (Fig. 1.21). Normal babies may starve for up to 4 days after birth as lactation becomes established, and during the first 72 hours after birth there is usually a weight loss of 5–10 per cent of body weight. During the first few days of life, when excess extracellular fluid is being excreted, the ability of the kidneys to produce a duiretic response to further fluid intake is limited, and although this response improves rapidly it is not fully developed until 2–4 weeks of age. This limited ability to excrete a water load in the newborn period, together with low renal clearance of sodium and chloride, may lead to the retention of undesirably large quantities of any fluid administered. On the other hand, fluid deprivation in the first 72 hours of life is relatively well tolerated in the full-term neonate with no abnormal

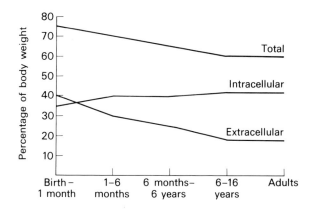

Fig. 1.21 Distribution of total, intracellular and extracellular water, expressed as a percentage of body weight related to age. (Reproduced, with permission, from Bush, 1971)

losses, and, despite the dilute nature of the urine, renal conservation of sodium and potassium is remarkably good. It will be seen below, however, that this does not apply in the premature neonate, where insensible water loss is greater, or in the presence of abnormal losses even in full-term neonates.

Water loss

Urine volume is limited mainly by the low GFR, especially in the first few days of life, although it is affected by variations in fluid intake and in solutes to be excreted. Most healthy infants pass urine in the first 24 hours of life and 99 per cent have micturated by 48 hours. Urine volume commences at about $25\,ml\cdot day^{-1}$ and rises to $100–200\,ml\cdot kg^{-1}$ body weight$\cdot day^{-1}$ by the end of the first week. The osmolality falls from $400–500\,mmol\cdot l^{-1}$ to about $100\,mmol\cdot l^{-1}$. Infants with water-losing renal disease are at great risk, for they may be unable to make up for their urinary water losses by drinking. Infants with abnormal kidneys may not have the usual antidiuretic and antinatriuretic response to surgery. The diuresis which follows the release of urethral valves may result in the passage of up to 1 litre of urine in 10 hours, together with a considerable loss of sodium.

Insensible fluid loss in newborn neonates weighing over 2 kg is between 0.7 and $1\,ml\cdot kg^{-1}\cdot h^{-1}$ under usual environmental conditions. In premature babies, however, insensible water loss is much greater, and values between 2.5 and $3\,ml\cdot kg^{-1}\cdot h^{-1}$ have been measured in neonates weighing less than 1 kg. Insensible water loss increases during exposure to radiant energy from overhead heaters, and also during phototherapy. The increase with radiant heaters varies from 50 to 200 per cent, depending on the maturity of the infant and the type of heater used; water loss during phototherapy can be minimized by careful temperature control of the infant. Insensible water loss also increases during pyrexia, when environmental temperature is excessively high, as in the tropics, and will be affected by changes in the humidity of ambient air, although the magnitude of such changes in normal circumstances is relatively small. Water loss in the faeces is also usually small, except in the presence of diarrhoea.

Metabolism

Liver function

Before birth, most of the functions of the liver are performed by the placenta or by the maternal liver, but at birth and shortly after, the liver must take on its major role in body homoeostasis. At this time there is considerable instability as enzyme functions develop, although the liver at birth weighs 4 per cent of total body weight compared to 2 per cent in the adult. Some aspects of liver function such as detoxication and carbohydrate metabolism are poorly developed at birth, particularly in prematurity, but others such as synthesis of albumin and coagulation factors are relatively normal.

Liver enzyme systems mature rapidly after birth and function at adult levels very early in the neonatal period, usually by 3 months of age.

Most of the amino acids essential for rapid growth of the fetus are supplied via the placenta. After birth, those amino acids which cannot be metabolized must be supplied in the diet and thus represent essential amino acids at this stage. For example, the last enzyme in the trans-sulphuration pathway for cystine synthesis is absent in the human fetal liver and thus cystine is an essential amino acid to the human neonate. It is readily available in breast milk (Table 1.5). Albumin synthesis in the liver begins at 3–4 months' gestation and increases towards term.

Alpha-fetoprotein (AFP) is an α_1-globulin sunthesized by the yolk sac and the fetal liver, with maximum production at about 13th week of fetal life. Although the source of the AFP in amniotic fluid is unknown, raised levels are a reliable detector of open neural tube defects of the fetus. Maternal serum levels of AFP are less reliable, although levels 2.5 times normal give a detection rate of 88 per cent for anencephaly and 79 per cent

Table 1.5   Essential amino acids

Adult	Infant
Isoleucine	*All those required by adult, plus:*
Leucine	Histidine
Lysine	Proline
Methionine	Alanine
Phenylalanine	Cystine
Threonine	
Tryptophan	
Valine	

for open spina bifida. There is little correlation between AFP levels from amniotic fluid or serum, which suggests that the mechanisms involved in its production are independent of each other. If it is detectable in the serum of babies after the neonatal period, it may be a sign of hepatoma or teratoma.

A major function of the liver is to metabolize bilirubin from the breakdown of red cells and cytochromes and to excrete conjugated bilirubin in the bile. Some drugs (such as sulphonamides) displace bilirubin from albumin, which increases the concentration of unbound lipid-soluble bilirubin, thus increasing the possibility of brain damage. Glucuronide conjugation—one of the main methods of detoxification in the liver—is very low at birth. The conjugation of bilirubin is very inefficient, as is that of exogenous substances (see below). The proportion of conjugated bilirubin is slightly less in the neonate than in the adult, but more significant is the fact that only 20 per cent of the bilirubin is found as the diglucuronide in the baby, the rest being the mono form. The second molecule of bilirubin is bound less freely than the first. This represents much less efficient conjugation, reflected in the low activity of the hepatic uridine diphosphoglucuronyl transferase system. Adult levels of activity are reached after about 70 days. Physiological jaundice is discussed on p. 70.

Carbohydrate metabolism

The liver plays a vital role in carbohydrate metabolism, which includes: the storage of carbohydrate as glycogen; the synthesis of glucose by the process of gluconeogenesis; the conversion of carbohydrate to fat; and the release of glucose from glycogen. There is rapid synthesis of glycogen by the liver as fetal life comes to an end (from 36 weeks). The carbohydrate reserves of the normal newborn are relatively low (about $11\,g\cdot kg^{-1}$ body weight) and one-third of this is available from liver glycogen. The low birth weight baby has proportionately lower carbohydrate reserves. Energy is derived from the use of fat and protein as well as carbohydrate. The amount and availability of each 'fuel' depend on constraints imposed by immaturity of metabolic pathways, caused by lack of specific enzymes or hormones in the first few days of life. The lower the birth weight, the poorer is the carbohydrate tolerance because of deficient insulin response. Thus the poor control of glucose metabolism in the preterm baby is caused partly by immaturity of the liver and also by a lack of gluconeogenic substrates due to inadequate fat stores and low total protein. In such infants, feeding within 4 hours of birth is essential, especially as the developing brain is affected adversely if nutrition is poor between the weeks 26 and 40 of postconceptual age. Until the 35th week the mechanism of swallowing is inadequate, and nasogastric or nasojejunal feeding is usually required. Total or partial parenteral nutrition may be necessary for low birth weight babies in whom the enteral route is impossible.

Glucose is the main energy source during the first few hours after delivery, and the blood sugar falls rapidly. Liver and muscle glycogen stores fall. Fat metabolism then takes over.

Blood sugar levels in the normal term baby average $2.7\text{--}3.3\,mmol\cdot l^{-1}$ ($50\text{--}60\,mg/100\,ml$). For a low birth weight infant, $2.2\,mmol\cdot l^{-1}$ ($40\,mg/100\,ml$) is an average random finding. Hypoglycaemia and its treatment are discussed on p. 78.

Drugs

There are marked differences from the older child or adult in the disposition of drugs in the newborn because after one dose of a drug the plasma concentration persists at a higher level for a longer time in the newborn and preterm than in older children. The major factors involved in the handling of drugs are, their bioavailability, pharmacokinetics and therapeutic actions: absorption, distribution, detoxication and excretion.

Absorption

In the newborn there is relative gastric achlorhydria, slow gastric emptying, slow transit through the intestine and a relatively large mucosal surface area. Water-soluble drugs, such as the antibiotics penicillin, tetracyclines and chloramphenicol, are all well absorbed after oral administration. Ampicillin may be better absorbed in the small baby than in the adult. Absorption after intramuscular injection may be variable because of the smaller muscle mass, reduced local blood flow and a limited capacity for muscle contraction.

Distribution

Distribution is affected by many factors such as tissue mass, blood flow, lipid solubility, permeability and protein binding. The neonate has a very high total body water and extracellular fluid volume, giving a greater proportion of the body weight as water, although the extent of this varies from baby to baby depending on such factors as the volume of the placental transfusion. There are smaller fat deposits than in the adult and the blood–brain barrier is less well developed. The markedly increased sensitivity of the newborn to the respiratory depressant effects of the opioid analgesics may be a result not only of greater quantities of the drug crossing the blood–brain barrier but also of the increased sensitivity of specific receptors in the brain related to poorer myelination. This also means that greater concentration of drugs such as antibiotics will reach the CSF by systemic administration.

Plasma protein binding is lower in the newborn, so the free fraction of any drug is significantly higher—up to 2.5 times that of the adult. Albumin binding is more likely to be altered by the presence of other substances in the plasma such as bilirubin or by acidotic changes. The consequence is a higher free fraction of drug in jaundiced or acidotic babies. This change in binding may be a more important factor than an actual reduction in the concentration of plasma proteins.

Detoxication

Detoxication takes place in the liver and relies mainly on the mechanisms of oxidation (e.g. barbiturates undergo side-chain oxidation as part of the detoxication process) and conjugation, usually with glucuronic acid. Such is the fate of morphine, salicylates, adrenal steroids, chloral hydrate, chlorpromazine and chloramphenicol. Because the enzyme activity involved in the metabolism of these drugs is poor in the early days of life, it is better to avoid their use where possible. Inefficient glucuronidation of chloramphenicol may lead to a build-up of its blood levels, resulting in the 'grey' syndrome of cardiovascular collapse and typical grey appearance.

As metabolic pathways become activated with improvement in liver function the half-life of drugs does decrease, but at a rate which is varied and usually unpredictable. It is therefore mandatory to monitor the levels of drugs, such as digoxin or gentamicin, with toxic side effects.

Excretion

The neonatal GFR is only 30–40 per cent of the adult value, although adult levels are attained in the first year of life. Thus drugs excreted unchanged by the kidneys will have a prolonged action because of the delayed excretion. Drugs such as digoxin and gentamicin treated in this way must have serum levels monitored carefully after several days of administration.

Acid-base state

Blood gases estimated from the cord blood show a combined respiratory and metabolic acidosis; for example, pH 7.26, Pa_{CO_2} 7.3 kPa (55 mmHg), Pa_{O_2} 2.7 kPa (20 mmHg).

After clamping of the cord, the Pa_{CO_2} falls to below normal and stays between 4.3 and 4.8 kPa (32–36 mmHg) for a few days before rising towards 5.3 kPa (40 mmHg) by 2–3 weeks of age (Fig. 1.22).

The pH rapidly rises from values found in cord blood to about 7.30 and stays for 2–3 weeks between 7.34 and 7.36 before values of over 7.38 are found. A mild metabolic acidosis may persist for weeks, especially in a premature baby fed on cow's milk. Full correction must wait for renal maturation. Changes in pH can be expected to influence potassium and calcium metabolism and the Pa_{CO_2}. A correction of base deficit greater than 5 should be undertaken using the formula:

$$\text{ml } 8.4\% \text{ sodium bicarbonate} = \frac{\text{kg wt}}{3} \times \text{base deficit}$$

The sodium bicarbonate solution has an osmolality of 2000 mmol·l^{-1}, and if given quickly may cause cellular damage, especially of the brain, and has been incriminated in the production of intraventricular cerebral haemorrhage. Sodium bicarbonate, except in a situation of severe or progressive acidosis, should be given slowly intravenously; perhaps a quarter of the calculated dose followed by the remainder over 1 hour.

Metabolic acidosis in the newborn commonly results from asphyxia or circulatory failure from a variety of causes. In asphyxial acidosis of the newborn, circulatory failure may occur because of interference with the breakdown of glycogen in the heart under anaerobic conditions. The effects on the brain can be equally disastrous and may be irreversible.

Monitoring of acid–base state must be frequent if adequate treatment is to be undertaken. Fresh arterial blood is preferable because it also gives information about alveolar ventilation and the alveolar–arterial oxygen difference (A–aD_{O_2}) may be calculated.

Calcium

Calcium is vital for the function of membranes, for coagulation and for bone growth. Homoeostasis of calcium is influenced by serum phosphate, parathyroid hormone, vitamin D and calcitonin, but relies on a balance between intake in the diet, calcium taken into bone and urinary excretion. The fetus acquires most of its calcium stores in the last 12 weeks of gestation, and at birth the calcium and phosphate levels are higher than in the mother. There is active transport of calcium ions from the mother to the fetus and the phosphate is high because of the relative hypoparathyroidism of the fetus. As expected, low birth weight babies have deficient stores of calcium, so hypocalcaemia is common in preterm babies in the first days of life.

After birth, plasma phosphate levels rise because of low GFR and parathyroid hormone deficiency which takes over 48 hours to rise to detectable

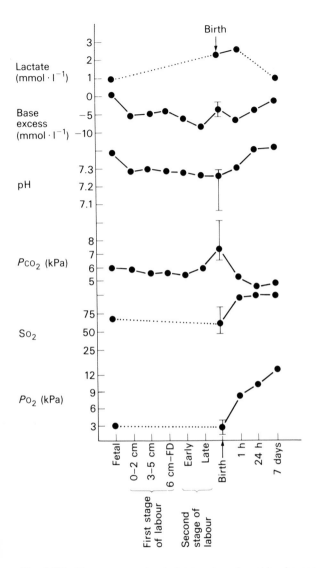

Fig. 1.22 Changes occurring in fetal and newborn blood over the perinatal period. Dotted lines indicate no data available. FD, full dilatation of cervix. (Reproduced, with permission, from Swyer, 1971)

levels. The high plasma phosphate depresses the serum Ca^{2+} level. Additional factors which may cause hypocalcaemia at birth are poor conversion of vitamin D to its active metabolite and poor absorption of calcium from the small and large intestine. High levels of glucocorticoids also depress serum calcium.

Hypocalcaemia is discussed further on p. 80.

References and further reading

General

Britton, S. B., Fitzhardinge, P. M., Ashby, S. (1981). Is intensive care justified for infants weighing less than 801 gm at birth? *Journal of Pediatrics* **99**, 937.

Davies, P. A., Robinson, R. J., Scopes, J. W., Tizard, J. P. M. and Wigglesworth, J. S. (1972). *Medical Care of Newborn Babies*. Clinics in Developmental Medicine, no. 44/45. Heinemann Medical, London.

Davis, J. A. and Dobbing, J. (1981). *Scientific Foundations of Paediatrics*, 2nd edn. Heinemann Medical, London.

Dawes, G. S. (1968). *Foetal and Neonatal Physiology*. Year Book Medical, Chicago.

Dubowitz, L. M., Dubowitz, V. and Goldberg, C. (1970). Clinical assessment of gestational age in the newborn infant. *Journal of Pediatrics* **77**, 1.

Halliday, H. L., McClure, G. and Reid, M. (1981). *Handbook of Neonatal Intensive Care*. Ballière Tindall, London.

Lubchenco, L. O. (1976). *The High Risk Infant*. W. B. Saunders, Philadelphia.

Mirkin, B. L. (1975). Perinatal pharmacology: placental transfer, fetal localization and neonatal disposition of drugs. *Anesthesiology* **43**, 156.

Roberton, N. R. C. (1979). Perinatal physiology. In: *Clinical Paediatric Physiology*. Ed. by S. Godfrey and J. D. Baum. Blackwell Scientific, Oxford.

Roberton, N. R. C. (1986). *A Manual of Neonatal Intensive Care*, 2nd edn. Edward Arnold, London.

Smith, P. C. and Smith, N. T. (1982). The special considerations of the premature infant. In: *Some Aspects of Paediatric Anaesthesia*, p. 273. Ed. by D. J. Steward. Elsevier/North-Holland Biomedical Press, Amsterdam.

Swyer, P. R. (1975). *The Intensive Care of the Newly Born. Physiological principles and practice*. Monographs in Paediatrics, vol. 6. S. Karger, Basel; Wiley, Chichester.

Symposium on the Neonatal Period. (1977). *British Journal of Anaesthesia* **49**, 1.

Respiration

Askin, F. O. and Kuhn, C. (1971). The cellular origin of pulmonary surfactant. *Laboratory Investigation* **25**, 260.

Auld, P. A. M. (1976). Pulmonary transition from fetal life. In: *Reviews in Perinatal Medicine*. Ed. by E. M. Scarpelli and E. V. Cosmi. University Park Press, Baltimore.

Avery, M. E., Fletcher, B. D. and Williams, R. G. (1981). *The Lung and Its Disorders in the Newborn Infant*, 4th edn. W. B. Saunders, Philadelphia.

Ceruti, E. (1966). Chemoreceptor reflexes in the newborn. *Pediatrics* **37**, 556.

Cook, C. D., Sutherland, J. M., Segal, S., Cherry, R. B., Mead, J., McIlroy, M. B. and Smith, C. A. (1957). Studies of respiratory physiology in the newborn infant. III. Measurements of mechanics of respiration. *Journal of Clinical Investigation* **36**, 440.

Darling, R. C., Smith, C. A., Asmussen, E. and Cohen, F. M. (1941). Some properties of human fetal and maternal blood. *Journal of Clinical Investigation* **20**, 739.

Dawes, G. S., Fox, H. E., Leduc, B. M., Liggins, G. C. and Richards, R. T. (1972). Respiratory movements and rapid eye movements during sleep in the foetal lamb. *Journal of Physiology* **220**, 119.

De Lemos, R. A., Shermata, D. W., Knelson, J. H., Kotas, R. and Avery, M. E. (1970). Acceleration of appearance of pulmonary surfactant in the fetal lamb by the administration of corticosteroid. *American Review of Respiratory Disease* **102**, 459.

Delivoria-Papadopolous, M., Roncevic, N. P. and Oski, F. A. (1971). Postnatal changes in oxygen transport of term, premature and sick infants. *Pediatric Research* **5**, 235.

Godfrey, S. (1981). Growth and development of the respiratory system: functional development. In: *Scientific Foundations of Paediatrics*, 2nd edn, p. 432. Ed. by J. A. Davis and J. Dobbing. Heinemann Medical, London.

Hellegers, A. E. and Schrueffer, J. J. P. (1961). Nomograms and empirical equations relating to oxygen tension, percentage saturation and pH in maternal and fetal blood. *American Journal of Obstetrics and Gynecology* **81**, 377.

Hislop, A. and Reid, L. (1981). Growth and development of the respiratory system: anatomical development. In: *Scientific Foundations of Paediatrics*, 2nd edn, p. 390. Ed. by J. A. Davis and J. Dobbing. Heinemann Medical, London.

Karlberg, P. and Koch, G. (1962). Respiratory studies in newborn infants. III. Development of mechanics of breathing during the first week of life. A longitudinal study. *Acta Paediatrica Scandinavica* Suppl. 135, p. 121.

Kulovich, M. V., Hallman, M. B. and Gluck, L. (1979). The lung profile. I. Normal pregnancy. *American Journal of Obstetrics and Gynecology* **135**, 57.

Liggins, G. C. and Howie, R. N. (1972). A controlled trial of glucocorticoid treatment for prevention of respiratory distress syndrome in premature infants. *Pediatrics* **50**, 515.

Mansell, A., Bryan, A. C. and Levison, H. (1972). Airway closure in children. *Journal of Applied Physiology* **33**, 711.

Mead, J., Whittenberger, J. L. and Radford, E. P. Jr (1957). Surface tension as a factor in pulmonary pressure volume hysteresis. *Journal of Applied Physiology* **10**, 191.

Meyrick, B. and Reid, L. (1970). The alveolar wall. *British Journal of Diseases of the Chest* **64**, 121.

Milner, A. D. and Vyas, H. (1982). Lung expansion at birth. *Journal of Pediatrics* **101**, 879.

Rigatto, H. and Brady, J. P. (1972). Periodic breathing and apnea in preterm infants. *Pediatrics* **50,** 202.

Sorbini, C. A., Grassi, V. and Solinas, E. (1968). Arterial oxygen tension in relation to age in healthy subjects. *Respiration* **25,** 3.

Stocks, J. (1977). The functional growth and development of the lung during the first year of life. *Early Human Development* **1,** 285.

Stocks, J. and Godfrey, S. (1977). Specific airway conductance in relation to post conceptional age during infancy. *Journal of Applied Physiology* **43,** 144.

Stocks, J., Thomson, A., Wong, C. and Silverman, M. (1985). Pressure flow curves in infancy. *Pediatric Pulmonology* **1,** 33.

Strang, L. B. (1977). Growth and development of the lung: fetal and postnatal. *American Review of Physiology* **39,** 260.

Strang, L. B. (1978). *Neonatal Respiration*. Blackwell Scientific, Oxford.

Vyas, H., Milner, A. D., Hopkin, I. E. and Falconer, A. D. (1983). Role of labour in the establishment of functional residual capacity at birth. *Archives of Disease in Childhood* **58,** 512.

Heart and circulation

Born, G. V. R., Dawes, G. S., Mott, J. C. and Widdicombe, J. G. (1954). Changes in the heart and lungs at birth. *Cold Spring Harbor Symposia on Quantitative Biology* **19,** 102.

Downing, S. E. (1970). Metabolic and reflex influences on cardiac function in the newborn. In: *Pathophysiology of Congenital Heart Disease*. Ed. by F. H. Adams, H. J. C. Swan and E. V. Hall. University of California Press, Los Angeles.

Drummond, W. H. (1983). Persistent pulmonary hypertension of the neonate (persistent fetal circulation syndrome). *Advances in Pediatrics* **30,** 61.

Kitterman, J. A. (1980). Patent ductus arteriosus: current clinical status. *Archives of Disease in Childhood* **55,** 106.

Kitterman, J. A., Phibbs, R. M. and Tooley, W. H. (1969). Aortic blood pressure in normal newborn infants during the first 12 hours of life. *Pediatrics* **44,** 949.

Macartney, F. J. (1979). Heart and circulation. In: *Clinical Paediatric Physiology*. Ed. by S. Godfrey and J. D. Baum. Blackwell Scientific, Oxford.

Mott, J. C. (1980). Patent ductus arteriosus: experimental aspects. *Archives of Disease in Children* **55,** 99.

Murphy, J. D., Rabinovitch, M., Goldstein, J. D. and Reid, L. M. (1981). The structural basis of persistent pulmonary hypertension of the newborn infant. *Journal of Pediatrics* **98,** 962.

Rigby, M. L. and Shinebourne, E. A. (1981). Growth and development of the cardiovascular system: functional development. In: *Scientific Foundations of Paediatrics*, 2nd edn, p. 373. Ed. by J. A. Davis and J. Dobbing. Heinemann Medical, London.

Rudolph, A. M. and Heymann, M. A. (1974). Fetal and neonatal circulation and respiration. *Annual Review of Physiology* **36**, 187.

Temperature control

Bennett, E. J., Patel, K. P. and Grundy, E. M. (1977). Neonatal temperature and surgery. *Anesthesiology* **46**, 303.

Cross, K. W., Flynn, D. M. and Hill, J. R. (1966). Oxygen consumption in normal newborn infants during moderate hypoxia in warm and cool environments. *Pediatrics* **37**, 565.

Dawkins, M. J. R. and Hull, D. (1964). Brown adipose tissue and the response of newborn rabbits to cold. *Journal of Physiology* **172**, 216.

Goudsouzian, N. G., Morris, R. H. and Ryan, J. F. (1973). The effects of a warming blanket on the maintenance of body temperature in anesthetized infants and children. *Anesthesiology* **39**, 351.

Heim, T. (1981). Homeothermy and its metabolic cost. In: *Scientific Foundations of Paediatrics*, 2nd edn, p. 91. Ed. by J. A. Davis and J. Dobbing. Heinemann Medical, London.

Hey, E. N. (1971). The care of babies in incubators. In: *Recent Advances in Paediatrics*, 4. Ed. by D. Gairdner and D. Hull. Churchill Livingstone, Edinburgh and London.

Hey, E. and Katz, G. (1970). The optimal thermal environment for naked babies. *Archives of Disease in Children* **45**, 328.

Silverman, W. A., Fertig, J. W. and Berger, A. P. (1958). The influence of the thermal environment upon the survival of newly born premature infants. *Pediatrics* **22**, 876.

Haematology

Bellingham, A. J. and Grimes, A. J. (1973). Red cell 2,3-diphosphoglycerate. *British Journal of Haematology* **25**, 555.

Burman, D. and Morris, A. F. (1974). Cord haemoglobin in low birth weight infants. *Archives of Disease in Childhood* **49**, 382.

Chessells, J. M. (1979). Blood formation in infancy. *Archives of Disease in Childhood* **54**, 831.

Glader, B. E. (Ed.) (1978). *Perinatal Haematology. Clinics in Haematology* **7**, no. 1.

Lubin, B. (1978). Neonatal anaemia secondary to blood loss. In: *Perinatal Haematology. Clinics in Haematology* **7**, no. 1.

Maisels, M. (1975). The management of hyperbilirubinaemia in newborn infants. In: *Neonatology: pathophysiology and management of the newborn*. Ed. By G. B. Avery. Lippincott, Philadelphia and London.

Stockman, J. A. and Oski, F. A. (1978). Physiological anaemia of infancy and the anaemia of prematurity. In: *Perinatal Haematology. Clinics in Haematology* **7**, no. 1.

Nervous system

Green, S. H. (1979). Neurophysiology. In: *Clinical Paediatric Physiology*. Ed. by S. Godfrey and J. D. Baum. Blackwell Scientific, Oxford.

Kidney

Barratt, T. M. (1974). The nephrological background to urology. In *Encylopaedia of Urology*, vol. 15, Suppl. Ed. by D. I. Williams, Springer Verlag, Heidelberg.

Bennett, E. J. and Bowyer, D. E. (1985). Fluid balance. In: *Paediatric Anaesthesia. Clinics in Anaesthesiology* **3**, no. 3.

Brodehl, J., Franken, A. and Gellissen, K. (1972). Maximum tubular reabsorption of glucose in infants and children. *Acta Paediatrica Scandinavica* **61**, 413.

Bush, G. H. (1971). Intravenous therapy in paediatrics. *Annals of the Royal College of Surgeons of England* **49**, 92.

Coulthard, M. G. (1983). Comparison of methods of measuring renal function in preterm babies using inulin. *Journal of Pediatrics* **102**, 923.

Coulthard, M. G. and Ruddock, B. (1983). Validation of inulin as a marker for glomerular filtration in preterm babies. *Kidney International* **23**, 407.

Edelman, C. M. Jr (1979). Physiologic adaptations required of a newborn's kidney. *Contributions to Nephrology* **15**, 1.

Guignard, J. P. (1982) Renal function in the newborn infant. *Pediatric Clinics of North America* **29**, 777.

Guignard, J. P. (1984). Clinical aspects of the developing kidney. Clinical implications of a low glomerular filtration rate. In: *Paediatric Nephrology* p. 60. Ed. by J. Brodehl and J. H. H. Ehrich. Springer-Verlag, Berlin.

Hey, E. N. and Katz, G. (1969). Evaporative water loss in the newborn baby. *Journal of Physiology* **200**, 605.

McCance, R. A. and Young, W. F. (1941). Secretion of urine by newborn infants. *Journal of Physiology* **99**, 265.

Roy, R. N. and Sinclair, J. C. (1975). Hydration of the low birth weight infant. *Clinics in Perinatology* **2**, 393.

Spitzer, A. (1978). Renal physiology and functional development. In: *Pediatric Kidney Disease* p. 25. Ed. by C. M. Edelmann. Little, Brown, Boston.

Ziegler, E. E. and Foman, S. J. (1971). Fluid intake, solute load and water balance in infancy. *Journal of Pediatric Surgery* **78**, 561.

Metabolism

Dawes, G. S. (1968). Fetal blood gas homoeostasis during development. Symposium on Life before Birth. *Proceedings of the Royal Society of Medicine* **61**, 1227.

Oliver, T. K., Demis, J. A. and Bates, G. D. (1961). Serial blood gas tensions and acid-base balance during the first hour of life in human infants. *Acta Paediatrica Scandinavica* **50,** 346.

Swyer, P. R. (1971). Special physiological and physiopathological considerations. In: *Care of the Critically Ill Child.* Ed. by R. S. Jones and J. B. Owen-Thomas. Edward Arnold, London.

2

The surgical neonate

Transportation

The regional care of critically ill newborn babies in modern intensive care units with physicians, surgeons and anaesthetists trained to deal with their problems has created a need for sophisticated transport systems. Transport incubators (Fig. 2.1) are now in common use and babies are daily transferred long distances, even in aircraft and helicopters.

Many regional centres for neonatal surgery and intensive care send out a team of doctor and trained nurse with a transport incubator to collect sick babies from peripheral hospitals. This system has the advantage that babies may be correctly assessed and prepared for the journey by those more familiar with transport techniques. Approximately 50 per cent of

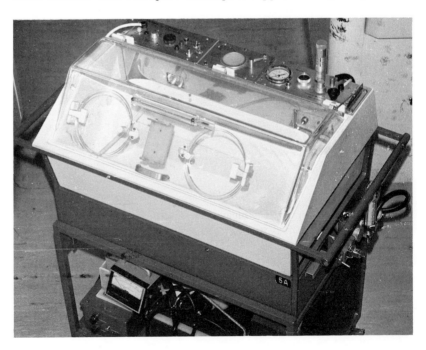

Fig. 2.1   A transport incubator. (Vickers Medical)

newborns transported in this way require some form of respiratory assistance. Medical and nursing care should be as thorough as if the baby were already in the regional intensive care unit.

Incubators must provide good visibility, immediate access and a constant neutral thermal environment. It must be possible to control the administration of oxygen, usually with a head hood.

If the thermal environment cannot be well maintained, the baby should be swaddled in a polyurethane-lined aluminium foil wrap which will give some protection against heat loss. The supply of compressed gas and battery power must be adequate for the journey.

A battery-driven air compressor or oxygen concentrator conveniently takes the place of bulky gas cylinders and is useful where mechanical ventilation is employed during the journey.

Before transfer, an intravenous cannula should be in place, providing secure access for intravenous administrations. A nasogastric tube must be passed in all babies with suspected intestinal obstruction, and the stomach contents aspirated at frequent intervals throughout the journey. The trachea of an infant with severe respiratory distress must be intubated before departure so that assisted ventilation may take place during the journey. The tracheal tube must be secured very firmly indeed, as it is extremely difficult to prevent dislodgement or kinking during transport. A clear airway is essential at all times, so suction catheters and suction apparatus must be at hand. A self-inflating manual bag system such as the Ambu is necessary, as is intubation equipment. It is usual to take a prepacked kit of equipment and drugs for resuscitation on all such journeys.

Ideally, monitoring of the baby should include ECG, as listening to the heart sounds using a stethoscope may be difficult because of the noise and motion of transport.

Monitoring of preterm babies having increased F_{IO_2} should also include transcutaneous oxygen monitoring. Maintenance intravenous fluids are given using a battery-driven syringe pump (e.g. Vickers IP5). Fluids should contain dextrose and regular Dextrostix estimations should be done on the journey. Continuous monitoring of the baby's temperature is also necessary.

Most commercial transport incubators have the optional facility for mechanical ventilation of babies in respiratory failure. Such equipment should have the same accurate control of F_{IO_2}, humidification and ventilator settings as any intensive care machine.

The incubator must have a means of securing the body inside it, and must itself be secured in case of sudden movements of the ambulance or aircraft.

With the help of this equipment and careful monitoring, it should be possible to transfer even the most sick infants long distances with the minimum of disturbance. It is usual for the baby to be accompanied by a qualified nurse and a member of the medical staff skilled in intubation and resuscitation techniques, including if necessary the placement of a chest drain for pneumothorax.

One published series (Blake *et al.*, 1975) describes 222 patients transported over a 50-mile radius: 40 per cent of the patients were clinically improved during the journey; 56 per cent were stable and only 4 per cent deteriorated.

There should be full co-ordination between the transport team and the receiving centre so that the staff are prepared with equipment and personnel for the new arrival. The extent to which respiratory support and monitoring are likely to be required should also be known.

Preoperative assessment and management

All neonates must be carefully assessed preoperatively by the anaesthetist. It may be necessary to explain to the parents what anaesthesia involves for patients in this age group. All babies are accurately weighed on admission and a full history is taken, including the method of delivery and the gestational age, and then a full clinical examination undertaken.

Many congenital defects are multiple, and a baby presenting for surgery for one defect could well have others with serious implications for the anaesthetist. One-third of patients with oesophageal atresia also have a cardiac defect. Fourteen per cent of babies with cleft lip and 33 per cent of those with cleft palate have other congenital abnormalities such as the Pierre Robin syndrome of micrognathia and glossoptosis; babies with Down's and Edwards' syndromes may have congenital heart diseases.

The anaesthetist will be alerted to obvious intubation difficulties as seen with Pierre Robin, Treacher–Collins or the Klippel–Feil syndromes.

Feeds may be given to the baby until 4 hours preoperatively, although the last feed is better given as clear dextrose rather than milk. A nasogastric tube should be passed in any sick baby, especially one with intestinal obstruction. Gastric distension is a very common problem in infancy, with acidosis and hypoxaemia as predisposing causes even in babies without intestinal obstruction, and increases the risk of regurgitation. Pulmonary aspiration, elevation of the diaphragm and basal atelectasis may all prejudice normal respiratory function.

Oesophageal motility is reduced in the newborn, especially in the lower third, so some degree of reflux occurs continuously. The cardio-oesophageal sphincter mechanism does not develop until the end of the first year. Gastric motility may be low and up to 40 per cent of any feed may still be in the stomach 2 hours later, depending on the type of fluid (breast milk passes into the intestine more rapidly), the position of the baby (more rapid emptying if the baby is prone) and the fitness of the baby. Gastric emptying times are markedly increased in premature and sick babies. The nasogastric tube should be left to drain freely and the equivalent volume of normal saline should be given intravenously to replace the loss. The tube must be aspirated before anaesthesia and left unclamped.

Too large a nasogastric tube (greater than 8 FG) can cause an increase in airway resistance or even respiratory obstruction in infants, as they are obligatory nose breathers.

If possible, the baby should be taken to theatre in optimum condition in an incubator when the body temperature is normal, adequate hydration and blood volume ensured, and when all the necessary investigations and x-rays have been performed.

The preterm infant

Twenty years ago very few preterm babies survived to need surgical treatment, but nowadays the survival rate of infants of less than 1000 g is at least 80 per cent. Because congenital defects occur more commonly in the preterm and this group is at risk from such conditions as hydrocephalus, inguinal hernia and necrotizing enterocolitis, the demand for surgery and anaesthesia is increasing. With the increase in survival has come a decrease in the number and severity of major neurological handicaps, which may be fewer than 6 per cent. The low birth weight preterm baby is not merely a small neonate, but is likely to have immature organs and enzyme systems with poor function which demand specialist medical, surgical and anaesthetic management.

It is important to have as exact an estimate of the gestational age as possible to predict how incomplete organ function is likely to be. Body weight is a poor guide to the assessment of gestational age, but it is important as a guide to survival as the mortality increases inversely with birth weight.

Clinical assessment of gestational age

There is an increase in muscle tone and a change in balance between extensor and flexor groups of muscles during the last 12 weeks of gestation. This forms the basis of the method of Amiel-Tison (1968) to assess gestational age (Fig. 2.2).

Prematurity

Most of the problems of prematurity are discussed elsewhere. These babies lose heat very easily because there is little subcutaneous fat. Metabolic heat production comes from brown fat, which can be used up within 48 hours in adverse conditions. A high neutral thermal environment is essential (up to 36°C for a 1000 g newborn)—especially during surgery. If a preterm baby is cooled there is an increased mortality and morbidity with increased susceptibility to RDS, acidosis and hypoxia, coagulopathy, intraventricular haemorrhage (IVH) and possibly a subsequently slower rate of brain growth.

Preterm babies may need total parenteral nutrition but glucose infusions should be reduced before surgery because stress, with cortisol secretion, causes insulin antagonism which may produce intraoperative hyperglycaemia and a hyperosmolar state which increases the risk of IVH. Reduced hepatic function is shown by jaundice and unstable levels of blood sugar. There are fewer functioning nephrons and renal clearances are diminished.

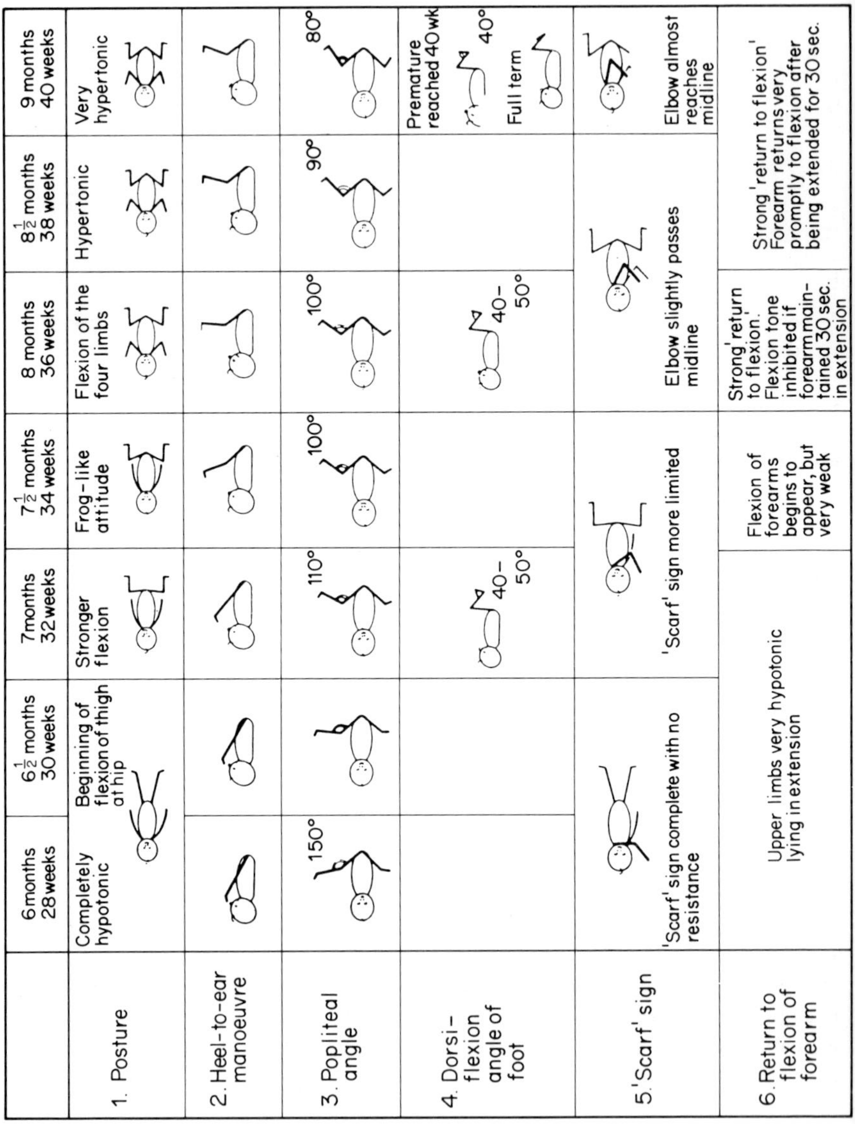

	6 months 28 weeks	6½ months 30 weeks	7 months 32 weeks	7½ months 34 weeks	8 months 36 weeks	8½ months 38 weeks	9 months 40 weeks
1. Posture	Completely hypotonic	Beginning of flexion of thigh at hip	Stronger flexion	Frog-like attitude	Flexion of the four limbs	Hypertonic	Very hypertonic
2. Heel-to-ear manoeuvre	150°						80°
3. Popliteal angle			110°	100°	100°	90°	80°
4. Dorsiflexion angle of foot			40–50°		40–50°		Premature reached 40 wk / Full term 40°
5. 'Scarf' sign	'Scarf' sign complete with no resistance			'Scarf' sign more limited	Elbow slightly passes midline		Elbow almost reaches midline
6. Return to flexion of forearm	Upper limbs very hypotonic lying in extension			Flexion of forearms begins to appear, but very weak	Strong' return to flexion. Flexion tone inhibited if forearm maintained 30 sec. in extension	Strong 'return to flexion' Forearm returns very promptly to flexion after being extended for 30 sec.	

Fig. 2.2   Clinical assessment of passive tone as it increases with maturity. (Reproduced, with permission, from Amiel-Tison, 1968)

Overhydration is very common, often because insensible water loss is difficult to measure, but also a haematocrit of more than 55 causes a deterioration in renal function. Fluid intake should be limited to not more than $90\,ml\cdot kg^{-1}\cdot day^{-1}$ for the first days of life; indeed, $100-120\,ml\cdot kg^{-1}\cdot 24\,h^{-1}$ may be all that is tolerated for several months by babies less than 1000 g. Relatively greater amounts of sodium are excreted than with full-term infants, and both hypo- and hypernatraemia are risks. All fluid volumes given, especially those involving intravenous anaesthetic drugs diluted for use, must be accounted for on fluid balance sheets.

Rhythmic respiration is not established because of immaturity of the nervous system causing what seems to be a failure of co-ordination of the stimuli which normally control respiration. About 40 per cent of premature babies have periodic respiration, including apnoea which is defined as cessation of breathing lasting for 20 seconds or more, resulting in bradycardia (less than $75\cdot min^{-1}$) and possibly cyanosis. The bradycardia itself may be caused not only by hypoxia but also by immaturity of the CNS. The tendency to apnoeic attacks is increased, even in the term baby, by RDS, sepsis, pneumonias, IVH and metabolic conditions such as hypocalcaemia and hypoglycaemia.

During apnoea the functional residual capacity (FRC) decreases to very low levels because the chest wall is even more compliant in the preterm baby and the gas exchange units are smaller ($75\,\mu m$ diameter compared to $150\,\mu m$ in the term baby) and tend to collapse at the end of expiration.

The resistance of the diaphragm to fatigue depends on the proportion of high oxidative type I muscle fibres in this dominant muscle of respiration. Before 30 weeks' gestation there are 10 per cent type I fibres, with 25 per cent at full term, whereas adults have 55 per cent. This paucity of high oxidative fibres in preterm babies must predispose to respiratory fatigue and reduce their ability to withstand respiratory demands. These babies may also have residual lung damage, oxygen dependency and reduced compliance after periods of time on mechanical ventilation.

The tendency to apnoea is increased in babies of low postconceptual age having general anaesthesia (these infants should not be treated on a day-stay basis), even for minor surgery such as repair of inguinal hernia. Babies below 44 weeks' postconceptual age are those at risk, and apnoea has been reported to occur as late as 12 hours postoperatively. Elective surgery should be postponed until the infant has passed 44 weeks' postconceptual age, but if surgery is necessary, close postoperative monitoring for apnoea and its effects is mandatory. The management of apnoeic spells includes constant distending pressure (continuous positive airway pressure, CPAP) and intravenous theophylline which may be given prophylactically in a dose of $6\,mg\cdot kg^{-1}$ (see p. 203).

Greater susceptibility to infections is a result of less efficient neutrophils and lower antibody titres than in term babies. Premature babies are particularly sensitive to sedatives and anaesthetic agents, including non-depolarizing muscle relaxants. Inhalational agents decrease tidal volume and increase Pa_{CO_2} as well as depressing the ventilatory response to CO_2. They predispose to apnoea and severely depress or even abolish the hypoxic stimulation to respiration. Nitrous oxide also depresses the ventilatory response to hypoxia.

The mechanisms whereby the trachea is protected from soiling by aspirated material are reduced.

The retina is vascularized from the nasal to the temporal side and is complete by the 44th week of gestation. If, during this process, the less mature side is exposed to high arterial Po_2, vascular spasm occurs, causing retinal tissue to become necrotic, which heals with fibrosis. New vessels are formed in the fibrotic areas and these proliferate through the vitreous, eventually causing retinal detachment— known as retinopathy of prematurity (ROP) or retrolental fibroplasia (RLF). Babies with the lowest post-conceptual age are the most likely to develop ROP. An exchange transfusion with adult blood may also increase the risk. It is recommended that arterial Pao_2 be maintained between 6.7 and 9.1 kPa (50 and 70 mmHg) by careful monitoring of inspired oxygen and arterial Po_2. The continuous use of a transcutaneous Pao_2 monitor is recommended because Pao_2 is not easy to predict for a given Fio_2, as changes in cardiac output and pulmonary shunting may vary, especially during anaesthesia. It is not known whether a short period of high Pao_2 or a longer period of lower Pao_2 carry the same risk, although there is a report of a baby developing ROP whose only exposure to increased Fio_2 was during anaesthesia. However, a type of ROP has been reported in babies who have never had an increased Fio_2 and also in patients with cyanotic congenital heart disease. Only 10 per cent of babies with ROP develop the cicatricial form. Animal work suggests that this form may occur when $Paco_2$ is raised, and in the presence of drugs such as salicylates.

Respiration

The signs of respiratory failure include dyspnoea with grunting, suprasternal, subcostal and intercostal retractions, increasing respiratory rate, oxygen dependency and the tendency to apnoeic attacks. The baby may be unable to feed or cry and there may be signs of circulatory failure. Auscultation of the chest may reveal pathology which is confirmed by chest x-ray and there may be changes in the blood gases.

A discussion of the detailed assessment of respiratory failure may be found on p. 196. Preoperative respiratory failure is usually a sign that respiratory support will be necessary postoperatively, and often this is most satisfactorily started before the operation. Oxygen therapy is discussed on p. 207, and respiratory support on p. 209 et seq.

Hyaline membrane disease

Perhaps the commonest medical condition involving pulmonary pathology in the neonate is hyaline membrane disease (surfactant deficiency, idiopathic respiratory distress syndrome). This is often seen as a complication of prematurity in the surgical neonate.

The condition occurs in 1 per cent of all live births and 30 per cent of all premature births, and is caused by a relative deficiency of lung surfactant associated with prematurity. The severity is increased by interference with surfactant synthesis in type II alveolar cells by immaturity or by hypoxia or asphyxia in the neonatal period. Up to 50 per cent of neonatal deaths are the result of RDS or its complications. Advances in respiratory care and general management of premature babies have greatly reduced the morbidity of this condition, although it is still considerable.

The incidence and mortality of RDS may possibly be reduced by the administration of corticosteroids to the mother (betamethasone 12 mg by intramuscular injection) every 24 hours for 1–3 days before delivery.

The main clinical features are tachypnoea, dyspnoea (with grunting respiration as the infant attempts to produce its own constant distending pressure), poor air entry, cyanosis and tachycardia. Signs of respiratory distress usually start within 6 hours of birth, with peak severity between 48 and 72 hours.

The chest x-ray shows a typical uniform opacity in the lung fields with an air bronchogram in more severe cases (Fig. 2.3), although for the first 24 hours the appearances may be relatively normal. Dipalmityl phosphatidylcholine is the major lipid component of surfactant, and the other phos-

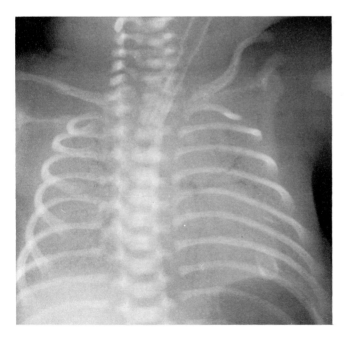

Fig. 2.3   Acute hyaline membrane disease. X-ray showing bilateral air bronchograms.

pholipid components are necessary for spreading and adsorption of surfactant in the alveoli.

Surfactant deficiency prevents the formation of a functional residual capacity of air by failing to stabilize small air spaces at the end of expiration and by delaying fluid clearance from alveoli. A disordered ventilation/perfusion ratio causes hypoxaemia, and pulmonary vascular resistance is raised by vasoconstriction, itself made worse by hypoxia, acidosis and hypercapnia. Tachypnoea, combined with stiffness of the lungs, increases the work of breathing by up to ten times. Right-to-left shunts through the ductus arteriosus or patent foramen ovale increase the arterial hypoxaemia. Reduced oxygenation to the heart impairs its function and consequently other organs suffer reduced perfusion. Metabolic acidosis will follow and a vicious circle is set up (Fig. 2.4). Hypoperfusion of the lungs allows in-

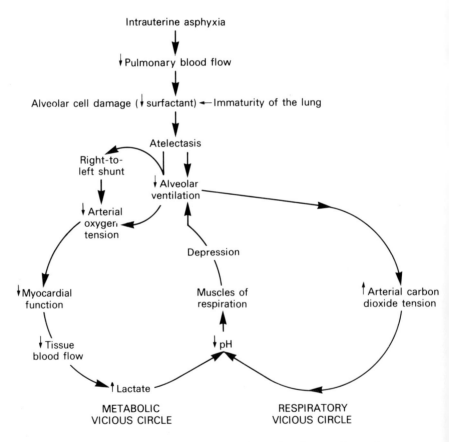

Fig. 2.4 Diagrammatic representation of the aetiology of hyaline membrane disease and its pathophysiological consequences. (Reproduced, with permission, from Swyer, 1975)

creased permeability of the pulmonary capillaries with leakage of plasma into the terminal bronchioles. Fibrin derived from the plasma constitutes the hyaline material seen at histology and from which the name hyaline membrane disease was formed.

Careful respiratory support usually begins with a trial of CPAP, perhaps with a nasal prong. Intubation and mechanical ventilation follow if pH is not maintained above 7.20, if Pa_{CO_2} is above 8 kPa (60 mmHg), Pa_{O_2} below 6.7 kPa (50 mmHg) with Fi_{O^2} above 0.7 or if there is persistent apnoea. Intermittent positive pressure ventilation (IPPV) may require reversed inspiratory/expiratory time ratios (up to 2:1) and positive end-expiratory pressure (PEEP). The use of square wave ventilation with a pressure-generating infant ventilator (e.g. Bourn BP 200), limiting inflation pressures to 30 cmH$_2$O and paralysis with the muscle relaxant pancuronium may reduce the risk of bronchopulmonary dysplasia (BPD). A patent ductus arteriosus (PDA) may also contribute to the risks of BPD, so attempts should be made to close the PDA pharmacologically using indomethacin (0.2 mg·kg^{-1} via nasogastric tube 12-hourly for three doses) or, if that fails, by surgical ligation when the acute phase of the condition has passed. In the future it may be possible to replace the surfactant using an artificial preparation, as has been achieved experimentally, but at the moment therapy is directed towards maintenance of cardiopulmonary function and normal acid–base status (Gitlin, Parad and Taeusch, 1984). Trials using heterologous natural surfactants are encouraging, although few patients have yet been treated. Because the mortality is now low with conventional therapy, the new treatment must not add to this. Sustained improvement in oxygenation and decreased need for ventilatory support have been seen after a single tracheal dose. If 'at risk' infants can be recognized, then this therapy may be used as a prophylaxis. PDA which requires closure seems to be a complication of artificial surfactant therapy.

During the course of the disease, nursing procedures should be kept to a minimum because of respiratory and cardiovascular instability. Pneumothorax with pneumomediastinum is a common complication. If pulmonary vascular resistance rises significantly, transitional circulation develops causing critical hypoxaemia, and this should respond to an infusion of tolazoline (1–2 mg·kg^{-1} over 1 hour).

Those patients who come to surgery will usually need IPPV and great attention to metabolic and respiratory functions postoperatively. Clinical recovery is usually complete by 2 weeks of life.

Perinatal pneumonia and meconium aspiration

Perinatal pneumonia is still the cause of 5–10 per cent of perinatal deaths and is found in up to 35 per cent of autopsies in this age group. The infection may be acquired transplacentally or by inhalation of infected amniotic fluids after prolonged rupture of the membranes or from another source of sepsis in the baby. Patients with cystic fibrosis (meconium ileus), congenital heart disease or prematurity are particularly susceptible. Aspiration pneumonitis, frequently complicated by infection, may be associated with inco-ordination of the swallowing mechanism, as seen in prematurity, with brain damage and with depression of the conscious level or with conditions such as tracheo-oesophageal fistula, cleft palate or hiatus hernia. The infant develops respiratory difficulties, oxygen dependency and a tendency to apnoea. There is no cough, and fever is variable. Changes on the chest x-ray will be present if the infection developed *in utero*, but changes of pulmonary atelectasis and consolidation commonly are not seen for 24–72 hours.

It is usually advisable to start therapy with antibiotics on clinical suspicion of infection, although bacteriological confirmation must be sought from sputum and blood cultures, and the antibiotic sensitivities determined. Urine and cerebrospinal fluid may also be sent for bacteriological examination as part of the initial septic-screening tests.

The infection must be dealt with properly and effectively before further lung damage ensues. The organisms involved are often the Gram-negative ones such as *E. coli*, Klebsiella or Pseudomonas, although pneumonia with *Staphylococcus aureus* is not uncommon.

Suitable antibiotics for the neonate to combat the common organisms found in this condition include cloxacillin $25\,mg\cdot kg^{-1}$ 6-hourly, gentamicin $2\,mg\cdot kg^{-1}$ 8-hourly and ampicillin 25–$50\,mg\cdot kg^{-1}$ 8-hourly.

Meconium aspiration may cause very severe respiratory failure, often complicated by transitional circulation (see Chapter 1).

It is important that the larynx be visualized in newborns who have passed meconium during delivery. If there is meconium in the pharynx this should be sucked out and the tracheal toilet with suction performed after intubation. If the aspirate contains meconium then bronchial toilet should be carried out, using 0.9% saline until the aspirate is clear. Massive aspiration blocks peripheral airways and causes overdistension of alveoli and secondary atelectasis. Gas trapping and pneumothorax are common sequelae. Respiratory support and the use of a pulmonary vasodilating drug such as tolazoline may be necessary. Antibiotics are used to prevent secondary infection but otherwise only supportive therapy is indicated.

Congenital viral infections are rare and usually involve those maternal viruses which cause a viraemia and direct placental infection with replication to spread to the fetus. Herpes simplex and cytomegalovirus (CMV) may also infect the fetus from the genital tract. Rubella has teratogenic effects of low birth weight, cataracts and retinitis, congenital heart disease and mental retardation with hearing loss. CMV causes microcephaly, encephalitis with seizures, pneumonia and liver damage. Herpes and respiratory syncytial viruses cause severe pneumonia.

Active acute or acute-on-chronic respiratory infections of any kind are an indication for delay of any but the most urgent operation. Lower respiratory infection is a very common sequel to upper respiratory tract infection after anaesthesia, as is a high incidence of laryngeal spasm during induction or emergence from anaesthesia.

Physiotherapy, humidity and antibiotics may be necessary before a baby is in optimum condition for surgery.

Near-miss sudden infant death syndrome (SIDS)

SIDS accounts for nearly 1500 unexpected deaths per year in the UK; in addition, there is a group labelled 'near-miss' SIDS who suffer a severe episode of apnoea and cyanosis, some of whom may subsequently die. This group, together with siblings of SIDS victims, has been extensively studied and may have increased morbidity associated with surgery and anaesthesia. Studies have centred on possible defective control of ventilation because abnormal respiratory responses occur in parents of SIDS victims and there is an increased incidence of apnoea in infants some of whom are SIDS victims later.

Gastro-oesphageal reflux is a common finding in these babies and acid flowing into the lower oesophagus may induce apnoea. The phase of active (REM) sleep is associated with depressed reflexes and therefore a vulnerability to asphyxia in infants. This is the sleep–apnoea theory for 'near-miss' SIDS, but in addition there may be a defect in the neurochemical control of respiration which allows non-arousal to occur during the apnoea.

Perrin et al. (1984) have found a ten-fold increase in dopamine concentration within the carotid bodies of infants with SIDS compared to those dying from other causes. It is postulated that this high dopamine concentration depresses the response of the infant to hypoxia. Home monitoring of ECG and/or apnoea may help to prevent SIDS in at risk babies—i.e. siblings of SIDS victims or those with 'near miss'. These babies should also have intense monitoring for 24 hours in hospital after even minor surgery.

Heart and circulation

The overall incidence of congenital heart disease is approximately 8 per 1000 births, although the incidence is higher in association with major chromosomal abnormalities such as Down's or Noonan's syndromes, congenital rubella or connective tissue disorders such as Marfan's or Ehlers–Danlos syndromes. Prematurity is 2.5 times more frequent in newborns with congenital heart disease and there is an association with conditions such as oesphageal atresia and cleft palate.

The medical and surgical management of newborn infants with congenital heart disease is mainly concerned with the treatment of central cyanosis and cardiac failure and, where possible, the prevention of pulmonary vascular disease.

Signs of failure

With few exceptions the right and left ventricles fail together, so congestive cardiac failure is associated with tachypnoea and tachycardia with a gallop rhythm. Normally the edge of the infant liver is palpable 1 cm below the costal margin, but, because it is such a distensible organ, enlargement is a very reliable guide to the severity of heart failure. It also means that a marked rise in venous pressure is a late sign of failure in infancy. By the same token, oedema is not an early sign of cardiac failure in the newborn, although fluid retention may be demonstrated by an unusual gain in body weight. The heart may be enlarged, with the cardio-thoracic ratio on the chest x-ray greater than 0.5. A chest x-ray may also show congested lung

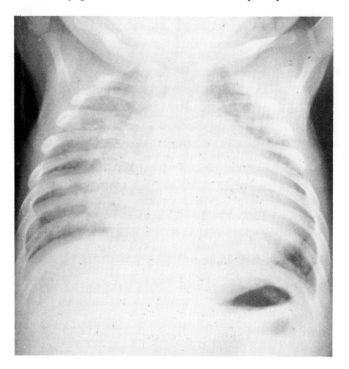

Fig. 2.5   Cardiac failure. X-ray showing large heart and congested lung fields.

fields with increased pulmonary vascularity (Fig. 2.5) where pulmonary blood flow is high (e.g. with VSD); or the lung fields may be oligaemic in patients with atresia of the pulmonary valve. Cardiac failure may also be seen with cardiac malformations of the cyanotic type, when cyanosis is unrelieved by an increased inspired oxygen concentration; i.e. there is a fixed intracardiac right-to-left shunt.

Causes of failure

Lesions presenting predominantly with cardiac failure include preductal coarctation of the aorta, ventricular septal defect, atrioventricular canal, aortic stenosis and patent ductus arteriosus, and those presenting with cyanosis and failure include transposition of the great vessels, total anomalous pulmonary venous drainage and persistent truncus arteriosus. (See Chapter 4 for discussion of cardiac surgery.)

Treatment of failure

Cardiac failure should be treated preoperatively, if necessary using digoxin $0.05\,mg\cdot kg^{-1}$ as a total digitalizing dose divided into three doses per 24 hours by intramuscular or intravenous injection. Maintenance is with digoxin, one-fifth of the total dose divided into two daily doses. Frusemide $1\,mg\cdot kg^{-1}$ i.v. as necessary may be given if the cardiac failure is severe. Because digoxin toxicity is intensified by hypokalaemia, digoxin levels and serum potassium should be measured during maintenance therapy. Potassium supplements are usually necessary.

The ECG should be checked before the third dose of digoxin is given. Other treatments include correction of acidosis, oxygen therapy and possibly inotropic support by infusions of dopamine or isoprenaline as described on p. 171.

All patients with cardiac disease require antibiotic cover for any surgical procedure which carries a risk of bacteraemia. Suitable antibiotics include penicillin $25\,m\cdot kg^{-1}$ i.v., ampicillin $25\,mg\cdot kg^{-1}$ i.v. or gentamicin $2\,mg\cdot kg^{-1}$ i.v., after induction of anaesthesia.

Sclerema neonatorum

Sclerema is a condition in which changes occur in the subcutaneous tissues of the neonate, making them feel hard and waxy. The first signs usually appear over the limbs and then extend to the trunk and the face. It may be present at birth if the mother is toxaemic, but is more usually seen by the fourth day in cases of severe asphyxia, hypothermia, sepsis, hyaline membrane disease or congenital heart disease. The differential diagnosis is peripheral oedema, but pitting can always be demonstrated with oedema even with very severe cases. The condition is related to peripheral circulatory failure, ischaemia and hypothermia. Its presence worsens the prognosis of the primary condition, especially if the sclerema is extensive, when the mortality may be as great as 75 per cent. Scleremic infants are very sick, lethargic, unable to suck and may develop respiratory failure—a contributing factor to which is the very great reduction in compliance of the chest wall. Pathological changes of inflammation, oedema and thickening of connective tissue bands are found. Corticosteroids are usually given (prednisone $1\,mg\cdot kg^{-1}$ 8-hourly) although it is uncertain if they affect the final outcome of the condition. Peripheral circulatory failure must be treated by intravenous infusions of crystalloid, blood or plasma. Exchange transfusion may be necessary to help the haemoglobin to give up oxygen in the periphery. Because of the association of sclerema with neonatal sepsis, an antibiotic regimen which includes gentamicin should be instituted.

In recent years, the incidence of sclerema has been reduced, possibly because resuscitation of the newborn is increasingly efficient and complete, and transport techniques have improved.

Haematology

Haemoglobin levels

The preoperative haemoglobin level should be at least $10 \, g \cdot dl^{-1}$, although higher levels are usually to be expected (see p. 30). Levels below $10 \, g \cdot dl^{-1}$ should be investigated.

A positive sickle test in the mother is an indication for electrophoretic studies of the baby's blood. Although for the first 8–12 weeks of life there is no problem with sickle haemoglobin and anaesthesia, early electrophoresis and complete diagnosis of the haemoglobinopathy may improve the management of those with sickle cell disease.

The aim of correcting anaemia should be to raise the level to $12 \, g \cdot dl^{-1}$ using a formula such as the following.

Subtract the patient's haemoglobin from the desired level (usually 12) to find the required amount of $Hb \cdot dl^{-1}$ of blood volume. This figure is multiplied by the blood volume to find the actual grams of haemoglobin required; $20 \, g \cdot dl^{-1}$ is the Hb concentration in packed cells and the volume to be transfused can then be calculated. For example, in a 4-kg infant with a Hb of $7 \, g \cdot dl^{-1}$ to be raised to $12 \, g \cdot dl^{-1}$:

$12 - 7 \, g \cdot dl^{-1}$	$= 5 \, g \cdot dl^{-1}$ increase necessary
Blood volume $(80 \, ml \cdot kg^{-1} \times 4)$	$= 320 \, ml$
$5 \, g \cdot dl^{-1} \times 320 \, ml$	$= 16 \, g \, Hb$
$16 \, g \div 20 \, g \cdot dl^{-1}$	$= 80 \, ml$ packed cells required

This can be transfused at a rate of $15 \, ml$ hourly. To avoid overloading the circulation it is common practice to give frusemide $1 \, mg \cdot kg^{-1}$ i.v. towards the end of the transfusion. If possible, a preoperative transfusion should be given at least 48 hours before surgery so that 2,3-DPG levels are normal by the time of surgery. All blood, except fresh donor blood, should pass through at least a $40 \mu m$ filter before transfusion.

Cross-matching

The viability of red cells in citrate–phosphate–dextrose (CPD) adenine storage is approximately 80 per cent after 5 weeks, but, because of increase in the number of microaggregates, decrease in 2,3-DPG and increase in potassium concentration with age, blood for transfusion to neonates should be as fresh as possible. Blood must be cross-matched for all major surgery and for operations where a blood loss of 10 per cent or more of the blood volume is anticipated. This includes most neonatal operations.

Haemorrhagic disorders

The cause of any haemorrhagic disorder in the newborn must be sought preoperatively and treated. The commonest cause of bleeding in the newborn is trauma during delivery. Since prophylactic treatment with vitamin K_1 is routine, haemorrhagic disease of the newborn caused by reduction in the levels of the vitamin K-dependent factors (II, VII, IX and X) is now uncommon. Bleeding will stop within 2-4 hours of administration of the vitamin. Water-soluble forms of the vitamin may cause haemolysis so that the natural form such as phytomenadione (Konakion) should be used.

A newborn may also have one of the rarer congenital deficiencies in the coagulation factors (e.g. haemophilia).

Sick neonates may develop disseminated intravascular coagulopathy (DIC) with a secondary platelet deficiency. The latter may also be caused by certain congenital infections such as rubella or primary bone marrow disease.

DIC occurs in association with serious neonatal disease with hypoxia, hypothermia, hypotension, acid-base disturbances and severe sepsis. Most patients have intravascular catheters and preterm babies are most at risk. DIC may be due to poor functioning of the reticuloendothelial system and the process of fibrinolysis. A low platelet count is found, together with deficiency of the consumed factors I, VII and fibrinogen which have been depleted by consumption. The diagnosis is confirmed when degradation products of fibrinogen are present.

There is diffuse haemorrhage and oozing from wounds as well as diffuse intravascular thrombosis. Fatal bleeding may occur into the lungs and the brain; in fact, most preterm babies which die with DIC have IVH and ischaemic necrosis of most organs. Treatment with heparin may be successful, giving 1 mg·kg^{-1} intravenously 4-hourly to keep the partial thromboplastin time below 100 seconds; this method is not used so often nowadays.

Initial screening tests must include a platelet count, prothrombin time and partial thromboplastin time, and treatment may involve the use of vitamin K, fresh-frozen plasma, fresh blood or plasma platelet concentrate. Administration of fresh platelet concentrate in a dose of $10-15 \text{ ml·kg}^{-1}$ provides all the necessary clotting factors as well as normally functioning platelets. If the platelets are normal, the same volume of fresh-frozen plasma may be given. Most neonates tolerate such transfusions at 8- to 12-hourly intervals as they may also be volume depleted by repeated haemorrhage. Close attention must be paid to the haematocrit and the haemoglobin level, and fresh blood given to maintain the Hb level at 12 g·dl^{-1} or above.

Septicaemia

Neonatal septicaemia carries a high mortality (up to 40 per cent) even with antibiotic therapy, and may affect as many as 1 in 500 newborns. Septicaemia may follow localized infection such as pneumonia or be a prelude to specific infections such as meningitis. *E. coli*, Pseudomonas, Klebsiella, *S. aureus* and Serratia are common organisms. Sick newborns, preterm infants, those with congenital heart disease and those from a low socioeconomic background are more likely to develop sepsis.

The clinical course may be rapid, starting with unusual lethargy, poor feeding and irritability, progressing to fall in body temperature, tachypnoea, apnoea, cyanosis, jaundice and bleeding and finally to complete cardiovascular and respiratory collapse. The very wide range of signs of sepsis in the newborn means that it should be suspected in the differential diagnosis of many conditions, such as RDS, heart disease, IVH and hypovolaemic shock. Cultures should be sought from samples of urine, blood, CSF and sputum. Specific therapy should be based on the results of sensitivity of the organism to a specific antibiotic, but before these are available it is usual to begin with penicillin $25\,\mathrm{mg \cdot kg^{-1}}$ i.v. 6-hourly, gentamicin $2\,\mathrm{mg \cdot kg^{-1}}$ 8-hourly and metronidazole $7.5\,\mathrm{mg \cdot kg^{-1}}$ 6-hourly i.v. Volume expansion of the circulation and respiratory support may be necessary. Approximately 30 per cent develop mild DIC which may need treatment with fresh-frozen plasma or platelet infusions.

Jaundice

Jaundice of the unconjugated hyperbilirubinaemia type is very commonly seen even in the normal neonate and many factors are involved. Liver enzymes associated with the conjugation of bile, particularly glucuronyl transferase, have low activity at birth, but there is also a large increase in bilirubin load. This larger load results from both increased enteric reabsorption of unconjugated bilirubin and also from the shortened life of macrocytic red cells of the newborn or increased resorption of red cells from haematomas caused by birth trauma. A high haemoglobin from placental transfusion increases the incidence of jaundice (up to 32 per cent with late cord clamping). In the full-term newborn, physiological jaundice is characterized by a progressive rise in serum unconjugated bilirubin from $34\,\mu\mathrm{mol \cdot l^{-1}}$ ($2\,\mathrm{mg}/100\,\mathrm{ml}$) to a peak of more than $100\,\mu\mathrm{mol \cdot l^{-1}}$ ($6\,\mathrm{mg}/100\,\mathrm{ml}$) at about 3 days of life and thereafter declines, at first rapidly and subsequently slowly to reach the adult value of $17\,\mu\mathrm{mol \cdot l^{-1}}$ ($1\,\mathrm{mg}/100\,\mathrm{ml}$) at the 10th day of life. The uncoupling of bilirubin from albumin is accelerated by hypoxaemia, acidaemia, hypoglycaemia, sepsis, a rapid rise of free bilirubin and immaturity. The preterm baby has low total protein levels and defects both in the binding activity of the albumin and in the binding capacity of albumin for bilirubin—a situation worsened by hypoxia, acidosis, drugs such as sulphonamides and sepsis.

In many preterm infants of less than 1000 g, serum levels of direct bilirubin may also rise because of intrahepatic cholestasis with slow excretion of bilirubin from the gut.

The danger of a high level of free unconjugated bilirubin is the damage it may inflict on the cells in the basal ganglia, midbrain and brain stem, known as kernicterus and manifest later in life by cerebral palsy, deafness and mental subnormality. All jaundiced babies tend to be sleepy, but those with bilirubin encephalopathy become very lethargic, develop a high-pitched cry and often suffer from convulsions. Unconjugated bilirubin of $340\,\mu\mathrm{mol \cdot l^{-1}}$ ($20\,\mathrm{mg}/100\,\mathrm{ml}$) may be the dangerous level, but lower levels can cause damage in the preterm babies, especially if they are acidotic, hypoxic, hypoglycaemic or hypoalbuminaemic.

Jaundice may also, of course, have a pathological basis which needs investigation; increased red cell destruction is the most common cause from factors such as bacterial infection or ABO incompatibility and congenital anaemias (Fig. 2.6).

Serum bilirubin $(mg \cdot dl^{-1})$	Birth weight	<24 h	24–28 h	49–72 h	>72 h
<5					
5–9	All	Photo-therapy if haemolysis			
10–14	<2.5 kg	Exchange if haemolysis	Phototherapy		
	>2.5 kg			Investigate if bilirubin >12 mg	
15–19	<2.5 kg	Exchange		Consider exchange	
	>2.5 kg			Phototherapy	
20 and +	All	Exchange			

☐ Observe   ▨ Investigate jaundice

Use phototherapy after any exchange

Fig. 2.6 The management of hyperbilirubinaemia in newborn infants. Guidelines are based on serum bilirubin concentration, birth weight, age and clinical status of the patient. In the presence of (1) perinatal asphyxia, (2) respiratory distress, (3) metabolic acidosis (pH 7.25 or below), (4) hypothermia (temperature below 35°C), (5) low serum protein (5 g·dl⁻¹ or less), (6) birth weight below 1.5 kg, or (7) signs of clinical or CNS deterioration: treat as in next higher bilirubin category. (Reproduced, with permission, from Maisels, 1975)

Phototherapy with a wavelength of 425–475 nm is used to decompose unconjugated bilirubin in the peripheral vessels and has effectively reduced the need for exchange transfusion, although side effects reported include damage to the eyes (conjunctiva and retina) and substantial increases in insensible water losses. Light in this blue range penetrates the skin, causing photoisomerism of bilirubin molecules mainly in extravascular tissues. The photoisomers diffuse into the blood to be excreted in the bile where they revert to bilirubin. There is a predictable non-linear correlation of the duration of therapy which is necessary with the plasma bilirubin concentration before treatment.

Babies undergoing phototherapy need protection for the eyes and an increase in maintenance fluids (Fig. 2.7).

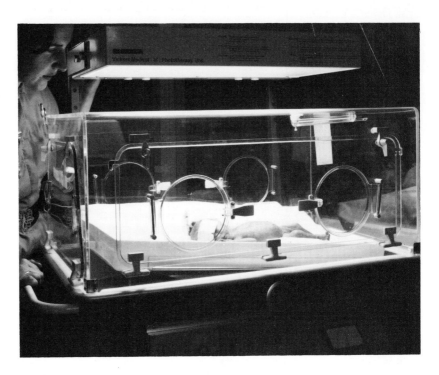

Fig. 2.7   A baby receiving phototherapy. Note the protective covering of the eyes.

Nervous system

Convulsions

Convulsions must be brought under control preoperatively. They are most frequent during the first 3 days of life, being related to birth asphyxia, trauma, intracranial haemorrhage, metabolic disorders such as hypoglycaemia and hypocalcaemia, and sepsis, particularly meningitis. The convulsions may vary from mild twitching to full grand mal seizures and coma.

The primary cause (e.g. hypocalcaemia or hypoglycaemia) must be sought and effectively treated. A severe seizure may prejudice the airway and increase the tissue oxygen demand, causing cyanosis; some form of artificial airway may therefore be necessary, as may an increased inspired oxygen concentration. The seizures must be controlled using diazepam (Valium) by incremental intravenous injection of up to 1 mg·kg^{-1} body weight or phenobarbitone 2 mg·kg^{-1} 8-hourly or 5 per cent paraldehyde infusion 2 mg·kg^{-1} body weight over 2-3 hours. If the seizures are poorly controlled with high doses of these agents it is occasionally necessary to institute mechanical ventilation with a muscle relaxant (e.g. pancuronium) as well as sedatives. If there is evidence of raised intracranial pressure (bulging fontanelle), a trial of dexamethasone 0.5 mg·kg^{-1} is indicated. Neonatal meningitis, like all neonatal infections, must be treated promptly and effectively. Antibiotic therapy (involving gentamicin and ampicillin) is usually continued for 3 weeks.

Myasthenia

Neonatal myasthenia gravis is found in 10-12 per cent of babies born to mothers with myasthenia, presumably caused by a factor transmitted via the placenta. The degree of ptosis and of weakness correlate well with the antiacetylcholine receptor titres present in the blood, the condition being an autoimmune phenomenon. This condition is transient and lasts an average of 24 days, but true congenital myasthenia gravis occurs in infants of normal mothers and in these cases the condition is lifelong.

Fluid and electrolyte balance

Abnormal water losses

Increased insensible water loss with prematurity, phototherapy and exposure to radiant heat has been mentioned on p. 42, as has increased urine volume in infants with water-losing renal disease. Perhaps the most critical pure water-losing situation in the newborn occurs with nephrogenic diabetes insipidus, in which case fluid replacement should be managed by a paediatric nephrologist.

In the presence of excess water loss, either through the skin as in very low birth weight babies or infants under radiant heat canopies or through the bowel, the urine output will fall. If adequate fluid replacement is not given, plasma osmolality may rise because of the limited ability of the neonatal kidney to concentrate the urine. On the other hand, when a high solute load is given, either intravenously or as unmodified cow's milk, plasma hyperosmolality may also occur because of the large amounts of urinary water required in which to excrete the solutes. The loss of saliva in patients with oesophageal atresia seldom causes much disturbance, but duodenal atresia may cause loss of gastric, duodenal, biliary and pancreatic secretions by vomiting. When obstruction occurs lower down the intestinal tract, both the volume and the complexity of the composition of lost fluid increase. In addition, lower intestinal obstructions are commonly associated with gross abdominal distension, which in turn causes increased capillary permeability and loss of crystalloid and colloid from the vessels in the bowel wall. As well as loss of alimentary secretions, intestinal obstruction is further complicated by starvation. It is reasonable to assume that the chemical composition of the neonate with congenital intestinal obstruction is normal at birth, but the fluid and electrolyte losses outlined above will become increasingly severe the longer diagnosis and treatment are delayed.

Sodium

It is rare to see pure sodium or pure water losses, and they are only discussed under separate headings for purposes of clarity.

Predominant loss of sodium usually leads to a loss in extracellular fluid volume, and this in turn may result in circulatory collapse, whereas pure water depletion tends to affect intracellular fluid volume, particularly in the brain. Similarly, sodium retention may lead to hypertension and oedema from expansion of extracellular fluid volume, whilst water retention causes the syndrome of water intoxication.

The concentration of sodium in the serum is determined by the relative amounts of sodium and water in the body. It is thus possible to have a normal serum sodium with severe salt depletion or overload if there are equivalent changes in body water. On the other hand, low serum sodium levels can occur with water overload even in the presence of normal body sodium. Sodium concentration in the serum of premature or term newborn infants is not significantly different from the normal adult range.

Potassium

Potassium concentrations above the normal adult range have been found on the first day of life by several workers. Potassium is the principal intracellular cation and may be lost from the body during starvation or injury in proportion to the loss of nitrogen. With renal or gastrointestinal loss of potassium, intracellular volume is maintained by sodium and hydrogen ions entering the cells. This causes a reduction in extracellular volume, intracellular acidosis and extracellular alkalosis. Impairment of potassium excretion as in advanced renal failure causes an increase in extracellular potassium concentration, with the risk of cardiac dysfunction. In acute renal failure, especially in neonates with their hypercatabolic metabolism, increase in potassium can be very rapid, and a knowledge of what is likely to happen to it in any individual clinical situation is probably more important in determining therapy than the actual serum level. A high potassium may decrease with the treatment of acidosis and dehydration, but could also indicate an aldosterone biosynthetic defect such as 21-hydroxylase congenital adrenal hyperplasia. Cardiac arrhythmias commonly occur when serum potassium levels are low, as for example during cardiac surgery.

Principles of intravenous therapy

Intravenous fluid therapy is indicated only if absorption by the oral route is inadequate. Preoperative starvation should not exceed 4 hours; even in cases of intestinal atresia or obstruction, early diagnosis and treatment may prevent long periods of fluid deprivation. Neonates should be kept on their normal feeding regimen until 4 hours before surgery, and they should be given priority on any operating schedule because if undue delays occur they will become progressively more water and salt depleted. In practice, an intravenous infusion is usually commenced preoperatively in this age group.

Bowel function usually returns fairly quickly after surgery in the neonate, and feeds of milk—preferably human—should be established as soon as possible, either orally or via a nasogastric or transanastomotic feeding tube.

Shock

In states of hypovolaemic shock, blood $20\,ml\cdot kg^{-1}$ body weight, plasma or 5% albumin should be infused rapidly, depending on the Hb and haematocrit. In severe cases, up to $40\,ml\cdot kg^{-1}$ is needed. This is sometimes the case in states of severe peritonitis. Central venous pressure monitoring is useful in ensuring the optimum right atrial filling pressure.

As dehydration is corrected, the peripheral circulation will improve and core/periphery temperatures will approximate. Indeed, the state of the peripheral circulation is a very sensitive guide to cardiac output and filling pressures in the baby.

The aim in preparation for surgery must be to achieve an optimal clinical state, but there should be as little delay as possible in operating on babies with severe peritonitis or possible gangrenous bowel.

Deficit replacement (Table 2.1)

An infant who is clinically dehydrated has probably lost $50-100\,ml\cdot kg^{-1}$ body weight (5–10 per cent). At 5 per cent dehydration there is loss of skin turgor, the fontanelles are slightly depressed and the baby is lethargic. At 10 per cent, the fontanelles and orbits are sunken, peripheral blood flow is poor and the body temperature may be high or low. Dehydration greater than 10 per cent affects the cardiovascular system and circulatory collapse is imminent.

If the deficit is severe, up to $20\,ml\cdot kg^{-1}$ of physiological saline may be given, and its effect judged clinically (improved skin elasticity, reduced pulse

Table 2.1 Contents of commonly used intravenous fluids

Solution	Na$^+$ (mmol·l^{-1})	Cl$^-$ (mmol·l^{-1})	K$^+$ (mmol·l^{-1})	Ca^{2+} (mmol·l^{-1})	Lactate (mmol·l^{-1})	Calories MJ·l^{-1}
0.9% Saline	154	154	—	—	—	—
0.45% Saline in 2.5% dextrose	77	77	—	—	—	0.4
0.18% Saline in 4% dextrose	31	31	—	—	—	0.63
Hartmann's solution	131	111	5.0	2.0	29	—
Half-strength Hartmann's solution	65.5	55.5	2.5	1.0	14.5	—
5% Dextrose	—	—	—	—	—	0.8

rate, increased venous pressure and urine output). Children with water-losing renal disease may require $200 \, \text{ml} \cdot \text{kg}^{-1} \cdot \text{day}^{-1}$ or more, and their sodium intake should be increased if there is combined salt and water loss. In nephrogenic diabetes insipidus water is required in large amounts, with only minimal salt, and even giving 0.9% saline can actually increase water losses to cover the excretion of the additional sodium.

Intestinal losses should be replaced with physiological saline, although if a metabolic acidosis is present, some of the sodium may be administered as bicarbonate. It is not usually necessary to give more than $2 \, \text{mmol} \cdot \text{kg}^{-1}$ of sodium bicarbonate in the first instance unless acidosis is severe.

Hypertonic and hypotonic dehydration should be appropriately corrected, the former with 0.18% saline or 5% dextrose, possibly after initial correction of any hypovolaemia with colloid. Care must be taken not to correct the deficiency too quickly or cerebral oedema will follow. Hypotonic dehydration is corrected with physiological saline.

Sodium deficits

Sodium deficits range from $0-4 \, \text{mmol} \cdot \text{kg}^{-1}$ in hypertonic dehydration to $8-12 \, \text{mmol} \cdot \text{kg}^{-1}$ in severe hypotonic dehydration. These should be replaced over a period of 6 hours, although more slowly in hypertonic states.

Treatment should be controlled by serum and urine electrolyte measurements. The osmolality ratio between plasma and urine should be 1:1.5. Normal serum osmolality is $270-285 \, \text{mmol} \cdot \text{l}^{-1}$; although values up to $310 \, \text{mmol} \cdot \text{l}^{-1}$ are still within the normal range, they do require an explanation. Urine osmolality varies with the fluid balance and the range of normal values is between 50 and $600 \, \text{mmol} \cdot \text{l}^{-1}$.

The amount of sodium required to restore the sodium content is largely related to the extracellular fluid volume, which is increased in the neonate to approximately 40 per cent of body weight. An amount equivalent to 20 per cent of body weight is commonly added to this to allow for intracellular requirements; this makes up the 'sodium space' of 0.6.

A useful formula for calculating the amount of sodium required to replace a deficit is:

Sodium required = deficit × body weight × 'sodium space'
   (mmol) $(\text{mmol} \cdot \text{l}^{-1})$ (kg)

A 3-kg neonate with a sodium deficit of $12 \, \text{mmol} \cdot \text{l}^{-1}$ would thus require $12 \times 3 \times 0.6 = 21.6 \, \text{mmol}$ of sodium. Since physiological saline contains $154 \, \text{mmol} \cdot \text{l}^{-1}$, this deficit would be corrected by infusion of $21.6/154 \times 1000 \, \text{ml} = 140 \, \text{ml}$ physiological saline.

Potassium deficits

Potassium deficit is more difficult to assess because the loss is mainly intracellular and only serum levels can be easily measured. The shift of potassium from the cells which occurs with the acidosis of birth and its return as the acidosis decreases have already been mentioned (p. 46). Similar shifts of potassium across the cell membrane occur with changes in acid–base state throughout life, and administration of bicarbonate will lead to a fall in plasma potassium.

Metabolic acidosis should be corrected using the formula:

$$\text{Dose required (mmol)} = \text{base deficit} \times \text{body weight (kg)} \times 0.3$$

It is usual to give half the calculated dose initially and then reassess the acid–base state.

Replacement of potassium deficit is not usually an urgent matter, although it may be in special circumstances such as open heart surgery. The concentration of potassium administered should not exceed $40\,\text{mmol·l}^{-1}$ and not more than $5\,\text{mmol·kg}^{-1}\text{·day}^{-1}$ should be given. Adequate urine flow should be present (at least $1\,\text{ml·kg}^{-1}\text{·h}^{-1}$) and deficit replacement should be spread over several days.

Maintenance requirements

The intravenous requirement for maintenance of fluid balance for the full-term neonate on the first day of life is met by the administration of 20–$40\,\text{ml·kg}^{-1}$ body weight·day^{-1} and increases by $20\,\text{ml·kg}^{-1}\text{·day}^{-1}$ until it reaches $120\,\text{ml·kg}^{-1}\text{·day}^{-1}$ towards the end of the first week. In very low birth weight babies (less than $1.5\,\text{kg}$) the maintenance fluid requirement at birth may be as much as double that at term, rising to $160\,\text{ml·kg}^{-1}\text{·day}^{-1}$. Because it is easier to give too much intravenous fluid than too little, some authorities in the past did not administer any fluid intravenously to full-term neonates in the first few days of life unless losses were abnormally high. It should be emphasized, however, that such losses almost always do occur in premature babies, mainly by insensible loss through the skin; in such babies the risks of hyperbilirubinaemia and hypoglycaemia can be minimized by infusion of appropriate quantities of 5% or 10% dextrose.

Intraoperative fluid requirements should be based on the maturity of the baby, the length of preoperative fluid deprivation and an estimation of the fluid lost into body cavities. Any fluid given in the injection of diluted muscle relaxants or other drugs should be included in the overall fluid balance. The normal maintenance requirements should be reduced by approximately 30 per cent in the first 24 hours after major surgery because of the antidiuretic response to the stress of anaesthesia and surgery, although infants with abnormal kidneys may not show this response. Post-operative fluid regimens should, however, include appropriate replacement for gastrointestinal losses and increased insensible loss associated with pre-maturity or the use of overhead heating canopies. Maintenance requirements for sodium and potassium in the neonate are $3\,\text{mmol·kg}^{-1}\text{·24 h}^{-1}$ and $2\,\text{mmol·kg}^{-1}\text{·24 h}^{-1}$, respectively, although sodium requirements are halved by the end of the first week of life. It should be remembered that premature babies of under 30 weeks' gestation require $5\,\text{mmol·kg}^{-1}\text{·24 h}^{-1}$, or more, whilst those between 30 and 35 weeks' gestation require at least $4\,\text{mmol·kg}^{-1}\text{·24 h}^{-1}$.

Potassium deficiency is not well reflected in measured serum levels; potassium should therefore be included in most solutions, although not at at a rate exceeding 3 mmol·kg^{-1} in 24 hours. Potassium should be withheld in cases of renal failure.

Renal failure

The choice of treatment depends to a great extent on the primary cause; vigorous treatment of underlying conditions such as septicaemia, for example, must be undertaken at once. Control of water and electrolyte changes must be sought and the circulating blood volume restored by plasma or blood if the baby is anaemic.

The decision to dialyse postoperatively is usually made if there is a frusemide-resistant oliguria (less than 0.5 ml·kg^{-1}·min^{-1}) or anuria following appropriate volume replacement. A urine/plasma urea ratio of less than 5 suggests a renal as opposed to prerenal problem. Dialysis would not depend on any specific potassium level, since, as already stated, potassium can rise rapidly in the neonatal period. Dialysis may be indicated in the presence of entirely normal biochemistry if the deteriorating clinical situation indicates it, or if imminent renal failure can be confidently predicted. What is more, one is often dialysing not so much to correct an obvious blood chemistry abnormality but to create space by removing salt and water so that bicarbonate, plasma and blood products can be given which would in other circumstances put the child into heart failure.

A temporary reduction in serum potassium may be achieved with 0.5–1 unit of insulin with 10–20 ml of 50% dextrose given intravenously. Administration of calcium resonium ion exchange resin 0.5 g·kg^{-1} orally or rectally may also be helpful.

Acidosis must be treated and monitored as described previously (p. 46). It is essential to maintain a normal pH if full benefit is to be obtained from any inotropic agents being administered.

Rapid deterioration in a vicious circle of falling cardiac output, hypotension, hypovolaemia, metabolic acidosis, hypoxia and further falls in cardiac output will occur unless the patient is treated vigorously. Terminal respiratory failure is a common sequel of renal failure in babies and is associated with their lower respiratory reserve.

Metabolism

Hypoglycaemia

Hypoglycaemia in the term baby is usually defined as 1.6 mmol·l^{-1} (30 mg/100 ml) or less, and in those of birth weights below 3 kg it is 1.1 mmol·l^{-1} (20 mg/100 ml) in the first 3 days of life. After this time the blood sugar should always be above 2.2 mmol·l^{-1} (40 mg/100 ml), and if found to be below this, it must be corrected. Unless the levels are very low, the hypoglycaemic baby may be asymptomatic, although symptoms such as tremors, apnoea, cyanosis, apathy, hypotonia, hypothermia and convulsions are all described. The possibility of hypoglycaemia must be anticipated to prevent avoidable brain damage; 25–50 per cent of babies with symptomatic hypoglycaemia develop neurological sequelae. Babies very likely to become hypoglycaemic include the premature and infants small for gestational age (SGA) with poor deposits of fat and glycogen, infants of diabetic mothers and those asphyxiated at birth. Very premature infants born before fat and glycogen deposits have been laid down may become hypoglycaemic at any time during the first week or two of life, especially if they are severely ill or if their calorie intake is inadequate. In SGA infants (less than 2.5 kg at term) the peak incidence of hypoglycaemia is usually found between 24 and 72 hours of age. At this stage glycogen stores have fallen whilst the infant, particularly if breast-fed, is still on a hypocaloric intake. There may be increased energy demands if the baby is nursed below the neutral temperature range. Infants of diabetic mothers have high insulin levels and may become hypoglycaemic within a few hours of birth. Since their homoeostatic mechanisms are usually working well, such infants seldom come to harm unless they are very ill or the mother was on sulphonylurea drugs. Infants with severe birth asphyxia may become hypoglycaemic shortly after resuscitation. Hypoglycaemia may, of course, be a symptom of some other condition such as glycogen storage disease or adenoma of the pancreas. By performing estimations with BM-Test strips (or Dextrostix) and/or laboratory blood sugar determinations every 4–6 hours in the first 3 days of life for SGA babies and others at risk, most cases of asymptomatic hypoglycaemia will be detected. If possible, early feeding should be undertaken; where this is not possible an infusion of 10% dextrose should be set up at a rate of $75-100 \, ml \cdot kg^{-1} \cdot 24 \, h^{-1}$. If the hypoglycaemia is unrelieved, the dextrose should be changed to 15%. If more immediate correction is required, $1-2 \, ml \cdot kg^{-1}$ of 50% dextrose should be given promptly. All intravenous fluids for infants should include dextrose. If the usual methods do not control the hypoglycaemia, steroids (prednisone $1 \, mg \cdot kg^{-1}$ 8-hourly) or ACTH (4 units 12-hourly) should be administered.

It is important to give concentrated dextrose solutions slowly to avoid reflex hypoglycaemia from the insulin released by the infusion. The need for repeated administration of such solutions is an indication for a line into a central vein.

Persistent symptomatic hypoglycaemia may be caused by the Beckwith–Wiedemann syndrome of postnatal gigantism, macroglossia and umbilical hernia or, rarely, by beta-cell nesidioblastosis. This latter condition causes a high insulin level and responds to subtotal pancreatectomy. Histology shows aberrant beta cells in small groups of two to six separate from the islets, spread throughout the pancreas. Continued hypoglycaemia is very often the cause of mental retardation.

Hyperglycaemia

Some infants having dextrose infusions develop hyperglycaemia, especially associated with prematurity and the stress of surgery possibly causing a release of cortisol. As the serum osmolality rises with the glucose load, osmotic diuresis occurs and the blood sugar level may rise as high as $44\,mmol\cdot l^{-1}$ $(800\,mg/100\,ml)$. Glucose infusions should not exceed $12\,g\cdot kg^{-1}\cdot 24\,h^{-1}$, and blood sugar should be very carefully monitored in the perioperative period.

Hypocalcaemia

Hypocalcaemia is commonest in the first 2 days of life in sick babies. It is possibly due to immaturity of the parathyroid glands, although it may appear at 5–7 days in babies fed on cow's milk, which has a high phosphate content. Hypocalcaemia may develop during an exchange transfusion with acid–citrate–dextrose. Hypocalcaemia is common in premature infants and 50 per cent may have a serum calcium below $2\,mmol\cdot l^{-1}$ $(8\,mg/100\,ml)$ in the first few days of life.

The signs of hypocalcaemia—which are mainly non-specific neurological signs such as irritability or failure to synchronize with a ventilator or, rarely, tetany or convulsions—are manifestations of a low ionized Ca^{2+} level, not necessarily fully reflected in total serum levels. The proportion which is protein bound can be estimated from the albumin level.

Treatment of hypocalcaemia is imperative and urgent if the total calcium level falls below $1.5\,mmol\cdot l^{-1}$ or if the ionized calcium level falls below $0.7\,mmol\cdot l^{-1}$. It is wise to treat ionized calcium levels below $0.95\,mmol\cdot l^{-1}$. If convulsions occur, calcium should be given without waiting for the results of serum calcium estimations ($1\,ml\cdot kg^{-1}$ of 20% calcium gluconate). In the absence of convulsions, hypocalcaemia should be treated by continuous infusion of a dilute (2%) solution of calcium gluconate at a rate of $5\,mg\cdot kg^{-1}\cdot h^{-1}$. Because calcium solutions are irritant, they should not be given into scalp veins, where tissue necrosis may occur. Indeed, calcium solutions more concentrated than this should not be given via any peripheral vein. Calcium is also incompatible with sodium bicarbonate.

Other metabolic disorders

Hypomagnesaemia may occur in association with hypocalcaemia, following exchange transfusion or following administration of diphenylhydantoin to the mother for the treatment of toxaemia of pregnancy. Treatment with 1% magnesium sulphate intravenously should not exceed 5–10 ml at a rate of less than $1\,ml\cdot min^{-1}$.

Inborn errors of metabolism occasionally require attention in the neonatal period. Galactosaemia may cause hypoglycaemia, and others such as hyperglycinaemia may cause acidosis. It is important to detect cases of phenylketonuria and maple syrup urine disease in order to take corrective measures to allow mental development to proceed normally.

Premedication

Atropine is the only drug commonly used for premedication in neonatal patients.

The dose of atropine is $0.02\,mg \cdot kg^{-1}$, although the standard dose given for many years at The Hospital for Sick Children, London, for infants weighing less than $2.5\,kg$ is $0.15\,mg$; for those between 2.5 and $8\,kg$, the dose is $0.2\,mg$ i.m. 30–45 minutes preoperatively. These larger doses are very well tolerated and abolish the bradycardia seen particularly with repeated doses of suxamethonium.

The antisialogogue action of atropine (and hyoscine) is less important nowadays since ether with its irritant effects on the tracheobronchial tree has been superseded, but its use remains more important in babies than in adults.

There is an increased risk of laryngeal spasm on extubation if the patient has excessive tracheobronchial secretions, and especially in those who have received halothane. Blockage of a narrow tracheal tube with secretions is also a possibility. All babies who are to receive suxamethonium, cyclopropane or halothane should be given atropine as a vagolytic drug. Excessive drying of secretions is undesirable, especially in patients with cystic fibrosis or those suffering from dehydration, and in these a reduced dose may be used.

Glycopyrrolate in doses of 0.004–$0.008\,mg \cdot kg^{-1}$ (maximum $0.2\,mg$) i.m. or i.v. is an alternative to atropine, although its antisialogogue effect may be weaker. However, it rarely produces such a marked tachycardia as atropine.

Some centres prefer the administration of atropine by intravenous injection during induction of anaesthesia to ensure immediate action, arguing that vagal tone tends to be low in newborn babies.

Competence of the cardio-oesophageal junction may be decreased with intravenous atropine, which may be important in patients with gastric emptying problems such as pyloric stenosis, although a large nasogastric tube and gastric washouts should ensure full drainage of the stomach in all such patients. Intramuscular atropine has little effect on lower oesophageal sphincter pressure.

Atropine has been incriminated in the production of febrile convulsions and although there are other factors involved such as hypovolaemia, atropine is best avoided in the pyrexial or toxic patient, or a lower dose should be used. It can be administered intravenously if necessary.

Hyoscine, which can cause excitation in the young, is not used in neonatal anaesthesia, and its excessive drying action on the mucosa is probably undesirable.

No sedation is required for neonates preoperatively although it may be given to those patients undergoing open heart surgery which may employ a technique of surface cooling before the chest is opened. For those babies it is essential to maintain, where possible, good peripheral perfusion. Babies are sensitive to all sedative drugs and their use must be limited to very special circumstances. Morphine given to neonates in doses of one-third of the adult dose on a weight-for-weight basis significantly reduces the ventilatory response to carbon dioxide.

Vitamin K $1\,mg$ i.m. should also be given because of its relative deficiency in the newborn and the immaturity of the liver enzyme system in synthesizing prothrombin.

References and further reading

Transport

Blake, A. M., McIntosh, N., Reynolds, E. O. R. and St Andrews, D. (1975). Transport of newborn infants for intensive care. *British Medical Journal* **4**, 13.

Hackel, A. (1975). A medical transport system for the neonate (*Anesthesiology* **43**, 258.

Preoperative assessment and management

Al-Dahhan, J., Haycock, G. B., Chantler, C. and Stimmler, L. (1983). Sodium homoeostasis in term and pre-term neonates. I. Renal aspects. *Archives of Disease in Childhood* **58**, 335.

Amiel-Tison, C. (1968). Neurological evaluation of the maturity of newborn infants. *Archives of Disease in Childhood* **43**, 89.

Arant, B. S. Jr (1982). Fluid therapy in the neonate—concepts in transition. *Journal of Pediatrics* **101**, 387.

Behrman, R. E. and Itsia, D. Y. Y. (1969). Summary of a symposium on phototherapy for hyperbilirubinemia. *Journal of Pediatrics* **75**, 718.

Bennett, E. J. (1975). *Fluids for Anesthesia and Surgery in the Newborn Infant*. Charles C Thomas, Springfield, Illinois.

Bennett, E. J. (1975). Fluid balance in the newborn. *Anesthesiology* **43**, 210.

Bennett, E. J. and Bowyer, D. E. (1985). Fluid balance. In: *Paediatric Anaesthesia. Clinics in Anaesthesiology* **3**, no. 3.

Betts, E. K., Downes, J. J., Schaffer, D. B. and Johns, R. (1977). Retrolental fibroplasia and oxygen administration during general anesthesia. *Anesthesiology* **47**, 518.

Brown, J. K. (1982). Fits in childhood. In: *A Textbook of Epilepsy*, 2nd edn. Ed. by J. Laidlaw and A. Richens. Churchill Livingstone, Edinburgh and London.

Bush, G. H. (1971). Intravenous therapy in paediatrics. *Annals of the Royal College of Surgeons of England* **49**, 92.

Chessells, J. M. and Hardisty, R. M. (1974). Bleeding problems in the newborn infant. In: *Progress in Hemostasis and Thrombosis*, vol. II. Ed. by T. H. Spaet. Grune & Stratton, New York.

Cooke, W. W. I. (1981). Factors associated with periventricular haemorrhage in very low birthweight infants. *Archives of Disease in Childhood* **56**, 425.

Cornblath, M. and Schwartz, R. (1976). *Disorders of Carbohydrate Metabolism in Infancy*, 2nd edn. Saunders, Philadelphia and Eastbourne.

Flynn, J. T. (1984). Oxygen and retrolental fibroplasia: update and challenge. *Anesthesiology* **60**, 397.

Gitlin, J. D., Parad, R. and Taeusch, H. W. (1984). Exogenous surfactant therapy in hyaline membrane disease. *Seminars in Perinatology* **8**, 272.

Gregory, G. A. and Steward, D. J. (1983). Life-threatening perioperative apnea in the ex-'premie'. *Anesthesiology* **59**, 495.

Haworth, J. C. (1974). Neonatal hypoglycemia. How much does it damage the brain? *Pediatrics* **54**, 3.

Herbst, J. J., Minton, S. D. and Book, L. S. (1979). Gastro-esophageal reflux causing respiratory arrest and apnea in newborn infants. *Journal of Pediatrics* **95**, 763.

Jeffery, H. E., Reid, I., Rahilly, P. and Read, D. J. C. (1980). Gastro-oesophageal reflux in 'near miss' sudden infant death infants in active but not quiet sleep. *Sleep* **3**, 393.

Kattwinkel, J. (1977). Neonatal apnea. Pathogenesis and therapy. *Journal of Pediatrics* **90**, 342.

Leading article (1984). Ventilatory dysfunction and sudden death syndrome. *Lancet* **2**, 558.

Levin, S. E., Bakst, C. M. and Isserow, L. (1961). Sclerema neonatorum treated with corticosteroids. *British Medical Journal* **2**, 1533.

Lister, J. (1977). Surgical emergencies in the newborn. *British Journal of Anaesthesia* **49**, 43.

Lorenz, J. M., Kleinman, L. I., Kotagal, U. R. and Reller, M. D. (1982). Water balance in very low birth-weight infants: relationship to water and sodium intake and effect on outcome. *Journal of Pediatrics* **101**, 423.

McDonagh, A. F. (1981). Phototherapy. A new twist to bilirubin. *Journal of Pediatrics* **99**, 909.

Maisels, M. (1975). The management of hyperbilirubinaemia in newborn infants. In: *Neonatology: pathophysiology and management of the newborn*. Ed. by G. B. Avery. Lippincott, Philadelphia and London.

Morley, C. J. (1984). Surfactant treatment for respiratory distress syndrome: a review. *Journal of the Royal Society of Medicine* **77**, 788.

Perrin, D. G., Cutz, E., Becker, L. E., Bryan, A. C., Madapallimatum, A. and Sole, M. J. (1984). Sudden infant death syndrome: increased carotid-body dopamine and noradrenaline content. *Lancet* **2**, 535.

Rickham, P. P., Lister, J. and Irving, I. M. (Eds) (1978). *Neonatal Surgery*, 2nd edn. Butterworths, London.

Roberton, N. R. C. (1979). Management of hyaline membrane disease. *Archives of Disease in Childhood* **54**, 838.

Rodriguez-Soriano, J. (1984). Sodium homoeostasis in the newborn kidney. In: *Paediatric nephrology*, p. 69. Ed by J. Brodhel and J. H. H. Ehrich. Springer-Verlag, Berlin.

Schaffer, A. J. and Avery, M. E. (1984). *Diseases of the Newborn*, 5th edn. Saunders, Philadelphia and Eastbourne.

Scopes, J. W. (1977). Management of respiratory distress syndrome. *British Journal of Anaesthesia* **49**, 35.

Silverman, W. A. (1981). Retinopathy of prematurity: oxygen dogma challenged. *Archives of Disease in Childhood* **57**, 731.

Sinclair, J. C., Driscoll, J. M., Heird, W. C. and Winters, R. W. (1970). Supportive management of the sick neonate. *Pediatric Clinics of North America* **17**, 863.

Spitzer, A. (1982). The role of the kidney in sodium homeostasis during maturation. *Kidney International* **21**, 539.

Stanbury, J. B., Wyngaarden, J. B. and Fredrickson, D. S. (Eds) (1983). *The Metabolic Basis of Inherited Disease*, 5th edn. McGraw-Hill, New York and Maidenhead.

Swyer, P. R. (1975). *The Intensive Care of the Newly Born. Physiological principles and practice.* Monographs in Paediatrics, vol. 6. S. Karger, Basel; Wiley, Chichester.

Waite, S. P. and Thoman, E. B. (1982). Periodic apnea in the full term infant: individual consistency, sex differences and state specificity. *Pediatrics* **70**, 79.

Young D. G. (1973). Fluid balance in paediatric surgery. *British Journal of Anaesthesia* **45**, 953.

3

Anaesthesia—basic principles

Anaesthetic equipment

Adult apparatus is rarely, if ever, suitable for use in neonates, because of its bulky nature and because of the anatomical and physiological differences between the neonate and the adult. Anatomical differences of the face and upper airway affect the design of masks, laryngoscopes and tracheal tubes, whilst the need to minimize resistance and dead space has design implications for breathing systems, connectors and tubes. The work of breathing, which is higher in the infant than in the adult, is further increased by turbulent gas flow, and total resistance should be less than $3.0\,kPa\cdot l^{-1}\cdot s^{-1}$ $(30\,cmH_2O\cdot l^{-1}\cdot s^{-1})$ during quiet breathing. Apparatus should be as light as possible, and the ability to humidify and heat the inspired gases and to scavenge expired gas is desirable.

Breathing systems

For neonatal anaesthesia the most commonly used circuit is the Ayre T-piece, introduced in 1937. In 1950, Jackson Rees modified the basic T-piece, increasing the length of the expiratory limb and adding an open-ended reservoir bag (Fig 3.1). Since then the circuit has been investigated extensively for controlled ventilation and spontaneous breathing in laboratory models and clinical anaesthesia for all age groups. It has been generally accepted for many years that a fresh gas flow (FGF) of two and a half to three times the patient's minute volume is required to avoid rebreathing with spontaneous ventilation. Recently, however, it has been suggested that FGF equal to or even lower than the minute ventilation can be used without significant rebreathing. Because of the practical difficulty of measuring minute volume in children, various formulae have been introduced for calculation of FGF necessary to avoid rebreathing. Froese and Rose (1982) have suggested that $3 \times (1000 + 100\,ml\cdot kg^{-1})\,ml\cdot min^{-1}$ will produce an arterial carbon dioxide tension of 4.9 kPa in children weighing 10–30 kg. An alternative formula—FGF $(ml\cdot min^{-1}) = 15 \times kg \times frequency$—has been derived from studies on infants down to 1 month of age, and acknowledges the importance of frequency as a determinant of minute volume. In neonatal anaesthesia controlled ventilation is virtually always used, and a fresh gas flow of $2–3\,l\cdot min^{-1}$ is sufficient. With mild hyperventilation normocapnia can be maintained even in the presence of some rebreathing of expired gas. If the

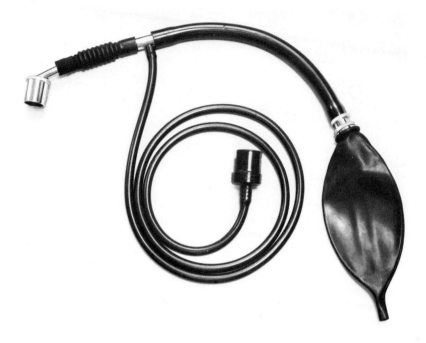

Fig. 3.1   The anaesthetic T-piece with face mask adaptor

system is to be use with spontaneous ventilation in neonates, it is essential that FGF is high enough to prevent rebreathing (at least $4 \, l \cdot min^{-1}$), since the ventilatory response of the newborn to CO_2 is reduced and hypercapnia is likely.

Many anaesthetists recommend manual ventilation when using the T-piece for neonatal anaesthesia, since this allows rapid detection of airway obstruction or disconnection from the 'feel' of the bag. This is particularly helpful during operations such as tracheo-oesophageal fistula, where surgical manipulations may interfere with the airway and air leaks can arise from the trachea. For operations where these problems do not arise, particularly those of long duration, the use of a mechanical ventilator has the advantage of producing predictable carbon dioxide levels as well as freeing the anaesthetist for the administration of drugs and fluids. The Penlon Nuffield 200 ventilator (Fig. 3.2) when fitted with the Newton paediatric valve is very useful in these circumstances, but it may lead to underventilation during surgical retraction on the lungs or if lung compliance decreases, since an increased amount of the driving gas will be lost through the fixed orifice leak in the Newton valve. T-piece occluders such as the Sheffield or Amsterdam ventilators can also be used (Fig. 3.3).

The Bain system, with coaxial tubing, behaves as a Mapleson D system, which has similar properties to the T-piece (Mapleson E). Scavenging is easier with this system, but accidents have occurred when the inner tube has become disconnected, causing a massive increase in apparatus dead

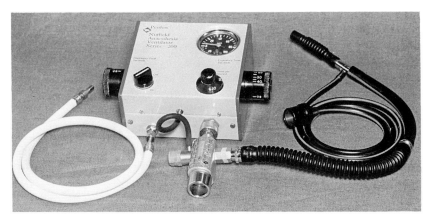

Fig. 3.2   The Penlon Nuffield ventilator series 200 with Newton paediatric valve.

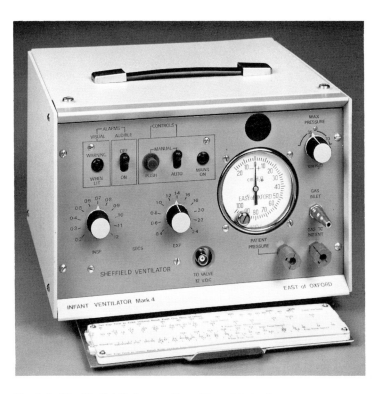

Fig. 3.3   The Sheffield infant ventilator (East of Oxford)

space. The system is widely used in children, but is more cumbersome than the T-piece for neonatal use.

Circle systems are widely used in adult anaesthesia where reduced losses of heat and water vapour and ease of scavenging are cited as advantages in addition to economy. Adult circle systems are unsuitable for young children because of their excessive dead space and high resistance. One-way valves increase resistance significantly, especially when wet, and may stick without warning. Circle systems specifically designed for children have not been particularly popular. Although there have been considerable advances in design, such as the introduction of electrically operated circulators and airway dividers to reduce dead space, they are not regarded as suitable for neonates, where the T-piece and Bain systems remain unchallenged.

Face masks

Face masks (Fig. 3.4) are not used for long periods in small babies because general anaesthesia almost invariably involves intubation (p. 98). A good fit on the face is of equal or even greater importance than very low dead space, which in practice is reduced by streaming effects of the FGF within the mask. The Rendell-Baker mask has the lowest dead space, but may not make a good air seal on the baby's face. The Rendell-Baker divided airway further reduces dead space.

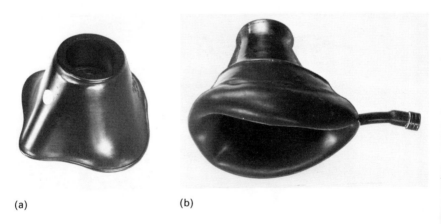

(a)   (b)

Fig. 3.4 Face masks suitable for neonatal use: (a) Rendell-Baker; (b) M & I E, with inflatable rim

Laryngoscopes

Because of the anatomy of the infant's upper airway, a straight-bladed laryngoscope is usually preferred, the blade being placed posterior to the epiglottis. There are many different designs of straight-bladed laryngoscopes available (Fig. 3.5). The Seward and Robertshaw blades are particularly useful for nasotracheal intubation because they allow more room for the

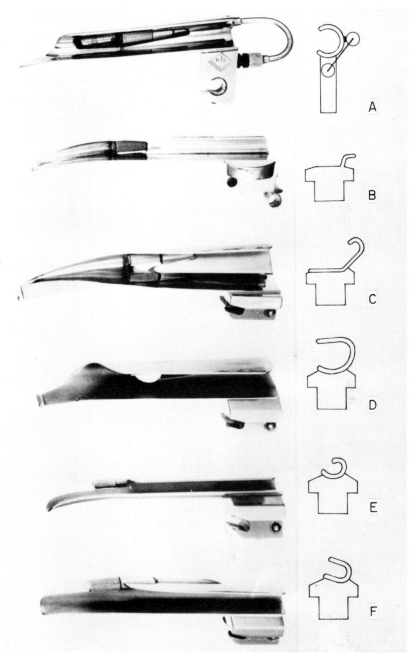

Fig. 3.5   Straight largyngoscope blades for infant use: A, Anderson–Magill; B, Seward; C, Robertshaw; D, Oxford; E, Miller; and F, Wisconsin

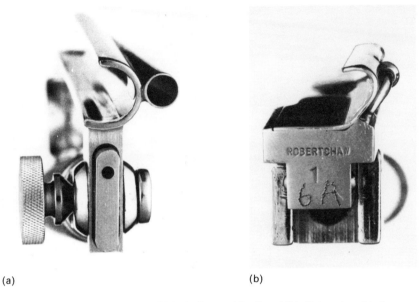

(a)   (b)

Fig. 3.6 Cross-sectional views of (a) Anderson–Magill and (b) Robertshaw blades, showing the larger area available for intubating forceps in the latter

introduction of Magill forceps into the mouth than most other blades (Fig. 3.6). The quality of the light source has improved significantly with the introduction of fibreoptics into this field.

Tracheal tubes (Fig. 3.7)

Plain tracheal tubes of the Magill type are available in implantation-tested rubber or polyvinyl chloride (PVC); 3 mm internal diameter is usual for the term baby and 2.5 mm for the premature (under 2 kg). The wall thickness of plastic tubes is highly reproducible, whereas the external diameter of rubber tubes may vary within quite wide tolerances. On the other hand, rubber tubes are thought by many to be easier to pass because of their greater stiffness. Both types of tube are satisfactory for short-term intubation, although PVC tubes are universally used for postoperative and intensive care. The wall thickness of silicone rubber (Silastic) tubes is at present too great to allow their use in the neonate.

The length to which a tube should be cut for oral intubation depends on the method of fixation. Values given in North American literature often refer to the practice of allowing a length of tube to protrude from the mouth. Tracheal tube lengths commonly required when the tracheal tube connector is strapped to the face as commonly practised in the UK are shown in Table 3.1. Because of the ease with which inadvertent bronchial intubation can occur, the chest should always be auscultated after intuba-

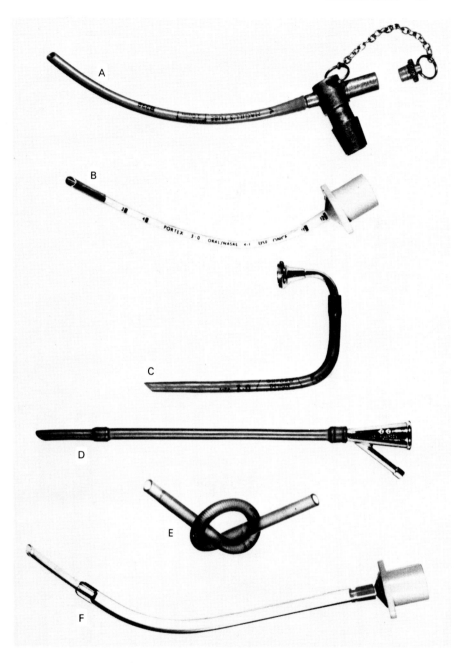

Fig. 3.7 Tracheal tubes commonly used in infancy: A, plain Magill; B, Portex;
C, Oxford; D, Magill armoured; E, latex armoured; and F, Cole pattern. (Reproduced,
with permission, from Hatch, 1981)

Table 3.1   Oral tracheal tube sizes for newborns

Patient's weight (kg)	Tube size (i.d.) (mm)	Tube length (cm)
0.7–1.0	2.5	7.0–7.5
1.0–1.5	2.5	7.5–8.0
1.5–2.0	3.0	8.0–8.5
2.0–2.5	3.0	8.5–9.0
2.5–3.0	3.0	9.0–10.0

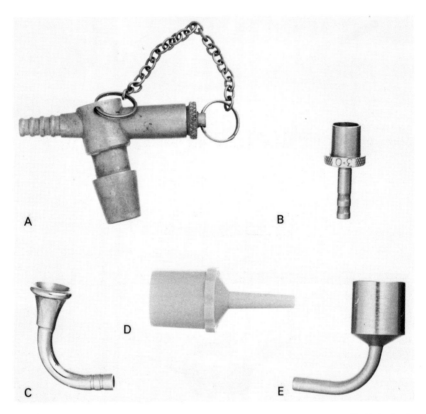

Fig. 3.8 Tracheal tube connectors used in neonatal anaesthesia: A, Cardiff; B, Oxford; C, Magill; D, Portex 15 mm; E, Penlon 15 mm.

tion to ensure ventilation of both lungs. Tracheal tube connectors in common use are illustrated in Figs. 3.8 and 3.9. A secondary fixation of a catheter mount to the forehead is recommended, as this stops rotational movement of the tube.

Magill flexometallic tubes (Fig. 3.10) are commonly used for neurosurgical procedures, as kinking will not occur with any position of the head.

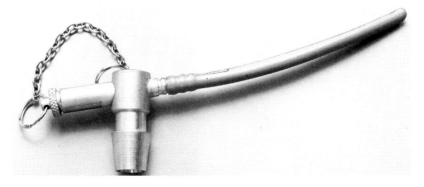

Fig. 3.9   Plain Magill tube with Cardiff connector.

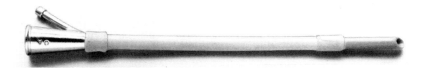

Fig. 3.10   Magill flexometallic tube.

Fixation of these tubes is not so easy and care must be taken not to allow the enlarged portion of the tube to pass between the vocal cords. A wire stilette is necessary to stiffen the tube for intubation. Firm fixation is particularly important for these tracheal tubes in neurosurgical anaesthesia, when access may be difficult. Fixation involving strips of plaster around the tube sticking down over the neck and up over the cheeks is recommended.

Oxford tubes (Fig. 3.11) are used in anaesthesia for oesophagoscopy, some otolaryngological procedures and plastic surgery of the head and neck. The Oxford tube has an ideal shape to prevent inadvertent kinking in the pharynx and, thus, respiratory obstruction. A curved Magill connection is used and intubation is most satisfactorily carried out with a small, lubricated, gum-elastic bougie through the tube. This technique surmounts the difficulty occasionally experienced with Oxford tubes in a patient with an anterior larynx where the tip of the tube cannot be angled forwards to reach the glottis. These tubes have a tapered outside diameter, so it is extremely important to use a tube of the correct size. If too large a tube is used, the larynx will be stretched as the tube is inserted, with subsequent oedema and stridor.

Preformed disposable tracheal tubes have become increasingly popular in recent years, as they allow the tracheal tube connector to be placed away from the surgical field. The Rae type tube is easier to pass than the Portex 'child's anatomical tube' (Fig. 3.12) and the shape of the latter tube may make it difficult to remove a suction catheter because of friction at the two acute bends. Care should be taken when using either of these tubes in the

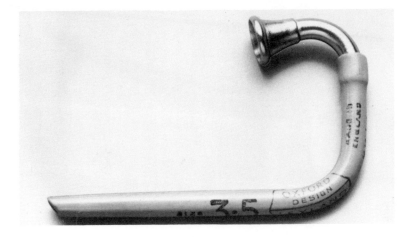

Fig. 3.11   Oxford tube with Magill curved connector.

presence of a mouth gag, as for palatal surgery, because pressure from the tongue plate can compress the tube.

Cole pattern tracheal tubes (Fig. 3.13) with a shouldered section are made of PVC, but the smallest sizes are unsatisfactory for spontaneous ventilation because of an unacceptably high resistance to breathing caused by turbulent air flow at the shoulder. The 8 French gauge (FG) size has an internal diameter of little more than 1 mm. They are unsuitable for prolonged intubation because fixation is not very firm and there is a tendency for the tube to move further into the trachea, thus dilating the glottis. If the shouldered part rests on the cricoid, the subglottic area will be damaged. Cases have been reported in which continued pressure by the oral tube has caused a cleft in the palate. Other cases have been reported in which accidental dislodgement of the tube has necessitated surgical removal from the oesophagus. However, these tubes are often used for neonatal resuscitation because they are easy for relatively inexperienced staff to use.

Anaesthetic apparatus should be sterilized between cases so that each patient has a clean circuit. Tracheal tubes and connections are autoclaved and kept sterile until use. If a lubricant is used then this should also be sterile.

Apparatus concerned with intraoperative monitoring and temperature maintenance is discussed on pp. 111 et seq.

Basic techniques

Induction of anaesthesia and intubation

The baby is transferred to a prepared operating theatre from the surgical intensive care unit in a heated incubator providing a neutral thermal en-

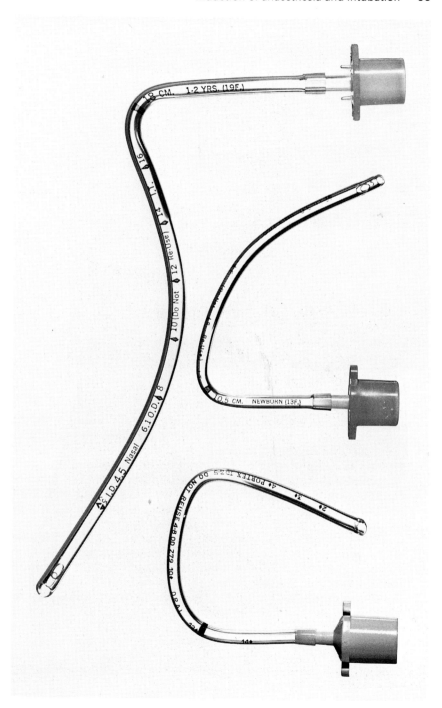

Fig. 3.12   Preformed tracheal tubes.

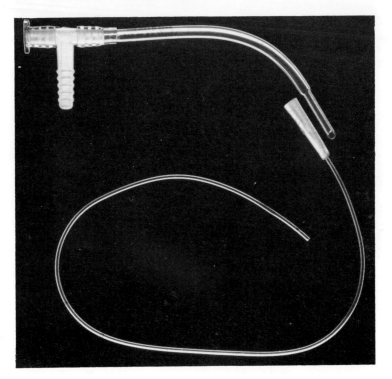

Fig. 3.13   Cole tube and suction catheter.

vironment. It is our practice to induce anaesthesia for neonates on the operating table itself, prepared with a prewarmed heating pad and warm coverings. Newly developed hot air mattresses have proved to be a very effective and safe alternative to other types of heated mattress and these are now in routine use at The Hospital for Sick Children (Fig. 3.14). The ambient temperature should not exceed 24°C, the room should be free of draught and it may be necessary to turn off any air-conditioning. Higher temperatures are not recommended, as discomfort of the staff will then become a consideration. An air mattress provides a warm atmosphere around the baby, so excessive room temperatures are no longer necessary. In the operating theatre, maximum heat loss is likely to occur in the period between induction of anaesthesia and the skin incision (Fig. 3.15). It is during this period with the insertion of intravenous and other lines that the neonate is most likely to become uncovered; this should be kept to an absolute minimum, especially if the baby is premature. At this stage an overhead heater may be used—possibly that from an open type of incubator used to bring the baby from the special care unit. It is advisable to wrap the limbs and cover the head with aluminium foil to minimize heat loss by radiation (Fig. 3.16).

Anaesthesia should not be induced until the surgeon is ready, as the neonate's metabolic response to cold is suppressed once general anaesthesia

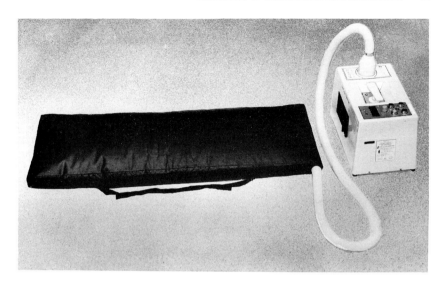

Fig. 3.14 Paediatric hot air mattress for use on the operating table. (Howarth Air Engineering, Bolton, Lancs.)

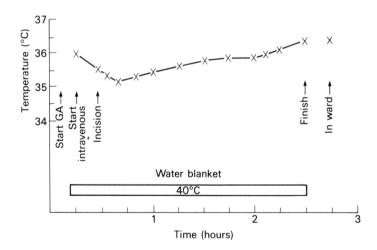

Fig. 3.15 Patient's temperature during surgery for repair of tracheo-oesophageal fistula in a baby aged 14 hours and weighing 2.1 kg.

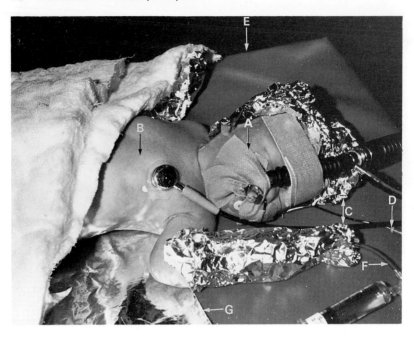

Fig. 3.16 The anaesthetized neonate prepared for surgery, showing: A, fixation of tracheal tube; B, precordial stethoscope; C, foil; D, thermistor; E, heating pad; F, intravenous line; and G, dry diathermy plate.

has been established. Skin preparation by the surgeon should not be prolonged and should preferably be with warm fluid. Drapes should be placed over the baby as soon as possible. Infusions of blood or fluid should be warmed before administration, and for prolonged cases the inspired gases should also be warmed and humidified. The baby should be covered with warm Gamgee or similar material as soon as the operation is finished, and should be returned to the ward in a preheated incubator.

Anaesthesia for neonates must involve intubation in the vast majority of cases, even for the most minor operations. The patency of the airway cannot be guaranteed with a face mask and spontaneous ventilation is rarely a part of neonatal anaesthesia. The respiratory system is so vulnerable to the depressant effects of inhalational anaesthesia and reduction in functional residual capacity (FRC) that controlled ventilation should be an integral part of the anaesthetic technique. This is only possible using a tracheal tube because the compliance of the chest is lower than that of the abdomen, and abdominal distension would tend to occur if assisted ventilation with a face mask were attempted.

In the newborn, tracheal intubation is most commonly performed before induction of anaesthesia but after a minute or two of preoxygenation from a face mask. The manoeuvre is easily performed without trauma even in vigorous babies because they have relatively little muscular strength. If the airway is secured before anaesthesia, there is less risk of aspiration of regurgitated gastric contents into the lungs. Moreover, if intubation difficulties are encountered (such as the small larynx sometimes associated with tracheo-oesophageal fistula, subglottic stenosis, laryngeal webs or other congenital airway problems), there is less difficulty in maintaining full oxygenation of the infant while a smaller tracheal tube is selected. On the

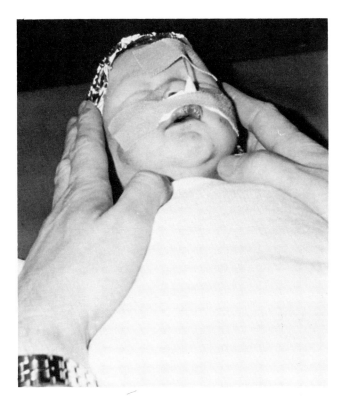

Fig. 3.17   Intubation: the correct way to hold the baby.

other hand, there may be great difficulty in maintaining an airway with a mask after induction of anaesthesia in the newborn and the risk of regurgitation is increased, especially if slight respiratory obstruction occurs. Laryngeal spasm is also a possibility.

After preoxygenation to help protect the infant from hypoxaemia during the breath-holding associated with awake intubation, laryngoscopy is performed. Correct holding of the baby is essential for easy intubation (Fig. 3.17). The head should not be extended at the neck, but at the atlanto-occipital joint, producing a 'sniffing' position. The arms are restrained within the warm covers and the assistant presses the baby's shoulders firmly onto the surface of the operating table with both his palms while his fingers hold the head steady on either side. The position of the head is crucial for successful intubation. The shoulders must not be allowed to rise from the table. The anatomy of the infant larynx is such that the best view is usually obtained using a straight-bladed laryngoscope, the tip of which picks up the epiglottis from its posterior surface (Fig. 3.18); however, if the

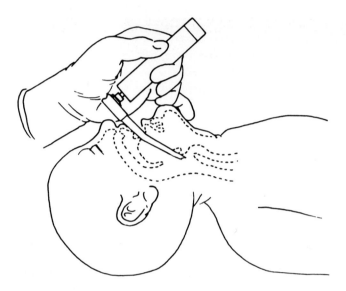

Fig. 3.18   Intubation of the neonate, showing the position of the tip of the straight-bladed laryngoscope in relation to the epiglottis.

epiglottis is very short, the best view of the larynx may be obtained with the tip of the blade in the vallecula.

The mouth is opened with the index finger of the right hand, and the laryngoscope blade is put into it from the right to keep the tongue over to the left and advanced into the pharynx beyond the glottis (Fig. 3.19). It is then withdrawn until the glottis is visualized and the vocal cords are seen moving as the baby takes a breath. If an Anderson–Magill blade is used, the hook should rest on the left index finger and the left little finger can then press the larynx back to improve the view. A plain Magill tube of rubber (autoclaved) or plastic (disposable) is gently inserted into the trachea as the baby takes an inspiratory breath. If firm resistance is met, a smaller tube should be used. Most neonates require a 3.0 mm or 2.5 mm (inside diameter) tracheal tube. The correct sized tube is that which is easily inserted and which has a small air leak around it, and is thus not too tight at the cricoid ring. This should be tested by light distension of the lungs with the T-piece bag, when an air leak should be audible. A tube which is too

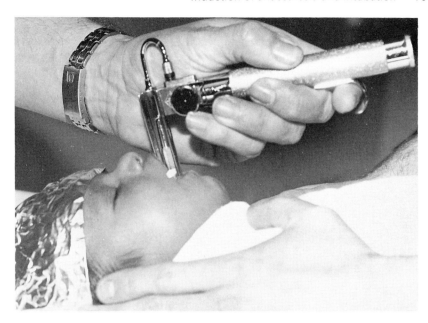

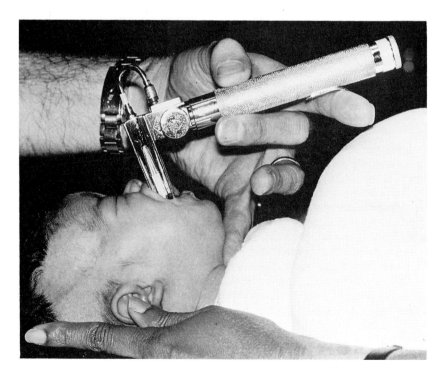

Fig. 3.19 Correct way to hold the laryngoscope.

tight may damage the mucosa at the cricoid and cause postoperative oedema and stridor. Ulceration of the mucosa may progress to subglottic stenosis. After auscultation of the chest to confirm that the tip of the tube has not passed into one or other main bronchus, it is firmly secured with strips of 2.5 cm wide stretch sticking plaster, and the catheter mount firmly fixed to the forehead (Fig. 3.20). An infant airway is inserted into the mouth

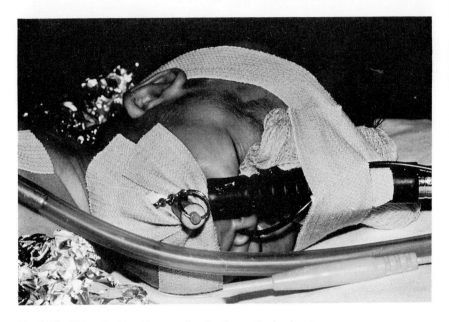

Fig. 3.20   The oral tube with secondary fixation to the forehead.

alongside the tracheal tube to splint it and prevent it from kinking. If an oesophageal stethoscope and/or a nasogastric tube are required, these are more easily placed before an oral airway is inserted.

Nasotracheal intubation is rarely used in the operating theatre except in cases already receiving respiratory support or for whom respiratory support is planned postoperatively. The technique is very well established indeed for prolonged airway management, but is technically more difficult to perform in the awake neonate because of the need for instrumentation in the mouth with intubating forceps. It is therefore safer to undertake oral intubation first and change to nasal intubation later if required.

For the sake of safety, awake intubation should be attempted in most babies under 21 days of life, as the ease of intubation is related to the muscular resistance rather than to the age of the baby. If the baby is very vigorous and the muscular resistance great, attempts at awake intubation should be abandoned and anaesthesia induced using the technique with which the anaesthetist is most familiar; for example, inhalational induction with oxygen/nitrous oxide/halothane, cyclopropane/oxygen (1 litre of each per minute) or intravenous induction with thiopentone $2-4\,mg\cdot kg^{-1}$ body weight. Induction of anaesthesia is followed by the intravenous administration of a muscle relaxant—commonly suxamethonium $1\,mg\cdot kg^{-1}$, or atracurium $0.5\,mg\cdot kg^{-1}$, or vecuronium $0.05-0.1\,mg\cdot kg^{-1}$.

Awake intubation causes a rise in intracranial pressure as measured by a transducer over the anterior fontanelle. This is acceptable for most patients, but for those whose ICP is already raised or in whom there is a risk of IVH such as the preterm or those with a coagulopathy, it may be advisable to use a conventional technique of induction of anaesthesia. However, the anaesthetist must be confident that he can achieve intubation without causing hypoxia.

The difficult intubation

The neonate may be more difficult to intubate than an adult or an older child because of the anatomical differences already described. In addition, there are certain conditions which may cause further difficulty: where there is immobility of the cervical spine as in Klippel-Feil syndrome, micrognathia with Pierre Robin syndrome, or macroglossia with Hurler's syndrome, laryngoscopy may be very awkward or even impossible. The presence of a cleft palate and an anteriorly placed premaxilla will hinder easy intubation and the blade of the laryngoscope may slip into the cleft. Babies with conditions such as cystic hygroma and haemangiomata of the head and neck with respiratory obstruction may also be very difficult to intubate.

In these situations awake intubation should be performed where possible, but if anaesthesia is necessary for an older neonate, only inhalational techniques are advisable. Success is best achieved with care and patience. A selection of sterile tracheal tubes down to 2.5 mm internal diameter should always be available. If a 2.5 mm tube will not pass into the trachea, the smallest Cole pattern tube may be required. A choice of straight- and curved-bladed infant laryngoscopes should be available and also a fairly stiff gum-elastic bougie. Laryngoscopy should be performed after preoxygenation; if visualization of the glottis is difficult, its whereabouts can be deduced by seeing bubbles of saliva as the baby breathes in and out. It may be possible to bring the glottis into view by pressing on the front of the neck. In particularly difficult cases it may help to thread the gum-elastic bougie through the tracheal tube and allow it to emerge by 2 cm or so at the tracheal end. The tip of the bougie can then be bent anteriorly and used to guide the tube into the trachea. Occasionally, it may be necessary to use the bougie alone to find the glottic opening. The chosen tracheal tube is then threaded over the bougie into the trachea. If the tracheal tube connector is curved, this is better inserted after the tube is in the trachea and the bougie has been removed.

The same techniques are also used when inhalational anaesthesia is necessary. Respiratory obstruction occurring after induction may be relieved by turning the baby on its side or even prone. Early insertion of an oral airway is less likely to provoke coughing and laryngeal spasm in this age group than in the older child. A nasopharyngeal airway is an alternative, although it carries the risk of an epistaxis. When the baby is sufficiently deeply anaesthetized (usually with oxygen and halothane), laryngoscopy and intubation are performed as described above. Muscle relaxants must not be used at this stage, as valuable evidence of the whereabouts of the glottis revealed by respiratory movements will be lost. Muscle relaxants must not be used in any case of respiratory obstruction until it has been proved possible to ventilate the lungs using a face mask. Inhalational induction of anaesthesia, especially in the presence of respiratory obstruction, may be aided by the application of some constant distending pressure on the lungs. This is achieved by maintaining a taut anaesthetic T-piece reservoir bag.

Intravenous cannulation

Intravenous access is mandatory for general anaesthesia in neonatal patients. Suitable veins may be found on the dorsum of the hand or at the wrist, on the feet or the scalp. Metal scalp vein needles are not satisfactory for prolonged use because they tend to cut out of the vein, although they may be easier to insert successfully; 20 and 22 gauge cannulae are available manufactured in polypropylene (Medicut) or Teflon (Abbocath, Jelco or Venflon). Teflon is less thrombogenic, but is softer than polypropylene so is more likely to kink unless fixation is meticulous and the arm or leg is securely splinted. Teflon cannulae are also available in 24 and 26 gauge. Correct holding of the limb is essential for successful venepuncture. If the wrist is squeezed too tightly, blood flow will be interrupted and the veins will collapse; if held too loosely, venous distension will not be achieved. The assistant holding the wrist must also slightly stretch the skin of the hand. After cleansing the skin with spirit, a hole beside the vein is made with a lancet. This is always necessary because, otherwise, Teflon cannulae buckle over the needle as they are advanced through intact skin. Some anaesthetists prefer to perform the manoeuvre single-handed and distend the vein by squeezing the wrist (or ankle) between the index and middle fingers of the left hand. Optimal venous distension and stretching of the overlying skin are achieved more easily in this way.

After successful venepuncture and careful fixation of the cannula, a three-way stopcock is fitted and the wrist (or foot) secured with a small arm splint. Intravenous fluids are usually given by means of a constant infusion pump, although these are strictly necessary only for intravenous alimentation or for the administration of inotropic agents. Care must be taken to watch for signs of extravasation around the vein when an infusion pump is used. A giving set incorporating a microburette is a suitable alternative, although it is a wise precaution to fill the chamber only with the requirements for 1 hour at a time.

Blood or plasma is required when the estimated blood loss has reached 10 per cent of the calculated blood volume (see p. 33). It is usual to transfuse with plasma (plasma protein fraction) up to 20 per cent of the blood volume if the haematocrit is over 45 per cent and the Hb over $15\,g\cdot dl^{-1}$. Blood should be as fresh as possible and in small packs to avoid waste. The blood may be administered through a standard giving set but is given by syringe, using a three-way tap for accuracy. Microfilters are not used routinely but are indicated where massive transfusion is expected or if the patient has pulmonary vascular disease. Standard warming coils are not used routinely, but some attempt must be made to raise the blood temperature from the storage level. Adequate warming of the blood is achieved if the standard tubing of the giving set is held in a thermostatically controlled water bath and blood drawn slowly through the tubing into the syringe.

The preterm baby

Preterm babies are particularly sensitive to intravenous and inhalational agents alike. They may need a high $F\text{io}_2$ and nitrous oxide may be contraindicated. The use of relaxants and 100% oxygen without anaesthesia is stressful and this technique should not be employed. Supplements, intermittently, of halothane or enflurane are effective, but fentanyl should be given only if postoperative mechanical ventilation is necessary.

Neuromuscular blocking agents

There is still controversy concerning the effects of the muscle relaxants on newborn babies. There are many reports of the sensitivity of the neonatal neuromuscular junction to tubocurarine and relative resistance to suxamethonium—the so-called 'myasthenic response'. It is generally agreed that some form of sensitivity to non-depolarizers does exist in the newborn for the first 7 days of life, although there is a wide variation in response. *In vitro* experiments show that increased sensitivity of the neonatal neuromuscular junction to these relaxants stems from its immaturity. At birth the muscle fibres are sensitive to acetylcholine throughout their length; only after a few weeks does the normal adult end-plate sensitivity develop, and then only if the innervation to the muscle is normal. At the same time that reduction of the sensitive area of the neuromuscular junction occurs there are changes in the frequency and amplitude of the miniature end-plate potentials. These are greater in amplitude but less frequent in the neonate than in the adult. These changes seem to correspond with the change in sensitivity to tubocurarine. The effective dose of tubocurarine to produce a 90 per cent block of thumb adduction in response to supramaximal single shock nerve stimulation has been shown to be $0.34\,\text{mg}\cdot\text{kg}^{-1}$ body weight in infants under 10 days of age—the same as infants of other age groups. What is different in the very young group is the wide variation in response, although all recovery times are comparable. Such differences in response could be related to the large extracellular fluid volume of the newly born and to the variability in size of this fluid compartment in which the drug is distributed. Evidence does seem to rule out quantitative changes in plasma protein concentration and, thus, bioavailability of the drug as a cause of the increased sensitivity of newborn babies to the non-depolarizers, but it does not necessarily preclude qualitative changes in binding to plasma proteins. One experimental series (Bennett *et al.*, 1976) showed that it is necessary to give an initial bolus injection of $0.25\,mg\cdot kg^{-1}$ tubocurarine for curarization in the first 7 days of life, $0.4\,mg\cdot kg^{-1}$ from days 7 to 14 and $0.5\,mg\cdot kg^{-1}$ thereafter. However, neonatal sensitivity has also been found to pancuronium compared with tubocurarine. At birth, pancuronium is nine times as potent as tubocurarine, although this drops to six times by 28 days of life. Because of this, pancuronium doses of $0.04\,mg\cdot kg^{-1}$ are safest in babies less than 7 days old, although after this $0.06\,mg\cdot kg^{-1}$ may be used. After the first 2 weeks of life, infants require similar doses to adults on a weight-for-weight basis (Fig. 3.21).

It seems that the development of normal adult response to tubocurarine is related more to the postnatal age than to the gestational age, and perhaps

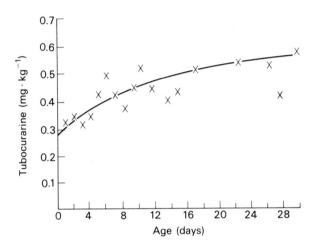

Fig. 3.21   Tubocurarine requirement during the neonatal period. (After data of Bush and Stead, 1962)

it is the greater neuromuscular activity after birth which stimulates the development of the mature end-plate characteristics.

Whether increased sensitivity to tubocurarine results from immaturity of the neuromuscular junction, differences in dilution of the drug or its binding by plasma proteins does not alter the need for careful titration of the drug dose against the response. Indeed the possibility of wide variations in patients less than 1 week old makes such a titration mandatory. Particular care must be taken in the premature if the patient is acidotic or hypothermic in the presence of certain of the antibiotics (amikacin and gentamicin) and anaesthetic agents such as halothane. Tubocurarine in clinical doses has little cardiovascular effect in the newborn, whereas pancuronium may provoke a tachycardia.

Tubocurarine should be diluted to a concentration of $0.5\,mg\cdot ml^{-1}$, and after intubation $0.5\,mg$ may be given intravenously. Premature babies should receive $0.25\,mg$. Increments of $0.25\,mg$ ($0.125\,mg$ in prematures) may be given to gain control of the ventilation, without exceeding a total dose of $1\,mg$ for the full-term newborn. It is our practice to supplement anaesthesia with low concentrations of halothane (0.25–0.5%) at the start of an operation, to avoid, where possible, the need for higher doses of relaxants. This should be discontinued at least 20 minutes before the end of the operation. Increments of tubocurarine may be given intraoperatively when necessary, in doses one-tenth of the original total dose. No such dose should be given within 20 minutes of the end of the operation.

The initial dose of pancuronium should be $0.1\,mg$, with increments of 0.05 or $0.025\,mg$ to achieve the desired control of ventilation.

The metabolism of atracurium is independent of renal and hepatic function but depends on pH and temperature. These features make the drug satisfactory for use in neonates in doses of $0.3\,mg$–$0.5\,mg\cdot kg^{-1}$ i.v. Vecuronium in doses of 0.05–$0.1\,mg\cdot kg^{-1}$ i.v. is also a very satisfactory drug and causes no histamine release. Neither of these relaxants produces significant changes in pulse rate or blood pressure. There has been increasing interest recently in the use of the newer non-depolarizing muscle relaxants atracurium and vecuronium in infancy, both because of their lack of cardiovascular effects and because of the possibility of using these agents by continuous infusion. Brandom et al. (1984) have shown that the dose required to produce 95 per cent twitch suppression (ED_{95}) in infants is similar to that for adolescents when expressed on a weight basis. When expressed in relation to surface area the ED_{95} for infants is about half that for children, suggesting that differences in response are related to differences in extracellular fluid volume. Goudsouzian (1985) has found no difference in the dose of atracurium required by infants and older children per unit body weight, but states that pharmacokinetic studies are needed to determine whether infants in fact require lower plasma concentrations than older children to achieve the same degree of neuromuscular blockade. The recovery times after intubating doses of $400\,\mu g\cdot kg^{-1}$ of atracurium or $80\,\mu g\cdot kg^{-1}$ of vecuronium in infants appear similar to those in adults. Studies in adults have suggested that infusion rates of $8\,\mu g\cdot kg^{-1}\cdot min^{-1}$ are required for atracurium (Gargarian et al., 1984) and $1.4\,\mu g\cdot kg^{-1}\cdot min^{-1}$ for vecuronium (Mirakhur, Ferres and Pandit, 1984) to maintain over 90 per cent twitch suppression with nitrous oxide, oxygen and narcotic anaesthesia. Clinical experience with older children suggests that similar infusion rates are required, but there has to date been little experience with the use of these infusions in the neonate. The technique must be used in conjunction with peripheral nerve stimulation, and the infusion rate should be adjusted to obtain the required degree of twitch suppression.

The effects of suxamethonium in the neonate are probably no different from those in the adult; reports of decreased sensitivity may relate to the larger extracellular fluid volume throughout which the drug is distributed, in spite of lower plasma cholinesterase activity in infants up to 6 months of age. It is suggested that there is an increased tendency for the newborn to develop a prolonged action of suxamethonium (phase II block), and doses in excess of $5\,mg\cdot kg^{-1}$ should be avoided. However, phase II block in neonates has seldom been reported in clinical practice.

Suxamethonium is diluted to a concentration of $2.5\,mg\cdot ml^{-1}$ and increments of 2.5 mg are given intravenously as necessary. The degree of muscular relaxation is best judged clinically from the abdominal musculature and the muscle tone in the fingers. An intermittent suxamethonium technique may be used for any neonatal operation (other than cardiac), but is probably better reserved for shorter operations to avoid the possibility of a phase II block. Again, it is our practice to supplement anaesthesia with low concentrations of halothane (0.25–0.5%) for short periods of time during controlled ventilation in such cases, but to discontinue it well before the end of surgery.

Both tubocurarine and suxamethonium must be given incrementally and the effects of each dose carefully assessed before more is given. Either drug is then extremely satisfactory and both have been used in neonatal anaesthesia for many years with great safety.

At least 20–30 minutes must elapse between the last dose of tubocurarine and the end of the operation if full reversal is to be achieved easily. A mixture of atropine ($0.025\,mg\cdot kg^{-1}$) or glycopyrrolate $0.01\,mg\cdot kg^{-1}$ and neostigmine ($0.05\,mg\cdot kg^{-1}$) is given intravenously, from the same syringe, for reversal of residual curarization. There may be a reduced requirement for neostigmine in the neonate.

Inadequate reversal, as judged by poor respiratory effort, poor muscle tone, tracheal tug, intercostal recession and possibly raised Pa_{CO_2}, may be caused by a variety of factors. There may have been actual overdose or the administration of an increment of drug too near the end of the operation. The dose may have been relatively too large because the effect of the drug has been potentiated by other agents, commonly halothane. Poor reversal will be seen in acidotic, hypothermic, hypoglycaemic babies and if the ionized calcium level is low. The last has a role in release of acetylcholine in the neuromuscular junction; if low levels are suspected, 10% calcium gluconate $15\,mg\cdot kg^{-1}$ should be given by slow intravenous injection.

Maintenance of anaesthesia

Controlled ventilation is the technique of choice, as respiratory depression easily occurs with spontaneous ventilation. After intubation it is our practice to induce light general anaesthesia with a 50% oxygen/50% nitrous oxide mixture and up to 0.5% halothane with gentle assisted ventilation while an intravenous cannula and temperature monitoring probes are inserted and ECG electrodes are applied. It is possible that a high Pa_{O_2} during the short duration of anaesthesia in a very low birth weight infant might cause retrolental fibroplasia, and the Pa_{O_2} should be monitored during anaesthesia in such infants. As soon as venous access is established, carefully titrated doses of relaxant are given as previously described. Arterial and central venous cannulation are undertaken at this stage if necessary.

The closing volume in the neonatal lung is greater than the FRC, so airway closure occurs within normal tidal respiration. Controlled ventilation ensures that adequate alveolar ventilation is taking place, and some positive end-expiratory pressure (PEEP) helps to maintain an adequate residual lung volume. Most paediatric anaesthetists feel it is safer to ventilate neonates by hand, rather than with a mechanical ventilator, except in special circumstances such as cardiac surgery or neurosurgery where a steady state is particularly important. A ventilatory rate of 30–40 per minute is employed (slower than the infant would be breathing spontaneously) with pressures of 25–30 H_2O and a fresh gas flow of 4 litres. It is usual to obtain a PEEP of about $5\,cmH_2O$ during manual ventilation, thus helping to preserve the FRC.

Inspired gases for neonatal anaesthesia should reach the patient fully humidified at a temperature not less than 33°C. This prevents damage to the mucosal lining of the respiratory tract by dry gases and therefore helps preserve mucociliary function and, possibly more important, minimizes heat loss from the baby. Certainly such gases, fully saturated at body temperature, will influence the thermal balance but there is an increased risk of infection from the humidifiers.

The aim is to produce mild hyperventilation—a safe procedure unless the patient is hypovolaemic from dehydration or haemorrhage. Great care must be taken with controlled ventilation in the presence of lung cysts because of the risk of tension pneumothorax, or with tracheo-oesophageal fistula because of gastric distension. Controlled ventilation is not contraindicated in these conditions, but extra vigilance is required and only gentle ventilation employed. For those unused to ventilating newborn babies by hand, a manometer may be incorporated in the T-piece circuit so that the actual pressures applied can be seen. Manual ventilation is the preferred technique for neonatal anaesthesia because minute-to-minute changes in compliance can be detected. This is especially important in thoracic surgery. Mechanical ventilators employing an electronic timing device to occlude the expiratory limb of a T-piece do exist (such as the Sheffield or Amsterdam) but are not as a routine used during anaesthesia for neonates. The Penlon Series 200 with a Newton valve is also an effective machine for use in theatre.

Whilst every attempt should be made to provide adequate anaesthesia for the neonate undergoing surgery, it must be stressed that excessive doses of inhalational agents are dangerously depressant to the cardiovascular, respiratory and central nervous systems.

Halothane is an ideal agent for use in children, even for repeated anaesthesia, as the adult problem of hepatic sensitization to this agent does not seem to arise, although reductive metabolism of this agent does occur in children. The level of anaesthesia is rapidly controlled and, at low doses, halothane has very little depressant effect on the cardiovascular system, except in patients with cardiac failure. The minimum alveolar concentration (MAC) is 1.1 for neonates (0.75 for adults).

Induction with halothane takes longer in a neonate than in an older child because of its effectively high dead-space/tidal volume ratio of up to 50 per cent and its increased physiological right-to-left shunt caused by the encroachment of the closing volume into tidal breathing.

Maintenance with intermittent halothane 0.25–0.5% with 50% oxygen/50% nitrous oxide gives excellent anaesthetic results, allowing lower doses of relaxants. If the halothane is discontinued 20 minutes before the end of the operation, the patient should be fully awake after reversal of the relaxant.

For preterm babies it may be necessary to use air/oxygen mixtures to give the required Fio_2.

Enflurane does not seem to have any particular advantages over halothane in this age group, although enflurane is less arrhythmogenic. Of necessity, clinical experience with this agent and with isoflurane is limited in this age group.

Intravenous analgesics have no place in neonatal anaesthesia except for those patients to be mechanically ventilated postoperatively such as after cardiac surgery.

Older, vigorous neonates undergoing short operations such as herniotomy may be allowed to breathe spontaneously a mixture of nitrous oxide, oxygen and halothane, although this is not recommended as a general rule. Anaesthesia for bronchoscopy also requires spontaneous ventilation (p. 187).

After the surgical procedure has finished and atropine and neostigmine have been given (in a dose of atropine $0.025\,mg\cdot kg^{-1}$, or glycopyrrolate $0.01\,mg\cdot kg^{-1}$, and neostigmine $0.05\,mg\cdot kg^{-1}$), controlled ventilation continues with 100% O_2, perhaps including 2–5% CO_2, until full spontaneous ventilation has been re-established. The baby is covered with fresh, warmed wrappings. Suction through the tracheal tube may be carried out using a fine sterile suction catheter if secretions are present, but not as a routine. As neonates are obligatory nose breathers, careful suctioning of the nostrils is done, using a soft rubber suction catheter.

Extubation

Extubation is carried out when the baby is fully awake (moving all limbs, eyes open) and respiratory effort is judged to be fully adequate in terms of depth, rate and absence of signs of distress such as intercostal recession and nasal flaring. The tube is withdrawn during compression of the T-piece reservoir bag so that the infant coughs the moment the tube leaves the trachea. The practice of extubating with a suction catheter down the tube is to be condemned because serious hypoxaemia may occur and there is a risk of aspiration of pharyngeal contents into the lungs as the first respiratory movement is inspiration.

There are many factors involved in poor respiratory function postoperatively, including pulmonary dysfunction such as hypoplasia occurring with diaphragmatic hernia or aspiration in tracheo-oesophageal fistula (see Chapter 4). Of the anaesthetic causes of postoperative respiratory insufficiency, inadequate reversal of the relaxant should be considered first. The dose of relaxant may have been excessive or increments may have been given too late, but the effects of normal doses are intensified in the presence of high concentrations of inhalational anaesthetics or diazepam transferred via the placenta from the mother. Reversal difficulties may be experienced if the patient is hypothermic, acidotic, low in ionized Ca^{2+}, very premature or has a low cardiac output. Such patients may need a period of mechanical ventilation while these abnormalities are corrected. Hypoventilation leads to pulmonary atelectasis, hypoxia, acidosis and circulatory failure.

After careful assessment, the baby is returned to its heated incubator for the journey back to the intensive care unit.

Patient care during anaesthesia

Careful and continuous monitoring of the clinical status of the patient is essential during any anaesthetic. Because of the high metabolic rate and reduced respiratory reserve of the neonate, the clinical condition can deteriorate very rapidly and no piece of apparatus has yet been designed which will replace the meticulously careful, well-trained clinical anaesthetist. There are, however, several devices available which help in patient monitoring, and the best are those which make the contact between the anaesthetist and the patient closer rather than more remote. In addition, a number of pieces of monitoring equipment are available which can give the anaesthetist information which cannot be obtained by direct clinical observation. It is also important to monitor not only the patient's well-being but also the function of the increasingly complicated pieces of anaesthetic equipment appearing in operating theatres.

Monitoring equipment must be reliable and easy to use, and should not by its size or design adversely affect the characteristics of the anaesthetic circuit or interfere with the safe conduct of the anaesthetic. Alarms should be fitted where appropriate, although these may fail or be set off by artefacts. Unnecessary bleeps and noises can be distracting both to the surgeon and anaesthetist.

Respiration

In the spontaneously breathing patient, monitoring of the airway and adequacy of respiration is carried out by observation of the movements of the reservoir bag of the anaesthetic T-piece. Almost all neonatal anaesthesia is carried out using controlled ventilation, however, and in this case the movements of the chest wall must be continuously watched. When manual ventilation is used, the anaesthetist can sense changes in compliance and resistance of the respiratory system or obstruction of the airway by changes in the 'feel' of the reservoir bag of the anaesthetic circuit with each breath. When mechanical ventilation is used, such changes are reflected by changes in the airway pressure dial of the ventilator, although these are less easily detected. The use of a precordial stethoscope is also helpful in monitoring inflation of the lungs but can only be used as a continuous monitor for long periods of time if employed in conjunction with a monaural earpiece. A Wright respirometer (Fig. 3.22) or similar respiration meter may be used on the expiratory port of a mechanical ventilator, and on some ventilators respiration is monitored by the incorporation of one or more pneumo-tachographs. Gross changes in oxygenation can be easily detected clinically but changes in carbon dioxide tension cannot; if an absolute assessment of blood gas status is required, arterial blood gas analysis is performed. The problems of blood gas measurements in the newborn are described on p. 198. In practice, arterial lines are used in neonatal anaesthesia for major

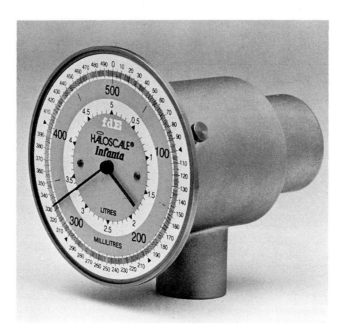

Fig. 3.22   Infant version of the Wright respirometer. (Ferraris Ltd, London)

surgery, particularly cardiac surgery, and also for any patient who requires respiratory support postoperatively. It may be difficult to obtain an arterial sample quickly in the operating theatre if an indwelling arterial line is not in place; if a central venous pressure line is available, a sample from this may be a helpful guide to a metabolic state and also to the blood gases. Serious arterial hypoxaemia is unlikely to be present if the oxygen tension of the venous sample is above 5.3 kPa (40 mmHg). The measurement of transcutaneous oxygen and carbon dioxide tensions is also feasible in the operating theatre, although the usefulness of this technique is limited in short operations by the fact that the electrodes may take up to 15 minutes to stabilize and may be adversely affected by anaesthetic gases. Monitoring of cutaneous oxygen tension is helpful, however, during anaesthesia in premature neonates where the risk of retinopathy of prematurity is high because the retinal vessels are susceptible to the effects of high arterial oxygen tensions. Usually the infant is transferred from the intensive care unit with a transcutaneous Po_2 (Tc Po_2) monitor already attached to him. In these cases the inspired oxygen concentration is adjusted to maintain an arterial oxygen tension in the upper part of the body (preductal) between 6.7 and 10.7 kPa (50–80 mmHg).

There has been increasing interest in recent years in the use of pulse oximetry during anaesthesia, and these devices have now been evaluated for use in infants and children. They function by producing light at two different wavelengths from light-emitting diodes. This light is transmitted through the tissues of the finger or ear, sensed by a photodetector, amplified and processed. The amplitude of the varying detected light depends on the size of the arterial pulse change, the wavelength and the oxygen saturation, and Beer's law allows continuous calculation of arterial oxygen saturation without interference from surrounding venous blood, skin or connective tissue. With improvements in the design of small sensors these devices are likely to be used increasingly in neonatal anaesthesia and intensive care.

Cuvettes for neonatal use are available for use with a capnograph (Hewlett-Packard) so that measurement of end-tidal CO_2 is now feasible and is a satisfactory technique for establishing the adequacy of ventilation during anaesthesia. However, indirect estimates of Pao_2 and $Paco_2$ should always be referred to direct measurement from blood gases.

Heart and circulation

It is more difficult to assess cardiovascular status clinically during anaesthesia than to assess respiration, although useful information can be obtained by careful observation of the peripheral circulation and by keeping a finger on the axillary or femoral pulse. The following apparatus is therefore frequently used in addition.

Precordial stethoscope

The precordial stethoscope (Fig. 3.23) provides useful information about the heart sounds and heart rate, and reduction in intensity of the heart sounds may indicate a fall in blood pressure or cardiac output. The chest piece should be sufficiently small to sit comfortably on the neonatal chest and should be securely fixed. The smallest available oesophageal stethoscope (12 FG) is sometimes too large to be used in the neonate, although it can be very useful especially when there is difficult access to the chest.

Blood pressure

The conventional measurement of blood pressure by auscultation of the Korotkoff sounds is often unsatisfactory during neonatal anaesthesia, due to difficulty of access. The recent introduction of the automated recording and display of blood pressure and pulse rate from these sounds is a signi-

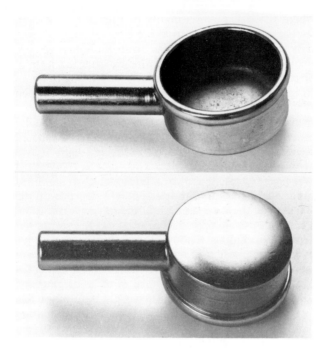

Fig. 3.23   The chest piece of a precordial stethoscope.

ficant advance, and there is now little excuse for not recording blood pressure regularly in all patients (Fig. 3.24). It should be remembered, however,
that accuracy still depends on using a cuff wide enough to cover two-thirds
of the upper arm, which in practice means a cuff width of 4 cm for neonates.
There have been reports of petechial haemorrhages appearing in the arm if
measurements are made too frequently, although this problem should be
lessened with the newer machines whose inflation/deflation time is shorter.
Doubts have been cast in adults on the accuracy of these automatic devices
when blood pressure is very low, and the additional clinical information
obtained from palpation of the axillary or femoral pulse should not be
ignored.

Other methods of blood pressure measurement include the use of Doppler
ultrasound flowmeters (which become useless when diathermy is used), am-
plification of the signal from a microphone placed under the cuff, visual
observation of the oscillations produced in an aneroid gauge as the cuff
deflates, and oscillotonometry.

Intra-arterial blood pressure monitoring is preferable when continuous
monitoring is necessary or when arterial blood samples are required. In the
newborn this can be obtained by catheterization of the umbilical artery. A
size 5 FG polythene cannula is inserted in infants weighing over 1.5 kg or
a size $3\frac{1}{2}$ FG for infants weighing less than 1.5 kg. Cannulae should be
radio-opaque, and the tip of the cannula should be passed into the descend-

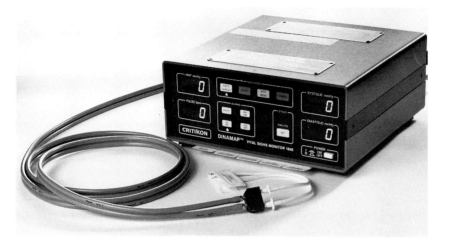

Fig. 3.24   Dinamap automated blood pressure-measuring device for use in all age groups.

ing aorta below the origin of the inferior mesenteric and renal arteries at the level of the L2 vertebra. In the older neonate the radial artery can often be cannulated percutaneously using a 22 or 24 standard wire gauge (s.w.g.) polythene or Teflon cannula. This should be connected to a pressure transducer by means of a short length of narrow-bore tubing and a three-way stopcock. Continuous flushing by means of a slow infusion pump using small volumes of heparinized dextrose or dextrose saline (1000 units of heparin per litre of fluid) minimizes the risk of thrombus formation and cannula blockage. Care must be taken to prevent the inadvertent injection of drugs into the artery. If the artery cannot be cannulated percutaneously, it may be necessary to expose it surgically and insert a similar cannula under direct vision. Although arterial cannulation is often followed by a temporary period of obstruction to blood flow, the incidence of long-term serious complications of radial and brachial artery cannulation in infants is very low.

Electrocardiogram

The ECG is a good monitor of pulse rate and disturbances of rhythm, although it provides no information about blood pressure or cardiac output. ECG recorders suitable for use in operating theatres should have a high common mode rejection ratio and therefore suppress unwanted signals from other pieces of electrical apparatus. It is useful to have an easily read trace, a rate counter and a freeze capacity on the oscilloscope. Lead 2 is likely to be the most useful for routine monitoring, although lead 3 will produce the most pronounced R-waves in cases of right axis deviation. Leads can be placed on the right and left arms or, preferably, on the right upper chest and left midaxillary line. A third lead is not always required but sometimes helps to reduce electrical interference and should be placed on the left flank or leg. A disposable back-plate is available with built-in electrodes.

It should be stressed that circulatory failure leading to hypoxic brain damage may occur before the ECG shows significant abnormalities.

Central venous pressure

Central venous pressure (CVP), which reflects right atrial filling pressure, expresses the relationship between peripheral vascular resistance, blood volume and right heart function. Although CVP measurement must be interpreted with caution, it can provide a useful monitor of blood loss or blood replacement in the short term.

The internal jugular vein can be cannulated percutaneously in the neonate without great difficulty, using the techniques described by English et al. (1964). The cannula is inserted through the junction of the medial one-third and lateral two-thirds of the sternomastoid muscle at a point midway between the mastoid process and the sternoclavicular joint, and directed towards the nipple. The vein, which is superficial in the infant, should be entered within 1–2 cm of the point of skin puncture, and can be made to fill and be more easily visualized by pressing over the liver. Care should be taken to avoid entering the common carotid artery, which lies just medial to the internal jugular vein at this point. If the cannula is inserted too far towards the thoracic inlet, puncture of the subclavian artery, the pleura or even the lung may result.

A lower approach to the vein at the apex of the triangle of the two heads of sternomastoid is also satisfactory. Suitable cannulae for use in neonates are the 18 s.w.g. Abbocath (51 mm long) or the Wallace 17.5 s.w.g. (53 mm long). The right vein is preferred because the pathway from right jugular vein to SVC is straight, whereas a cannula in the left may not easily cross the midline and may not function well.

If there is need for a constant infusion of a drug such as dopamine or sodium nitroprusside, a second cannula may be inserted into the same vein. After the cannula has been inserted it is mandatory to test with a water column that the pressure is in fact venous. Free aspiration of blood must be possible at all times; if it is not, then the cannula should be repositioned. Unsatisfactory position may be the cause of late perforation of the vessel, resulting in hydrothorax.

The subclavian vein has been safely cannulated by a percutaneous technique in the neonate. A skin incision is made below the clavicle, just lateral to its midpoint, and the needle is aimed at a point 1–1.5 cm above the sternal notch. The angle between the needle and the chest is initially about 45 degrees, enabling the needle to pass beneath the clavicle, when the angle is reduced to 15–20 degrees. If the infant has a prominent chest, the hub of the needle must be flattened against it during entry.

A Seldinger technique is very useful for subclavian cannulation, and packs such as Vygon Leadercath contain a needle, guide wire and venous catheter.

It is not usually possible to pass a central venous cannula percutaneously up the arm from the antecubital fossa in the neonate, although this can be done following surgical exposure.

The central venous cannula may be connected either to a simple water manometer or, via a short length of narrow bore tubing, to a pressure transducer. It should be remembered that 1 mmHg = 1.36 cmH₂O.

Left atrial pressure or pulmonary capillary wedge pressure

As a rule, in paediatric patients if cardiac failure occurs, both ventricles fail together and so left and right filling pressures are usually similar. However, measurement of left atrial pressure is essential following repair of many congenital heart lesions in the neonate because left atrial pressure gives a more reliable indication of blood loss or adequate replacement than right atrial or CVP pressure in this situation—especially after surgery on the mitral valve. Left atrial pressure lines can be inserted under direct vision at the time of operation by the surgeon, but care must be taken to ensure that air is not injected into them because this will be passed into the systemic circulation and may pass into the cerebral vessels. Following non-cardiac operations, pulmonary wedge pressure may be measured using the Swan–Ganz catheter inserted via the right internal jugular or subclavian vein. This measurement is occasionally used to monitor the effect of pulmonary vaso-dilating drugs in such conditions as congenital diaphragmatic hernia. It is, however, a difficult, invasive and potentially dangerous technique in the neonate, and the indications for it are few and probably confined to those patients who have crises of pulmonary hypertension.

Fluid balance and blood replacement

The most accurate method of transfusion of blood or fluid in the newborn is by syringe, and the volume of fluid injected as diluent for muscle relaxants or other drugs should be included in the total fluid balance. The baby may arrive in the operating theatre with 100 ml measuring sets attached to the intravenous cannula, but these do not allow a rapid change from the administration of crystalloid fluids to that of blood.

Monitoring of blood loss is best achieved by weighing small numbers of swabs before they dry out. The experienced anaesthetist should also be able to make an approximate estimate of the blood loss from visual observation of the swabs. Allowance should be made for loss on drapes, and the volume of blood contained in the suction bottle should be measured directly. Color-imetric techniques are time consuming and do not allow the anaesthetist to obtain an estimate of blood loss at the time when it is occurring. Urine output may be monitored by the use of adhesive collecting bags, but in major surgery (such as cardiac surgery) catheterization should be performed.

Adequacy of volume replacement during surgery can be assessed by blood pressure, peripheral circulatory state or, in cases of massive blood replacement, by CVP monitoring. A core–peripheral temperature difference greater than 2°C is a reliable and sensitive sign of a reduced cardiac output.

Biochemical estimations

Biochemical estimations are seldom required during neonatal anaesthesia, although estimation of the blood glucose level is valuable in premature or small-for gestational-age infants. Dextrostix, or BM-Test strips are simple to use and reasonably reliable as long as they are fresh. In the sick hypoxic acidotic newborn, levels of serum calcium, sodium and potassium should be measured before surgery; blood gas and acid–base estimations may be needed, especially if cardiovascular or respiratory failure ensues.

Temperature

Temperature should always be measured during neonatal surgery because of the increased susceptibility of the newborn to heat loss, and because hypothermia significantly increases morbidity and mortality. Nasopharyngeal, oesophageal or rectal temperatures can be most easily monitored and are all reliable although the rectal temperature probe may become displaced during anaesthesia without the anaesthetist being aware of it.

Monitoring of theatre equipment

Anaesthetic machines

Anaesthetic machines and related equipment such as suction devices, upon which the patient's life may depend, must be thoroughly checked before anaesthesia is induced. This check includes inspection of the gas supply and breathing circuits, ensuring that pipeline probes are firmly inserted, that cylinders are full and are operating properly, a check of flowmeters and vaporizers, and a test to make sure there are no leaks in the circuit. Every anaesthetic machine should be equipped with an oxygen-failure alarm, and, in view of the fact that retrolental fibroplasia has been reported in a premature infant whose only exposure to an increased inspired oxygen fraction (F_{IO_2}) occurred during surgery, it is wise to monitor F_{IO_2} at all times.

If a heated humidifier is to be incorporated into the breathing system it should conform to accepted standards of electrical safety and a fail-safe cut-out device should operate in case of thermostat failure. The performance of the humidifier should be monitored by measurement of the temperature of the inspired gas at the patient end of the system.

Oxygenation

Significant periods of hyperoxaemia and hypoxaemia have been detected during paediatric surgery by the use of transcutaneous oxygen electrodes, and it is probable that their use during neonatal anaesthesia will soon become routine. Halothane and nitrous oxide are both reduced by these electrodes, falsely elevating the $Tc\,Po_2$, but this effect can be overcome by offsetting the applied voltage, changing the electrolyte or avoiding these agents. Pulse oximeters may become the most useful monitors of oxygenation.

If serious oxygenation problems are expected during surgery, it is wise to insert an arterial cannula beforehand, as described on p. 198.

Mechanical ventilators

Many mechanical ventilators are fitted with airway pressure gauges, volume meters, and disconnection and overpressure alarms, and for those without these monitors there is a fairly wide range of 'add-on' modules available. The recent introduction of the Infanta version of the Wright anemometer, with three times the sensitivity of the adult version, allows the anaesthetist to monitor tidal and minute volume with ease, even in the neonate.

As with anaesthetic machines, all neonatal ventilators should be fitted with oxygen analysers, particularly since the commonly used oxygen blenders cannot always be relied upon to deliver the preset Fio_2 accurately.

Heating devices

Because of the increased susceptibility of the newborn to heat loss, additional heat must be provided during anaesthesia and this is conventionally achieved by lying the baby on a heated electric or water blanket. These appliances must be electrically safe and must also be accurately monitored. Water mattresses must have an easily adjusted thermostat and a fail-safe cut-out device to prevent the water temperature rising above 42°C in the event of the thermostat failure. The temperature difference between the heating unit and the water in the mattress depends on the length of connecting tubing and the circulating flow rate. It is therefore wise to monitor the temperature of the blanket by means of a thermistor probe placed between it and the skin surface of the neonate.

Because there is less risk of burns with hot dry air than with water, the hot air mattress described on p. 96 is probably the safest as well as the most efficient method of providing heat during anaesthesia. Patient temperature should, however, be carefully monitored, as hyperpyrexia can occur during long operations.

Electrically heated blankets can rapidly overheat and cause serious burns, and their use should probably be discontinued.

Environmental monitoring

Temperature

It is essential to monitor both the temperature and the rate of air change in the operating theatre during neonatal anaesthesia. The theatre should be draught-free and the temperature should be as high as can be tolerated by the staff. This latter is unlikely to be above 25°C.

Pollution

Increasing attention is being paid to the problems of pollution of the operating theatre by volatile and gaseous anaesthetic agents discharged from breathing circuits. The removal of these agents from the paediatric T-piece presents a particular problem. Although scavenging systems have been described which involve the insertion of collecting devices into the expiratory limb of the reservoir bag, or the modification of the circuit to include scavenged expiratory valves, these devices alter the basic simplicity of the T-piece, often make it more cumbersome to use and, in some cases, increase the danger of obstruction to expiratory gas flow. A scavenging dish (Fig. 3.25) for the anaesthetic T-piece which does not alter its characteristics

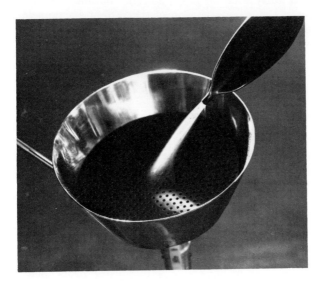

Fig. 3.25   A scavenging dish. Smoke is used to illustrate the effect of the scavenger on gas flow from the open tail of the T-piece bag. (Reproduced, with permission, from Hatch, Miles and Wagstaff, 1980)

has been described by Hatch, Miles and Wagstaff (1980). The dish removes large volumes of contaminated air and, if placed close to the open-tailed bag of the T-piece, provides a safe and convenient scavenger. It has been incorporated into a scavenging system which can also be used with a standard antipollution valve or ventilator exhaust port (Fig. 3.26). Measurements before and after installation have shown it to be capable of reducing nitrous oxide levels in the operating theatre to acceptable levels. Levels of other anaesthetic gases or vapours such as halothane are known to follow nitrous oxide levels closely. Nitrous oxide is used in almost every anaesthetic given in the UK and levels are reasonably easy to measure because of the large volumes involved.

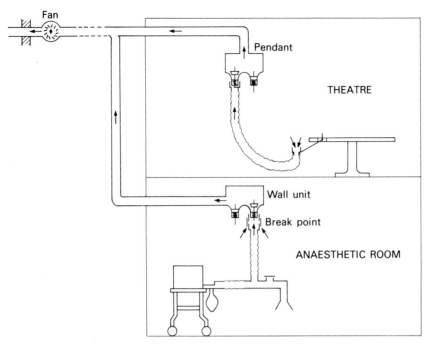

Fig. 3.26 Diagram of a typical scavenger installation. The theatre pendant is shown connected to the scavenging dish, whilst the anaesthetic room wall unit is shown with a standard antipollution valve. (Reproduced, with permission, from Hatch, Miles and Wagstaff, 1980)

References and further reading

Anaesthetic equipment

Bain, J. A. and Spoerel, W. E. (1977). Carbon dioxide output and elimination in children under anaesthesia. *Canadian Anaesthetists Society Journal* **24**, 533.

Fisher, D. M. (1983). Anaesthesia equipment for pediatrics. In: *Pediatric Anesthesia*, p. 347. Ed. by G. A. Gregory. Churchill Livingstone, New York.

Fisk, G. C. (1973). Equipment for inhalation anaesthesia for children. *Anaesthesia and Intensive Care* **1**, 468.

Froese, A. B. and Rose, D. K. (1982). A detailed analysis of T-piece systems. In: *Some Aspects of Paediatric Anaesthesia*, p. 101. Ed. by D. J. Steward. Elsevier/North Holland Biomedical Press, Amsterdam.

Hatch, D. J. (1978). Tracheal tubes and connectors used in neonates—dimensions and resistance to breathing. *British Journal of Anaesthesia* **50**, 959.

Hatch, D. J. (1981). Anaesthetic equipment for neonates and infants. *British Journal of Hospital Medicine* **26**, 84.

Lindahl, S. G. E., Hulse, M. G. and Hatch, D. J. (1984). Ventilation and gas exchange during anaesthesia and surgery in spontaneously breathing infants and children. *British Journal of Anaesthesia* **56**, 121.

Nightingale, D. A., Richards, C. C. and Glass, A. (1965). An evaluation of re-breathing in a modified T-piece system during controlled ventilation in anaesthetized children. *British Journal of Anaesthesia* **37**, 762.

Rayburn, R. L. and Graves, S. A. (1978). A new concept in controlled ventilation of children with the Bain anesthetic circuit. *Anesthesiology* **48**, 250.

Rees, G. J. (1958). Neonatal anaesthesia. *British Medical Bulletin* **14**, 38.

Rickham, P. (1954). An investigation of blood loss during operations on the newborn infant. *Archives of Disease in Childhood* **29**, 304.

Rose, D. K. and Froese, A. B. (1979). The regulation of Pa_{CO_2} during controlled ventilation of children with a T-piece. *Canadian Anaesthetists Society Journal* **26**, 104.

Seeley, H. F., Barnes, P. K. and Conway, C. M. (1977). Controlled ventilation with the Mapleson D sysrem. A theoretical and experimental study. *British Journal of Anaesthesia* **49**, 107.

Symposium on Pediatric Anesthesia. (1975). *Anesthesiology* **43**, 141.

Willis, B. A., Pender, J. W. and Mapleson, W. W. (1975). Rebreathing in a T-piece: volunteer and theoretical studies of the Jackson Rees modification of the Ayre's T-piece during spontaneous respiration. *British Journal of Anaesthesia* **47**, 1239.

Maintenance of anaesthesia

Diaz, J. H. and Lockhart, C. H. (1979). Is halothane really safe in infancy? *Anesthesiology* **51**, S313.

Gregory, G. A. (1983). Anaesthesia for premature infants. In: *Pediatric Anesthesia*, p. 579. Ed. by G. A. Gregory. Churchill Livingstone, New York.

Lerman, J., Robinson, S., Willis, M. M., Gregory, G. A. (1983). Anesthetic requirements for halothane in young children 0–1 month and 1–6 months of age. *Anesthesiology* **59**, 421.

Lomaz, J. G. (1965). Halothane and jaundice in paediatric anaesthesia. *Anaesthesia* **20**, 70.

Robinson, S. and Gregory, G. A. (1980). Fentanyl–Air/oxygen anesthesia for PDA ligation in infants less than 1500 grams. *Anesthesia and Analgesia* **59**, 556.

Salanitre, E. and Rackow, H. (1969). The pulmonary exchange of nitrous oxide and halothane in infants and children. *Anesthesiology* **30**, 388.

Salem, M. R., Wong, A. Y. and Collins V. J. (1973). The pediatric patient with a full stomach. *Anesthesiology* **39**, 435.

Smith, P. C. and Smith, N. T. (1972). Anaesthetic management of a very premature infant. *British Journal of Anaesthesia* **44**, 736.

Steward, D. J. and Creighton, R. E. (1978). The uptake and excretion of nitrous oxide on the newborn. *Canadian Anaesthetists Society Journal* **25,** 215.

Sumner, E. and Patrick, E. K. (1980). The paediatric patient. In: *Preparation for Anaesthesia*, p. 359. Ed. by A. J. Stevens, Pitman Medical, Tunbridge Wells.

Vivori, E. and Bush, G. H. (1977). Modern aspects of the management of the newborn undergoing operation. *British Journal of Anaesthesia* **49,** 51.

Wark, H. J. (1983). Postoperative jaundice in children—the influence of halothane. *Anaesthesia* **38,** 237.

Way, W. L., Costley, E. C. and Way, E. L. (1965). Respiratory sensitivity of the newborn infant to meperidine and morphine. *Clinical Pharmacology and Therapeutics* **6,** 454.

Relaxants

Bennett, E. J., Ramanamurthy, S., Dalal, F. Y. and Salem, M. R. (1975). Pancuronium and the neonate. *British Journal of Anaesthesia* **47,** 75.

Bennett, E. J., Ignacio, A., Patel, K., Grundy, E. M. and Salem, M. R. (1976). Tubocurarine and the neonate. *British Journal of Anaesthesia* **48,** 687.

Brandom, B. W., Woelfel, S. K., Cook, D. R., Fehr, B. L. and Rudd, G. D. (1984). Clinical pharmacology of atracurium in infants. *Anaesthesia and Analgesia* **63,** 309.

Bush, G. H. and Stead, A. L. (1962). The use of *d*-tubocurarine in neonatal anaesthesia. *British Journal of Anaesthesia* **34,** 721.

Churchill Davidson, H. C., Way, W. L. and de Jong, R. H. (1967). The muscle relaxants and renal excretion. *Anesthesiology* **28,** 540.

Gargarian, M. A., Basta, S. J., Savarese, J. J., Ali, H. H., Sunder, N., Scott, R., Gionfriddo, M. and Batson, A. G. (1984). The efficacy of atracurium by continuous infusion. *Anesthesiology* **61,** A291.

Goudsouzian, N. G. (1985). Relaxants in Paediatric Anaesthesia. *Clinics in Anaesthesiology* **3,** no. 3, 539.

Goudsouzian, N. G., Donlon, J. V., Savarese, J. J. and Ryan, J. F. (1975). Re-evaluation of dosage and duration of action of *d*-tubocurarine in the pediatric age group. *Anesthesiology* **43,** 416.

Mirakhur, R. K., Ferres, C. J. and Pandit, S. K. (1984). Muscle relaxation with an infusion of vecuronium. *Anesthesiology* **61,** A293.

Nightingale, D. A. and Bush, G. H. (1973). A clinical comparison between tubocurarine and pancuronium in children. *British Journal of Anaesthesia* **45,** 63.

Nightingale, D. A. and Bush, G. H. (1983). Atracurium in paediatric anaesthesia. *British Journal of Anaesthesia* **55,** 115.

Salem, M. R., Toyame, T., Wong, A. Y., Jacobs, H. K. and Bennett, E. J. (1977). Haemodynamic responses to antagonism of tubocurarine block with atropine prostigmine mixture in children. *British Journal of Anaesthesia* **49,** 901.

Watts, C. F. and Dillon, J. B. (1969). The response of newborn to succinylcholine and *d*-tubocurarine. *Anesthesiology* **31**, 35.
Zsigmond, E. K. and Downs, J. R. (1971). Plasma cholinesterase activity in newborns and infants. *Canadian Anaesthetists Society Journal* **18**, 278.

Patient care and monitoring during anaesthesia

Battersby, E. F. (1980). Monitoring during anesthesia for pediatric surgery. In: *International Anesthesiology Clinics.* Ed. by G. Gerson. Little, Brown & Co., Boston, Mass.
Betts, E. K., Downes, J. J., Schaffer, D. B. and Johns, R. (1977). Retrolental fibroplasia and oxygen administration during general anesthesia. *Anesthesiology* **47**, 518.
Clark, C., Gibbs, J. A. H., Maniello, R., Outerbridge, E. W. and Aranda, J. V. (1981). Blood transfusion: a possible risk factor in retrolental fibroplasia. *Acta Paediatrica Scandinavica* **70**, 535.
English, I. C. W., Frew, R. M., Piggott, J. F. and Zaki, M. (1964). Percutaneous catheterisation of the internal jugular vein. *Anaesthesia* **24**, 521.
Filston, H. C. and Grant, J. P. (1979). A safer system for percutaneous subclavian venous catheterization in newborn infants. *Journal of Pediatric Surgery* **14**, 564.
Furman, E. B., Hairabet, J. K. and Roman, D. G. (1972). The use of indwelling radial artery needles in paediatric anaesthesia. *British Journal of Anaesthesia* **44**, 531.
Gothgen, I. and Jacobsen, E. (1978). Transcutaneous oxygen measurement. II. The influence of halothane aand hypotension. *Acta Anaesthesiologica Scandinavica* suppl., **67**, 71.
Gregory, G. A. (Ed.) (1983). Monitoring during surgery. In: *Pediatric Anesthesia*, p. 381. Churchill Livingstone, New York.
Hatch, D. J., Miles, R. and Wagstaff, M. (1980). An anaesthetic scavenging system for paediatric and adult use. *Anaesthesia* **35**, 496.
Hutton, P., Dye, J. and Prys-Roberts, C. (1984). An assessment of the Dinamap 845. Anaesthesia **39**, 261.
Rickham, P. P. (1954). An investigation of blood loss during operations on the newborn infant. *Archives of Disease in Childhood* **29**, 304.
Saidman, L. J. and Smith, N. T. (1978). *Monitoring in Anesthesia.* Wiley, New York and Chichester.
Welle, P., Hayden, W. and Miller, T. (1980). Continuous measurement of transcutaneous oxygen tension in neonates under general anesthesia. *Journal of Pediatric Surgery* **15**, 257.

Patient care and monitoring

Yelderman, M. and New, W. Jr (1983). Evaluation of pulse oximetry. *Anesthesiology* **59**, 349.

4

Anaesthesia — specific conditions

Surgical emergencies in the newborn

Almost all surgery in the neonatal period is performed on an emergency basis, and early diagnosis and treatment are essential if reasonable survival rates are to be achieved. The problems of transportation, preoperative assessment and general anaesthetic management of the neonate have already been discussed, and this chapter is devoted to specific surgical emergencies and their management.

Refinements in ultrasound diagnosis and its very widespread use in pregnancy allow many fetal abnormalities to be discovered before birth. Abdominal wall defects, hydrocephalus, oesophageal atresia, diaphragmatic hernia and hydronephrosis are all readily seen with ultrasound. Such early diagnosis raises the possibility of fetal surgery, for example for hydrocephalus or urinary tract obstruction, and this has already started in certain centres. It also allows the delivery of the baby at an optimal time for reception in the regional neonatal surgical unit.

Oesophageal atresia

Oesophageal atresia, with or without fistula, occurs in between 1 and 3000 and 1 in 3500 live births. In this condition the main danger to life comes from the risk of aspiration of secretions into the bronchial tree, with subsequent pulmonary infection together with possible spillover of acid gastric juice through the fistula. Although other factors will affect survival, particularly birth weight and the presence or absence of major congenital abnormalities, early diagnosis and treatment before aspiration and contamination of the lungs has occurred are where survival rates are improved by good management. In the 5-year period 1979–1983 at The Hospital for Sick Children, London, there were a total of 200 neonates treated for oesophageal atresia, with or without fistula, and 179 (89.5%) of these have survived.

The diagnosis should be suspected in any case of polyhydramnios and premature labour. At birth the baby is often seen to produce excess saliva which may drool from the mouth. The presence of oesophageal atresia can be confirmed by the inability to pass a 10 FG catheter down the oesophagus and into the stomach. If the catheter is too soft, it may coil in the upper pouch and the diagnosis may be missed. If a radio-opaque catheter is used,

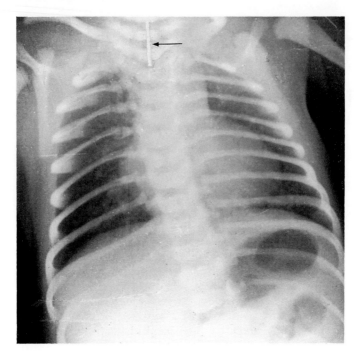

Fig. 4.1 Oesophageal atresia with fistula. X-ray showing opaque catheter in the upper pouch, aspiration pneumonitis and gas in the stomach.

X-ray confirmation of the length of the blind-ending upper pouch can be obtained. A plain x-ray of the chest and abdomen will also disclose the presence of a fistulous communication between the tracheobronchial tree and the lower oesophageal pouch, as any gas bubble seen in the stomach must have entered through such a communication (Fig. 4.1). Since the common anomaly is this combination of blind-ending upper pouch and lower pouch fistula (Fig. 4.2), the majority of cases of oesophageal atresia should be diagnosed easily soon after birth. The use of contrast medium is

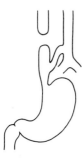

Fig. 4.2 Oesophageal atresia/fistula: the common anomaly (85 per cent incidence).

to be condemned because of the risk of pulmonary aspiration, compounding the pneumonitis and increasing the morbidity and mortality.

If no gas bubble is seen, the most likely diagnosis is atresia without fistula. The rare occurrence of upper pouch fistula (Fig. 4.3) should be excluded or confirmed by the surgeon at the time of operation, whether or not a lower pouch fistula is present.

Perhaps the most difficult diagnosis to make is that of isolated tracheo-oesophageal fistula without oesophageal atresia. Prominent gaseous distension is sometimes the presenting sign in the newborn but the diagnosis may be delayed for several months, when the infant usually presents with a history of recurrent attacks of chest infection. The differential diagnosis includes cystic fibrosis of the lungs, other causes of repeated aspiration such as inco-ordinated swallowing or hiatus hernia, and rare lung diseases. In

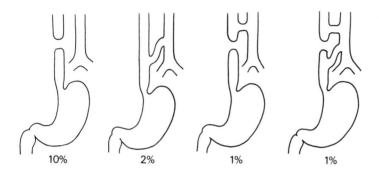

Fig. 4.3 Oesophageal atresia/fistula: the rarer anomalies (the approximate incidence is indicated under each).

this case diagnosis is usually made with the use of contrast medium by cineoesophageal swallow. The films are sometimes difficult to interpret and they should be seen by an experienced radiologist. Aspiration of feeds into the airway can sometimes be confirmed by the finding of fat-laden macrophages in tracheal aspirate.

Once the diagnosis of oesophageal atresia has been made, steps should be taken to protect the lungs from aspiration. The most satisfactory way of doing this is by the passage of a double-lumen Replogle tube into the upper pouch. Continuous low pressure suction is applied to one lumen and the second lumen entrains air, thus preventing the tube becoming stuck to the wall of the pouch. Alternatively, the upper pouch can be kept empty by intermittent suction. Gastro-oesophageal reflux is discouraged in the upright position but this position does not prevent the collection of mucus in the upper pouch and it may be preferable to nurse the baby prone. A delay of at least several hours with appropriate antibiotic therapy and physiotherapy may be justified before surgery, and has been shown to be of particular value where there has already been aspiration and contamination of the bronchial tree before the diagnosis has been made.

Associated anomalies

About 30–50 per cent of babies presenting with oesophageal atresia have associated congenital anomalies. The most common are congenital heart disease, particularly atrial or ventricular septal defects, patent ductus arteriosus, Fallot's tetralogy, and coarctation of the aorta, vascular anomalies and upper airway problems such as laryngo- or tracheomalacia. Severe tracheomalacia may require prolonged intubation or even tracheostomy, and the operation of aortopexy is now performed for this condition. The most severe cases may be incompatible with life.

Cleft lip and palate may be found in association with oesophageal atresia, as may vertebral, renal and anorectal defects. The VATER syndrome combines vertebral (or ventricular septal defect), anal, tracheal, (oesophageal and renal (or radial) anomalies. Plain x-ray of the abdomen may help in screening for some of these defects. The presence of gas in the small bowel, for example, will exclude the possibility of duodenal atresia. Vertebral anomalies may also be detected on plain x-ray. If serious congenital heart disease is suspected, echocardiography may be helpful prior to oesophageal repair.

These babies are commonly of low birth weight, and Waterston in 1962 showed that mortality rose steeply with low birth weight, the presence of other major anomalies and the severity of pneumonia (Waterston, Bonham Carter and Aberdeen, 1962). They described three groups of patients with differing survival rates classified according to these factors. Group A, with lowest mortality (5 per cent), comprised babies of birth weight over 2.5 kg who were well. Group B, with a mortality of 32 per cent, comprised babies weighing 1.8–2.5 kg and those of higher birth weight with moderate pneumonia or congenital anomalies. Group C, with the highest mortality at 94 per cent, comprised babies weighing under 1.8 kg and those of higher birth weight with severe pneumonia or congenital anomalies.

Anaesthetic management

Because of the importance of gestational age in relation to mortality, this should be carefully assessed before surgery, and steps should be taken to treat any hypoglycaemia or respiratory distress.

It is not necessary for tracheal intubation to be performed before arrival in the operating theatre; this is usually carried out awake as for any other neonatal surgical emergency, although the upper pouch should be aspirated immediately before intubation. When the tracheal tube has been secured in place, the lungs should be gently inflated and careful auscultation of the chest carried out to ensure that adequate air entry is achieved in both lungs. The stethoscope should also be placed over the stomach to check that the anaesthetic gases are not inflating it via the fistula. This is usually situated on the posterior wall of the trachea, and is often just proximal to the carina.

In the majority of cases the lungs can be adequately inflated without distension of the stomach, but if the position of the tracheal tube is not satisfactory, it is usually because the tip is pointing towards the fistula. It is extremely unusual to intubate the fistula itself, although this has been reported. If a significant amount of gas is passing through the fistula, the tracheal tube should be repositioned, either by passing it further down the trachea or by turning it on its connector so that its bevelled tip is pointing in a different direction. It is unusual not to be able to find a position where the lungs can be satisfactorily inflated without a significant amount of air passing through the fistula, and controlled ventilation can normally be commenced with the use of muscle relaxants. In the unlikely event of it not being possible to inflate the lungs adequately, or if the stomach is being significantly distended, the surgeon would be informed and the patient allowed to continue to breathe spontaneously. Many surgeons would perform gastrostomy before thoracotomy in this rare situation, and some surgeons prefer to do this with every case, as it prevents the theoretical risk of the enlarging stomach splinting the diaphragm and impeding respiration further. The most important task is to ligate the fistula. When the chest is opened, controlled ventilation must be commenced, and if adequate inflation of the lungs is not achieved the surgeon should control the leak through the fistula as soon as possible—if necessary, using his finger to do this in the first instance. The normal approach to the fistula is extrapleural, although this takes longer and cannot be used in the emergency described above.

The other problem which the anaesthetist is likely to face is surgical retraction during the thoracotomy, which may obstruct ventilation. If the lungs are already stiff with severe pneumonia, it may be difficult to detect complete obstruction, but in most cases the sudden change in pressure required to inflate the lungs is easily detected by the hand. For this reason, manual ventilation is preferred to mechanical ventilation. The use of the precordial stethoscope is extremely valuable in these cases, particularly for the information it provides about the amount of air entering the lungs. It should be positioned over the left side of the chest, or even in the left axilla, well away from the surgical field. Occasionally the trachea can be seriously damaged during the surgery and large air leaks may occur.

Anaesthesia can be maintained with nitrous oxide, oxygen and muscle relaxation, with the addition of minimal amounts of an inhalation agent such as halothane if required. Care must be taken not to increase the inspired oxygen fraction above that necessary to prevent hypoxia, especially in the preterm neonate who is particularly at risk from retrolental fibroplasia. Transcutaneous oxygen electrodes are being increasingly used during anaesthesia in these high-risk babies.

Blood should be available for transfusion, but with experienced surgical care it is seldom required. Usually, sufficient crystalloid solution is given with the various diluted drugs administered to satisfy maintenance requirements, which are low in the first few days of life (as described on p. 77). The upper pouch should be sucked from time to time and occasionally tracheobronchial suction may be required. Monitoring of blood pressure, ECG and temperature is essential.

Postoperative care

Postoperatively, if the chest is not seriously contaminated and the patient is awake and moving vigorously with no residual effects of muscle relaxation, extubation can be performed. If there is any doubt about the adequacy of ventilation, if the oesophageal anastomosis is tight or if the lungs are seriously contaminated, it is probably wiser to continue controlled ventilation for at least 24 hours. These babies all need intensive postoperative care; approximately 25 per cent of them will need some period of postoperative ventilation, and it is wise in those suffering from severe aspiration pneumonitis, with very low birth weight or life-threatening associated anomaly to monitor direct arterial and central venous pressure. Transcutaneous oxygen tension (Tc Po_2) should be monitored in preterm infants. Chest physiotherapy will be required together with appropriate antibiotic therapy. Intragastric feeding is commenced as soon as possible, either via a transanastomotic feeding tube or by gastrostomy.

If, for anatomical reasons, primary anastomosis of the two ends of the oesophagus cannot be achieved, a feeding gastrostomy will be performed and continuous suction to the upper pouch or oesophagostomy will be required until a delayed repair can be carried out.

Anaesthesia for oesophagoscopy

After primary anastomosis of oesophageal atresia, repeated oesophageal dilatations may be necessary for actual or incipient strictures.

Premedication is with atropine, and awake intubation with a preformed tube, Oxford tube or plain tube with curved Magill connection is performed after preoxygenation. If anaesthesia is required in an older baby, the use of cricoid pressure must be considered to prevent aspiration of regurgitated upper oesophageal contents. The T-piece comes down over the baby's chest. A relaxant technique with controlled ventilation is most satisfactory. Suxamethonium (succinylcholine) has often been used for this procedure, but newer relaxants such as atracurium or vecuronium may have a place. The eyes must be protected by taping them shut, and heart beat and respiration monitored with a precordial stethoscope. The passage of the oesophagoscope may compress the trachea and obstruct the ventilation. Coughing on the tracheal tube when the oesophagoscope is in place has been responsible for oesophageal perforations, so perfect immobility should be produced throughout. After the endoscopy the patient is allowed to awaken fully, suction is carefully applied to the pharynx and extubation performed with the infant in the lateral position.

Congenital diaphragmatic hernia (Table 4.1)

Congenital diaphragmatic hernia (CDH) is a rare but serious emergency in the newborn period, with an incidence of approximately 1 in 4000 live births, although in terms of perinatal mortality this may be closer to 1 in 2000 as some continue to occur as stillbirths.

Table 4.1   Congenital diaphragmatic hernia, 1979–1983, at The Hospital for Sick Children, Great Ormond Street, London

Age at GOS	Number	Survived
0–6 hours	93	49 (53%)
6–24 hours	21	20 (95%)
Over 24 hours	24	24 (100%)
Total	138	93 (67%)

There are several types of anomaly, the commonest (about 80 per cent) occurring through a posterolateral defect in the left side of the diaphragm at the foramen of Bochdalek. Failure of fusion of the pleuroperitoneal folds and septum transversum by the 12th week of fetal life or premature return of the intestines from their extracoelomic position to the abdominal cavity allows the posterior portion of the dividing membrane to stay open. Closing of the right side is usually completed before the left, which may explain the

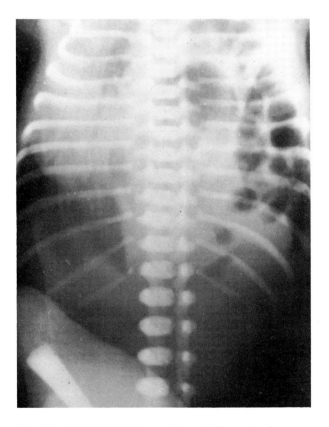

Fig. 4.4   Left-sided diaphragmatic hernia. X-ray showing gross mediastinal displacement caused by gas-filled intestine in the left chest.

greater incidence of left-sided hernias. The hernia usually consists of the whole of the midgut, and may include the stomach, part of the descending colon, the left kidney, the spleen and the left lobe of the liver. The midgut fills with air soon after birth—usually at the time of the first feed—causing further displacement of the mediastinum to the right and compression of the right lung (Fig. 4.4).

The onset of respiratory distress depends largely on the degree of pulmonary hypoplasia present, which is usually bilateral since the development of the contralateral lung is hindered by shift of the mediastinum in fetal life. Mortality of up to 50 per cent is confined to that group of babies who develop severe respiratory distress within the first 4 hours of life. At post-mortem the lung weights on the affected side may be found to be as low as 2 g compared with a normal individual lung weight of from 17–35 g in full-term babies. Survival is unlikely if the combined lung weights are less than 50 per cent of normal. Babies dying of CDH do have hypoplastic lungs in terms of weight and branching of bronchial generations, the distal airways being the greatest affected. The cell types, however, are normal for the gestation of the fetus. Together with this is a decreased pulmonary vascular bed causing an increased pulmonary vascular resistance. Increase in the muscular content of the media of the arterioles predisposes to the development of transitional circulation in these patients. In some babies, congenital diaphragmatic hernia causes little respiratory embarrassment,

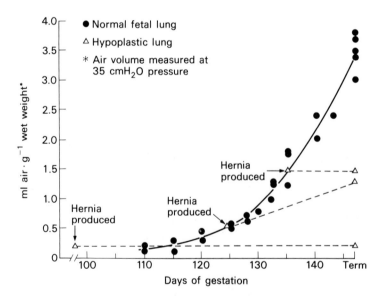

Fig. 4.5 Air capacity of lungs of lambs at gestational ages 110–147 days. The lungs of lambs with diaphragmatic hernia had air capacities equivalent to lungs at the gestational age at which the hernia was produced. (Reproduced, with permission, from de Lorimer, Tierney and Parker, 1967)

and occasionally the diagnosis is not made until early childhood or even later. These children presumably have little or no pulmonary hypoplasia. The reason why some cases of diaphragmatic hernia have severe pulmonary hypoplasia and others apparently very little is not clear. Work in animals suggests that it depends upon the gestational age at which herniation of the intestinal contents into the chest actually occurs (Fig. 4.5). If lung maturation is arrested by the herniation, it is clear that when this occurs early in intrauterine life there is a greater chance of pulmonary hypoplasia than when it occurs later.

Associated anomalies

The problem of associated pulmonary hypoplasia is discussed above. Other lung anomalies such as sequestrated pulmonary lobes may also occur.

The commonest anomalies associated with diaphragmatic hernia are intestinal, and malrotation of the gut is almost a universal finding. Congenital heart disease and renal anomalies are less common.

Diagnosis

Increasingly, CDH is diagnosed in fetal life by ultrasound or fetography, although the condition should be suspected in any case of respiratory distress occurring soon after birth. Examination of the chest may reveal reduced movement and reduced breath sounds on the affected side, dullness to percussion, mediastinal displacement and a scaphoid abdomen. A straight x-ray will usually confirm the diagnosis, although this can occasionally be confused with congenital pulmonary lobar emphysema.

Anaesthetic management

The early onset of respiratory distress with severe hypoxia demands urgent treatment, usually by tracheal intubation and careful ventilation, and deflation of the stomach via a *large* nasogastric tube keeps the stomach and intestines from distending in the chest. This, together with venous access should precede transfer of the infant to a regional centre for neonatal surgery. The lungs should not be inflated with a face mask because this will increase the amount of air passing into the stomach and intestines, increase mediastinal displacement and predispose to pneumothorax. The hypoplastic lungs always rupture before they are fully expanded, usually in areas of more normal lung development and frequently on the contralateral side.

The aim of treatment for those presenting early with symptoms is the achievement and then maintenance of cardiopulmonary stability with direct monitoring of arterial pressure, preferably from the right radial artery (preductal blood) and right atrial pressure via right internal jugular vein. Mechanical ventilation is continued using pancuronium $0.1\,\mathrm{mg\cdot kg^{-1}}$ with morphine $0.2\,\mathrm{mg\cdot kg^{-1}}$ or fentanyl $5\,\mu\mathrm{g\cdot kg^{-1}}$ i.v. as necessary. Postductal Po_2 can be estimated using a transcutaneous electrode over the lower half of the body. In some instances surgery has been delayed for up to 48 hours in an attempt to achieve stability, as it is recognized that the operation in itself is not curative as long as the gut is not allowed to become distended within the chest and also that a stable cardiopulmonary state is of the greatest importance.

The surgical correction is via a laparotomy because of the associated malrotation of the bowel and anaesthesia may comprise relaxant, high FiO_2 if necessary and supplementation with fentanyl. Because of the pulmonary hypoplasia, great care should be taken not to use excessive pressures when ventilating the lungs as these may cause pneumothorax. If possible, inflating pressures should be kept below 25–30 cmH$_2$O, using hand ventilation. The possibility of a pneumothorax on the contralateral side should always be borne in mind and drainage of the pleural cavity should always be considered if the baby's condition suddenly deteriorates. No attempt should be made to expand the ipsilateral lung at the end of the procedure, as this will invariably cause a pneumothorax. The monitoring of ECG, arterial pressure, nasopharyngeal temperature and TcPo_2 should be continued throughout the operation. The use of a precordial stethoscope may be impracticable if there is severe mediastinal shift and may interfere with the surgical field.

There is no agreement on the best arrangement for the chest drain. Some surgeons do not put one in but balance the mediastinum by putting a scalp vein needle into the left chest and allowing air to escape underwater—the needle is then removed. Another possibility is to put a chest drain into the left side but to clamp it and unclamp every 8 hours to maintain stability of the mediastinum. Whatever the arrangement, the possibility of pneumothorax must always be borne in mind.

Postoperative care

Babies who present with respiratory distress within a few hours of birth need preoperative, intraoperative and postoperative mechanical ventilation, and in many cases this is necessary for several days. Postoperative respiratory support should also be considered for any baby operated on within 24 hours of birth. Older babies who have not required preoperative respiratory support and who are breathing satisfactorily at the end of surgery may be extubated, but it is wise to return all babies to the ward breathing an oxygen-enriched mixture.

Many of the patients in the early presenting group will remain hypoxic postoperatively despite mechanical ventilation with high FiO_2 because of the degree of pulmonary hypoplasia. Other discouraging signs are the need for high inflation pressure (greater than 40 cmH$_2$O), CO$_2$ retention and progressive metabolic acidosis. The mortality in this group is as high as 50 per cent because the degree of pulmonary hypoplasia may be incompatible with life, so that no amount of intensive care will save the child. In addition to these patients, approximately 15 per cent develop signs of transitional circulation within 48 hours, usually with evidence of right-to-left shunting through the ductus (difference between pre- and postductal Pao_2) but also at atrial level which may be demonstrated by contrast echocardiography. Transitional circulation is so common an event in CDH because the pulmonary vascular bed is reduced and the small pulmonary vessels remain unusually active because of failure of the smooth muscle of the media to regress in the normal way after birth and thus vasoconstrict readily in response to acidosis, hypercarbia and hypoxaemia or to a sympathetic stimulus. Most patients who develop transitional circulation will die with critical hypoxaemia unless attempts are made to reduce the reversible component of the pulmonary vascular resistance. The pH should be normal or greater than 7.4 and hyperventilation is usually impossible in these patients because of low lung compliance. Many drugs have been used to reverse this situation—chlorpromazine, nitroprusside, phentolamine and phenoxybenzamine—but tolazoline is undoubtedly the most specific agent for this purpose. Animal work has shown that this drug, although an α-adrenergic blocking agent, has its main action as a histaminergic agonist acting at H_2 receptors. This is the main action also in man as shown by the extraordinary 'lobster' red colour of the peripheries, by lack of response if histamine stores are already depleted by drugs such as morphine or curare, and by the effect on the secretion of gastric acid to cause mucosal erosions or hypochloraemic alkalosis. Tolazoline should be given to those patients with evidence of transitional circulation, but in practice it is also given to those patients who arrive deeply cyanosed and continue to be so in spite of normal resuscitative measures. Tolazoline may be given, cautiously, as a bolus of $1-2\,\mathrm{mg\cdot kg^{-1}}$ followed by an infusion of $1-2\,\mathrm{mg\cdot kg^{-1}\cdot h^{-1}}$, with close monitoring of central venous pressure, as they may need volume-blood or plasma. The arterial pressure also should be closely watched, as these patients may need inotropic support, either dopamine $5-10\,\mu\mathrm{g\cdot kg^{-1}\cdot min^{-1}}$ or a similar dose of dobutamine as dopamine is thought to have a pulmonary vasoconstrictive action in infants.

If cardiac output and thus renal blood flow are maintained, renal failure is avoided. Gastric bleeding is avoided by instillation of antacid, such as magnesium trisilicate mixture, down the nasogastric tube. As with inotropes, weaning from tolazoline should be done very slowly, and only after the circulation has been stable for at least 24 hours (Fig. 4.6).

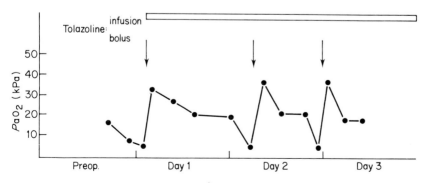

Fig. 4.6 Changes in Pa_{O_2} as tolazoline reverses a transitional circulation.

Tolazoline will act as a predictor of the outcome because if there is no response then the mortality is 100 per cent, whereas the mortality in the group that does respond is approximately 30 per cent.

If extracorporeal membrane oxygenation becomes widely practised, it might be considered for those patients who initially respond to tolazoline, and hence have shown the ability for normal gas exchange, but who later relapse to become unresponsive.

Attempts should be made to keep Pao_2 between 8 and 10.7 kPa (60–80 mmHg) and $Paco_2$ as near as 5.3 kPa (40 mmHg) without excessive inflation pressure as hypoplastic lungs are especially prone to developing bronchopulmonary dysplasia. Weaning from the ventilator may be prolonged in severe cases and tachypnoea may persist for several weeks.

Exomphalos and gastroschisis

Exomphalos is a herniation into the umbilical cord, and gastroschisis is a defect of the abdominal wall lateral to the umbilicus, usually on the right side. The exomphalos sac may be intact or may rupture before, during or after birth with prolapsed abdominal contents coming through it; on the other hand, gastroschisis is always ruptured *in utero* and has no covering membrane. Exomphalos, with an incidence of between 1 in 5000 and 1 in 10 000 live births, is more common than gastroschisis, which has an approximate incidence of 1 in 30 000 live births. There is evidence that gastroschisis is becoming more common.

Associated anomalies

Many of these babies are of low birth weight, especially those with gastroschisis. Common anomalies particularly associated with exomphalos are other gastrointestinal or craniofacial anomalies, including hare-lip and cleft palate, or genitourinary anomalies. Severe congenital heart disease may be present and is one cause of the high mortality with this condition (e.g. pentalogy of Cantrell—exomphalos, short sternum, anterior diaphragmatic hernia, left ventricular diverticulum, VSD, pulmonary stenosis). Some patients with exomphalos have a very narrow 'dog-type' chest (Fig. 4.7) with underlying hypoplastic lungs and may die early with respiratory failure or later with cor pulmonale. Exomphalos forms part of the Beckwith-Wiedemann syndrome (p. 252).

Anaesthetic management

Surgical treatment is usually by excision of the sac when present and complete repair of the anterior abdominal wall usually after this has been stretched manually to enlarge the abdominal cavity. Most anaesthetic problems arise from impaired ventilation if closure of the abdominal wall compresses the intestinal contents, pushing the diaphragm upwards and restricting its downward movement on inspiration. This may occur even with full

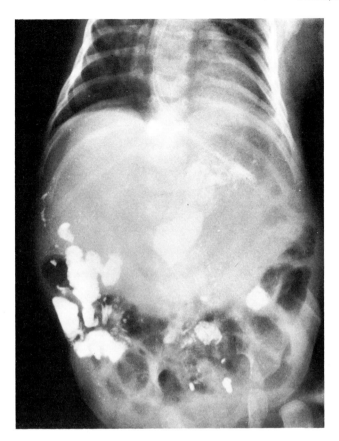

Fig. 4.7 Exomphalos. X-ray showing the narrow chest.

muscular relaxation. If the chest is small and the compliance of the lungs is low and thus falls further when attempts are made to close the abdomen, then it may be wiser to use a pouch of silicone rubber (Silastic) for the abdominal contents. This augments the abdominal wall temporarily in these severe cases and the intestinal contents are gradually returned to the abdominal cavity during the course of the first few days of life. There is a risk, however, that the edges of the Silastic pouch may tear away from the abdominal wall, or may become infected, and the use of Silastic can now often be avoided by manual stretching of the abdominal skin.

Other anaesthetic problems arise from severe fluid and electrolyte disturbances resulting from loss of fluid from the bowel surface and heat loss from the large exposed visceral surfaces.

Postoperative care

Although the mortality from gastroschisis remains fairly high, it has been reduced by advances in surgical and postoperative treatment. If the abdomen has been closed, mechanical ventilation is usually necessary for at least 48 hours because the abdomen becomes even more taut on the second postoperative day. The bowel wall has usually become thickened because of its exposure to amniotic fluid, and the onset of peristalsis is often delayed. Continuous intravenous feeding is often required for up to 6 weeks or so in this condition and this has significantly improved survival rates, although there is a risk that central feeding lines may become infected, leading to septicaemia, particularly from organisms such as Candida. Continuous nasogastric suction should be performed during this period, and electrolyte and acid-base status regularly checked.

Relatively few caes of exomphalos require postoperative respiratory support, and mortality in this condition is due to associated major cardiac or respiratory abnormalities.

Intestinal obstruction

Intestinal obstruction is one of the commonest surgical emergencies in the newborn, amounting to approximately 25 per cent of all neonatal emergency operations. Although the chemical composition of the neonate with congenital intestinal obstruction is normal at birth, delay in diagnosis will cause increasing fluid and electrolyte disturbances. In addition, increasing abdominal distension may lead to respiratory embarrassment and the risk of aspiration. Aspiration pneumonitis has been a common early cause of death, which may occur before other complications have time to arise. The passage of a gastric tube before transfer to a neonatal surgical unit is mandatory. Dehydration, shock and acidosis may complicate the picture, together with the possibility of intestinal perforation and septicaemia due to ischaemic necrosis of obstructed bowel. Finally, the high incidence of associated major congenital anomalies also increase the mortality and morbidity. The fact that a low overall mortality can be achieved in this group of patients (Table 4.2) is largely related to early diagnosis and treatment.

The possibility of intestinal obstruction should be borne in mind in cases

Table 4.2 Admissions to the neonatal surgical units, 1979–1983, The Hospital for Sick Children, London

Diagnosis	Number	Deaths
Abdominal surgery:		
General	893	61 (6.8%)
Exomphalos	69	15 (21.7%)
Gastroschisis	44	5 (11.4%)
Necrotizing enterocolitis	94	16 (17%)
Tracheo-oesophageal fistula/atresia	200	21 (10.5%)
Diaphragmatic hernia	168	45 (26.8%)
Miscellaneous	148	23 (15.5%)
Total	1616	186 (11.5%)
Meningomyelocele	101	— (0)

of toxaemia of pregnancy, polyhydramnios and premature labour, and where there is a family history of such diseases as mucoviscidosis or Hirschsprung's disease. The likelihood of obstruction—organic or functional—becomes very high when there is green-stained vomiting by the baby or failure to pass meconium for 24 hours.

Duodenal atresia

Duodenal obstruction may be due to complete atresia, stenosis, intraluminal diaphragm or annular pancreas. The reported incidence is between 1 in 6000 and 1 in 20 000 live births. The stomach and proximal duodenum dilate rapidly, giving rise to the classic 'double bubble' on erect x-ray (Fig. 4.8). Vomiting usually occurs early, and becomes copious and forceful. If the obstruction is below the ampulla of Vater, vomiting will become bile-stained, but many cases of duodenal atresia are supra-ampullary. Later, hypochloraemic alkalosis, weight loss and dehydration may occur. Gastric perforation has been reported.

Associated anomalies. About 70 per cent of cases have one or more associated congenital anomalies. One-third have Down's syndrome (mongolism), often itself associated with congenital heart disease; 15 per cent have cystic fibrosis. Other intestinal anomalies, such as malrotation, oesophageal atresia, imperforate anus and Meckel's diverticulum, are fairly common, as are renal anomalies. Fifty per cent of these neonates weigh less than 2.5 kg at birth, and 20 per cent less than 2 kg.

Anaesthetic problems. Since these neonates are generally operated upon within 3 days of birth, their general condition is usually quite good. They may, however, have evidence of pneumonitis or atelectasis from pulmonary aspiration. Gastric distension may be splinting the diaphragm and should be relieved with a nasogastric tube. The surgical procedure, usually duodeno-duodenostomy, requires full muscle relaxation but otherwise presents few problems to the anaesthetist. Blood loss is usually slight, and transfusion seldom required.

Late cases may present with dehydration, hypothermia, shock and severe metabolic and electrolyte disturbances.

Other atresias

With an incidence of between 1 in 1500 and 1 in 3000 live births, other atresias are usually jejunal or ileal, and occasionally colonic. Multiple atresias occur in about 10 per cent of cases. In some the intestine is arranged in a spiral around a central mesenteric vessel, and is known as 'apple peel' or 'maypole' atresia. These cases tend to have a familial incidence.

Whatever the cause, the proximal intestine dilates enormously and this may interfere with venous return from the bowel, causing bowel wall congestion or necrosis. Bile-stained vomiting occurs earlier with high

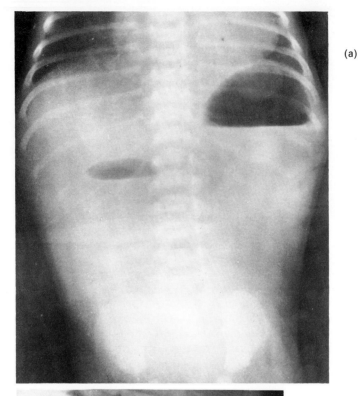

(a)

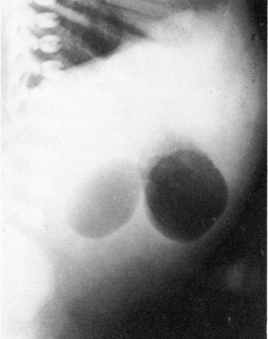

(b)

Fig. 4.8 Duodenal atresia. (a) Posteroanterior and (b) lateral erect x-rays showing the classic 'double bubble'.

lesions. Meconium peritonitis is present in approximately 30 per cent of cases, probably secondary to bowel infarction.

Associated anomalies.   These are mainly other intestinal abnormalities such as volvulus. Birth weights are often within the normal range.

Anaesthetic problems.   The main anaesthetic problems are respiratory embarrassment or aspiration from the gross distension that sometimes occurs, particularly with atresias low in the intestinal tract. The volume and complexity of the composition of fluid lost are also greater with low atresias. Intestinal losses should be replaced with physiological saline, although bicarbonate may also be needed to correct any metabolic acidosis. Increased capillary permeability causes loss of crystalloid and colloid from vessels in the bowel wall; if shock is present, colloid up to $20\,ml\cdot kg^{-1}$ should be infused rapidly. This is more likely to occur with low obstructions where the diagnosis may have been delayed and bowel infarction, meconium peritonitis or bacterial peritonitis may be present. Gaseous distension may be made worse by the use of nitrous oxide, and severe metabolic derangement may potentiate the action of the muscle relaxants.

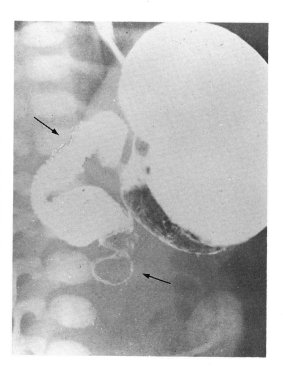

Fig. 4.9   Volvulus. Barium x-ray showing obstruction to the second part of the duodenum by Ladd's bands and the classic twisted ribbon sign.

Malrotations and volvulus

Considering how complicated the process of rotation of the intestine is in the normal fetus, it is perhaps not surprising that things may go wrong and the gut may take up a number of abnormal positions. The commonest one is for the duodenum to lie behind or to the right of the superior mesenteric artery with the caecum in front of it. Folds of peritoneum, known as Ladd's bands, attach the caecum to the posterior abdominal wall, in the right hypocondrium, and these tend to obstruct the second part of the duodenum (Fig. 4.9). Malrotations are, however, surprisingly rare.

If intestinal strangulation occurs due to volvulus, blood may be passed per rectum, and abdominal distension will ensue as with other causes of intestinal obstruction.

Associated anomalies.   Exomphalos and duodenal atresia are sometimes associated with malrotation, as is diaphragmatic hernia.

Anaesthetic problems.   The problems are either those of partial duodenal obstruction or of volvulus, where distension and fluid and electrolyte losses secondary to vomiting occur early. The situation may be complicated by pyrexia, bowel infarction or septicaemia. Surgery usually only involves division of Ladd's bands, derotation and fixation of the bowel, but occasionally resection of non-viable bowel and creation of a double-barrelled enterostomy is required. In the worst cases the amount of viable bowel left may be incompatible with life.

It has been claimed that the incidence of bowel necrosis can be reduced by the use of low molecular weight dextran. Similar claims have been made in animals for the use of hyperbaric oxygen, but these have not been substantiated in man.

Meconium ileus

Between 10 and 15 per cent of patients with cystic fibrosis (mucoviscidosis) present with meconium ileus, which has an incidence of about 1 in 20 000 live births. In this condition, the distal ileum is obstructed by inspissated meconium with a consistency similar to chewing gum. Atresias, volvulus, perforation, gangrene and meconium peritonitis are common complications.

A Gastrografin enema, containing the wetting agent polysorbate 80, may relieve obstruction in selected uncomplicated cases, but since complications are sometimes hard to detect surgery is usually preferred in all cases. At laparotomy, the distal ileum is often found to be distended, and surgery may involve resection of non-viable segments of bowel and the creation of an ileostomy. In addition, polysorbate 80 injected into the bowel lumen may enable some of the sticky meconium to be milked out of the cut end of the bowel, but too much handling of the bowel may make the situation worse.

Anaesthetic problems.   These are related to the degree of obstruction and the presence of the complications mentioned above. The use of atropine is controversial, as it may increase the viscid nature of tracheal secretions. In addition, the respiratory problems of cystic fibrosis mean that careful attention must be given to humidifying the respired gases, especially in the postoperative period.

Meconium perforation

Intestinal obstruction may occur in the neonatal period following an intrauterine bowel perforation, with leakage of meconium causing an intense peritoneal reaction. The bowel is usually bound in extremely dense adhesions and specks of calcification may be visible radiologically. The perforation usually occurs proximal to an obstruction (e.g. from volvulus).

Anaesthetic problems.   Intraoperative blood loss may be very heavy, equal to or even exceeding the entire blood volume in rare cases.

Milk plug obstruction

This rare cause of lower ileal obstruction is due to a mass of inspissated milk, and is seen only in babies reared on artificial feeds. The baby is normal at birth, passes normal meconium and stools, and then develops intestinal obstruction, possibly due to transient reduction in bile acid excretion.

Surgery is usually required, but seldom involves more than milking the obstruction through the ileocaecal valve into the caecum.

Meconium plugs

Meconium plugs are often associated with Hirschsprung's disease, and are usually removed by rectal washouts.

Duplication cysts

These are rare, but can occur anywhere from the tongue to the anus. Intrathoracic duplications may cause respiratory distress and mediastinal shift as they fill with secretions. Perforation or ulceration into the oesophagus or bronchus has been reported, but this seldom occurs in the neonatal period.

Abdominal duplications may mimic pyloric stenosis, become the starting points of an intussusception, cause intestinal obstruction by ribboning or by volvulus, perforate or bleed.

Hirschsprung's disease

This disease involves a functional obstruction due to lack of ganglia in the distal colon and rectum. The incidence is probably between 1 in 5000 and 1 in 10 000 live births, although varying figures have been reported.

In most cases vomiting, reluctance to feed and abdominal distension begin within 48 hours of birth. There is commonly failure to pass meconium, and erect x-ray shows multiple fluid levels typical of low intestinal obstruction (Fig. 4.10). Barium enema or anorectal manometry studies may

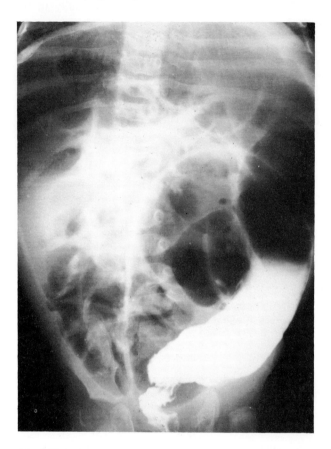

Fig. 4.10 Hirschsprung's disease. X-ray using radio-opaque medium to demonstrate the zone of transition at the sigmorectal level.

help in establishing the diagnosis, but rectal suction biopsy is required for confirmation.

Rectal washouts may temporarily relieve the obstruction, but colostomy is usually performed in the neonatal period, followed by a 'pull-through' operation 6–9 months later to bring the ganglionated bowel through the preserved sphincteric mechanisms to the perineum.

Anaesthetic problems. In the neonate there are usually few anaesthetic problems, although occasionally older children may present for surgery with gross abdominal distension and general debility. Neonatal problems are related to recurrent intestinal obstruction and the development of potentially fatal complications such as necrotizing enterocolitis.

Intussusception

Intussusception rarely occurs in the neonate, except in the presence of duplication cysts. Intrauterine intussusception has been reported as a cause of intestinal atresias.

Anorectal anomalies

These result from an embryological failure of differentiation of the cloaca and urogenital sinus. They are divided into 'high' anomalies (rectal agenesis) when the rectum ends above the levator muscle, and 'low' anomalies (covered anus) when it passes through the muscle to end close to the perineum. High anomalies, often accompanied by a rectourethral fistula are commoner than low anomalies in the male. In the female, high anomalies, often accompanied by a rectovaginal fistula, are rarer than low ones.

Associated anomalies.   Over 60 per cent of babies with anorectal anomalies, particularly high ones, have one or more associated anomalies. Genitourinary anomalies are most common, because of the closely integrated embryology of the two systems. Vertebral and skeletal anomalies and congenital heart defects are also common, as are alimentary tract anomalies, particularly oesophageal atresia and Hirschsprung's disease.

Anaesthetic problems.   Most of the anaesthetic problems are related to the associated anomalies. The surgical management of the covered anus is by the relatively simple procedure of anal 'cut-back' performed in the lithotomy position, whilst high rectal agenesis is usually treated by colostomy at birth followed by a definitive 'pull-through' procedure 6–9 months later.
    Caudal analgesia has been recommended for these procedures, using 0.25% bupivacaine without adrenaline (1 ml·kg^{-1}). Onset of analgesia takes 15–20 minutes, but is more rapid if 1% lignocaine is added to the bupivacaine.

Congenital pyloric stenosis

This is one of the commonest malformations of the digestive tract, its incidence having been estimated at between 1 in 300 and 1 in 400 live births. It is also one of the commonest of conditions in the first few weeks of life to be treated outside specialist neonatal surgical centres.
    Approximately 85 per cent of affected infants are male and between 40 and 60 per cent are firstborns. The pathological abnormality is a gross thickening of the circular muscle of the pylorus, which forms a hard tumour and causes an increasing degree of obstruction to the passage of food from the stomach. The presenting symptom is vomiting, which does not usually start before the 10th day but increases in severity and generally becomes

projectile. The infant loses weight and becomes dehydrated, and loss of chloride from the stomach may produce hypochloraemic alkalosis and even tetany. The physical signs which confirm the presence of pyloric stenosis are visible gastric peristalsis, especially after feeds (although this is an unreliable physical sign) and the presence of a palpable tumour usually felt just to the right of the umbilicus. The absence of a palpable tumour does not, however, exclude the diagnosis, and radiological examination can also be misleading. Whilst medical treatment has been advocated in this condition, it is now standard practice to recommend surgical correction by pyloromyotomy in virtually every case. This operation is not, however, an emergency procedure and must be preceded by complete correction of fluid and electrolyte abnormalities. Sodium, potassium and chloride ions are lost in the acid vomitus, and the renal response to this is twofold. First, bicarbonate is excreted (combined with sodium) in an attempt to restore the pH, and, secondly, potassium is excreted and sodium retained in order to minimize the reduction in extracellular fluid. The first of these renal responses tends to produce an alkaline urine, and the second an acid one.

The extent of the K^+ loss is not usually well reflected in serum levels. A compensatory respiratory acidosis is also seen with hypoventilation, possibly to the point of apnoea. Extremes of dehydration are rare nowadays, but would be seen with prolonged vomiting when pH falls with ketoacidosis and when a vicious circle develops with falling cardiac output, increasing acidosis and hypoxia.

No surgery should be undertaken until the chloride is at least $90\,\mathrm{mmol\cdot l^{-1}}$, the bicarbonate $24\,\mathrm{mmol\cdot l^{-1}}$ and the sodium $135\,\mathrm{mmol\cdot l^{-1}}$; 0.9% sodium chloride may be given and up to 400 ml may be necessary. (Giving 0.9% NaCl $2\,\mathrm{ml\cdot kg^{-1}}$ will raise the chloride by $1\,\mathrm{mmol\cdot l^{-1}}$.) Although surgery is not urgently required, correction of any degree of shock definitely is and a urine flow of $1-2\,\mathrm{ml\cdot kg^{-1}\cdot h^{-1}}$ should be established as soon as possible.

Most cases are diagnosed early nowadays, however, and little fluid or electrolyte replacement therapy is required.

Maintenance fluids should be $2\,\mathrm{ml\cdot kg^{-1}\cdot h^{-1}}$ of 4% dextrose in 0.18% saline. Mild cases do not need potassium supplements, but in others it should be given at a rate not exceeding $3\,\mathrm{mmol\cdot kg^{-1}\cdot 24\,h^{-1}}$. A large gastric residue is drained off and 4-hourly washouts of the stomach with physiological saline are carried out until the aspirate is clear and odourless (a secondary gastritis is often present).

Atropine premedication is given and the nasogastric tube aspirated before induction of anaesthesia. The tube will be left in place because it does not reduce the effectiveness of cricoid pressure and will act as a 'blow-off' valve if the intragastric pressure should rise.

The patients are usually too old and too lusty for awake intubation so consideration must be paid to a possible risk of regurgitation of stomach contents and their subsequent aspiration during the induction of anaesthesia. This is unlikely if the nasogastric tube is left open after aspiration.

Induction of anaesthesia is by an inhalation or an intravenous method. Cricoid pressure is as effective in babies as it is in adults and may be applied

after suxamethonium has been given for relaxation. Intermittent suxamethonium (increments of 5 mg) has been described as the relaxant of choice
for the operation of pyloromyotomy, but equally good condtions can be
obtained using a non-deplorizing relaxant.

The surgical procedure involves delivering the pylorus, splitting the
muscle and then closing the abdomen. It is important that the child does
not cough or strain at the time of muscle splitting, as the surgeon is attempt-
ing to cut down to but not through the mucosa. Postoperative morbidity
increases if the mucosal layer is incised. The baby should be extubated
awake in the lateral position.

Postoperative care

Oral feeding with clear fluids can usually be started 4–6 hours after the
operation, but an intravenous infusion of 4% dextrose in 0.18% saline
($3 \, ml \cdot kg^{-1} \cdot h^{-1}$) should be maintained for the first 12–24 hours until a
normal oral intake has been re-established.

Biliary atresia

Biliary atresia may be extrahepatic or, more commonly, intrahepatic, and
other major anomalies such as congenital heart disease may be associated.
The differential diagnosis is with neonatal hepatitis. Surgical exploration of
the bile ducts and intraoperative cholangiography are usually required to
confirm the exact nature of the anomaly and to assess the feasibility of
surgical correction by some form of anastomosis between the porta hepatis
or biliary passages and the intestinal tract—the Kasai operation. The operation is most likely to be successful if it is performed early, before the liver
is too damaged. The postoperative course may be complicated by ascending
cholangitis.

Anaesthetic management

Because of reduced hepatic function these babies may have coagulation
abnormalities, and haematological studies should be carried out before
surgery. It is probably wise to administer vitamin K_1 intramuscularly prior
to surgery, as hypoprothrombinaemia is common. The operation may be
prolonged, so maintenance of normothermia is important; also, blood loss
may be heavy, so a reliable intravenous line must be inserted and adequate
supplies of blood must be available for transfusion, if required. Hepatorenal
failure does not seem to be a problem in infancy, so the administration of
mannitol is probably unnecessary. Halothane is not contraindicated in anaesthesia for biliary atresia.

Inguinal hernia

Inguinal hernias may present towards the end of the neonatal period;
because these may become incarcerated, repair should not be delayed. The

hernia is usually the result of a patent processus vaginalis and repair is by simple herniotomy. Most hernias can be reduced easily at this age and it is unusual for the patient to develop significant intestinal obstruction, provided diagnosis and treatment are carried out without delay. Inguinal hernia is especially common in low birth weight babies and is found in up to 15 per cent of such patients.

Anaesthetic management

If strangulation has occurred the baby may be shocked and dehydrated with loss of water and electrolytes by vomiting. Such babies must be treated by nasogastric suction and intravenous therapy before surgery. The main problem arising at operation is that traction on the peritoneum is extremely stimulating to the child and may cause laryngeal spasm if tracheal intubation has not been performed. For this reason intubation is recommended, but the procedure can be conducted using spontaneous or controlled ventilation. The child should be allowed to wake up before extubation is performed. For babies of less than 5 kg a relaxant technique using atracurium or vecuronium is very satisfactory.

Postoperative care

If the child's general condition is satisfactory, a graduated feeding regimen can be started as soon as he is fully awake, as for pyloric stenosis.

Postoperative analgesia is seldom required at this age but intramuscular codeine phosphate in a single dose of $1 \, mg \cdot kg^{-1}$ can be safely used. Patients below 44 weeks postconception should not be treated on a day-stay basis as there is significant risk of apnoeic problems postoperatively.

Necrotizing enterocolitis

Necrotizing enterocolitis (NEC) is the commonest acquired lesion of the gastrointestinal tract in the neonatal intensive care unit, affecting up to 8 per cent of such patients, although the incidence is up to 12 per cent of preterm babies. The disease affects the terminal ileum and ascending colon, although in severe cases the entire bowel may be involved. NEC is characterized by abdominal tenderness and distension with ileus, blood in the stools and, in 85 per cent of cases, a typical x-ray appearance of gas within the bowel wall (Fig. 4.11). This 'pneumatosis intestinalis' is often preceded by thickening of the bowel wall with oedema. The portal venous system within the liver may be outlined by gas. Stages I–III of the disease are described, ranging from non-specific symptoms with mild gastrointestinal upset and increasing ileus to an advanced stage with cardiorespiratory collapse, peritonitis and septicaemia, usually with gut perforation. The onset commonly is between the 3rd and 10th day of life but may occur even before enteral feeding has started.

There has been a considerable increase in the incidence of necrotizing enterocolitis in recent years. It is now thought that ischaemic damage to

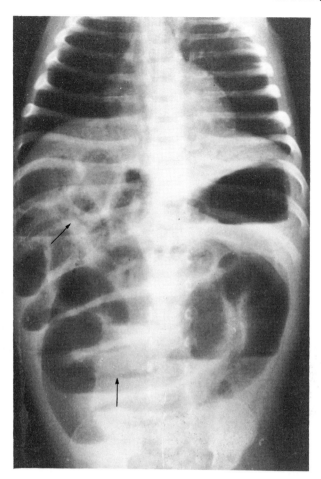

Fig. 4.11   Necrotizing enterocolitis. Erect x-ray showing distended loops of bowel, with fluid levels, intramural gas and gas in the portal venous system.

the bowel related to peri- or postnatal asphyxia and the diversion of blood flow from the gut to other more vital organs actually plays little or no role in the pathogenesis of NEC in man, although in experimental animals such haemodynamic changes can result in necrosis in the gut causing perforations and peritonitis. The condition is probably caused by the opportunist infection of the bowel wall by Gram-negative gut organisms after defence mechanisms have broken down. NEC may occur in epidemics, and strict isolation of cases is mandatory. Organisms such as *Clostridium perfringens* or *C. difficile*, *E. coli* or Klebsiella are implicated. The disease may start with direct bacterial invasion, helped by malabsorption, mucosal injury and an abnormal environment for the gut microflora. Local mucosal injury, for example from hyperosmolar feeds in the presence of milk formula feed rather than breast milk, and a relative immune deficiency as in the preterm, allows the disease to progress. A further risk factor for NEC is polycythaemia after birth, and 60 per cent of cases have had umbilical artery or venous catheterization.

Mortality is related to low birth weight, the onset of septicaemia and the incidence of disseminated intravascular coagulation (DIC), and may be as high as 40 per cent in some series.

After diagnosis, the babies must start a regimen of intravenous fluids and nasogastric suction. Any umbilical catheters should be removed. Penicillin, gentamicin and metronidazole should be given intravenously; the cardiovascular system must be closely monitored and if the peripheral circulation is poor, blood or plasma should be transfused. Respiratory failure, hypoxia and apnoea are indications for respiratory support, and this is especially likely postoperatively.

At any stage, surgical intervention may be necessary if it is possible that perforation has occurred as suggested by fluid or free gas in the abdominal x-ray. After the acute stage is over, fibrotic healing causing bowel strictures may occur, again bringing the patient to the operating theatre.

Urogenital abnormalities

Renal agenesis may occur, for example as part of Potter's syndrome, characterized by oligohydramnois, pulmonary hypoplasia, talipes and characteristic facies. The commonest lesions causing urinary tract obstruction in the newborn are pelvic hydronephrosis and posterior urethral valves.

Hydronephrosis

The cause of hydronephrosis is not fully understood but occurs by obstruction at the pelvi-ureteric junction; considerable damage to the renal parenchyma may result, to a degree proportional to the length of time of obstruction. The condition is commonly diagnosed by prenatal ultrasound and some centres have undertaken surgery to the fetus. However, an isotope scan often shows good renal function and not all patients with hydronephrosis have an obstructed ureter so that fewer than half require surgery early in life. There seems to be no difference in the results between patients operated on before birth and those whose surgery is delayed until after birth—especially as some may need no urgent surgery at all. The commonest presenting postnatal symptoms are a palpable abdominal mass and non-specific symptoms such as failure to thrive associated with urinary tract infections. Investigations include ultrasound and isotope scan procedures, and surgery consists of pyeloureteroplasty or bilateral nephrostomies if drainage is urgent. The babies occasionally have severe electrolyte and fluid disturbances which need to be corrected preoperatively.

Urethral valves

Posterior urethral valves which cause obstruction in the neonate usually present because of uraemia, acidaemia and the toxic effects of severe urinary infection. The diagnosis should be suspected when there is vomiting and failure to thrive as these are common presenting symptoms; in a severe case, cardiorespiratory collapse may occur following a vicious circle of vomiting, dehydration, reduced renal function, acidosis and, eventually, a fall in cardiac output. Abnormalities of micturition may go unnoticed.

The valves, which may be thick and rigid, tend to pass downwards and laterally, extending around the lumen of the urethra, and fuse together at a lower level. Catheterization and instrumentation are easily carried out, but the valve cusps obstruct the flow of urine. The obstruction to urine flow can have a very severe effect on the developing urinary tract, often before birth. The long-term prognosis must depend on the degree of renal damage; in one older series, 22 of 54 boys presenting within 3 months of age died. Now, no patients die in the early stages, but many develop chronic renal failure with the growth spurt of adolescence and eventually only 20 per cent have completely normal kidneys. The amount of irreversible kidney damage cannot be assessed from the initial degree of uraemia, which is caused also by dehydration, obstruction to urine flow and infection in a very sick baby.

Initial treatment must include fluids intravenously for dehydration, sodium bicarbonate to correct acidosis, antibiotics and urinary catheterization. Surgery is indicated only when metabolic correction has taken place. Definitive diagnosis requires radiography (retrograde cystogram). The great majority of urethral valves may be destroyed by fulguration throughout their length, using a cystoscope. When the instrument cannot be passed through a small anterior urethra, a urethrostomy in the perineum is created to enable the cystoscope to enter the posterior urethra.

Anaesthesia should follow the basic principles for neonatal patients; if adequate medical treatment has been carried out initially, then no additional problems should ensue. After relief of the obstruction, a large fluid intake may be required, depending on the urine output and its osmolality. Up to 1 litre of fluid may be required over the first 12 hours postoperatively in severe cases. Potassium supplements are often necessary for these cases, although serum electrolyte values are unhelpful as a guide for intravenous doses of potassium.

Prune belly syndrome

The prune belly syndrome (Fig. 4.12), which involves defective muscularization of the anterior abdominal wall and the urinary tract, is only seen in its full extent in males. The full syndrome is a complex with several developmental errors. The severity of the muscular defect varies and may involve one or both sides of the abdominal wall. The skin over the abdomen is classically wrinkled like a prune, although it may merely have abnormal transverse creases. The costal margin is flared and the sternum is usually prominent. The upper parts of the recti and the oblique muscles of the abdomen are usually present.

Abnormalities of the gastrointestinal tract may include volvulus and intestinal obstruction, but changes in the genitourinary system are commonly

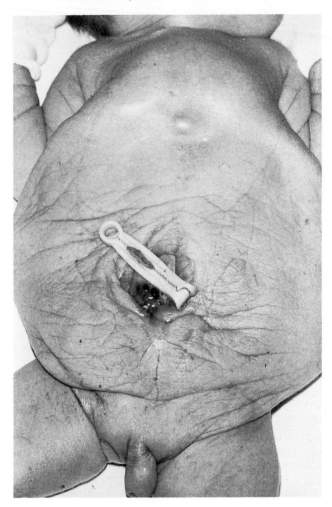

Fig. 4.12   The prune belly syndrome.

seen and their severity is proportional to the deficiency of the abdominal musculature. The bladder is large and the urachus patent as far as the umbilicus. The ureters are dilated and the pelvices of the kidneys may be similarly affected; the degree of dysfunction depends on the back-pressure effect of the urine and subsequent urinary tract infection. The testes are always undescended.

These babies may have renal failure, acidosis and dehydration and may also be septicaemic. Because of the absent abdominal musculature, they may have reduced pulmonary function, with an inability to cough and clear the chest of secretions.

Surgery is designed to restore function of the urinary tract, to improve emptying of the bladder and to preserve or improve renal function.

The anaesthetist must take into account the possibility that renal function may be impaired, so care must be taken with those drugs known to be excreted in the urine. There is usually a history of repeated chest infections, and any infection of the chest or urinary tract should be vigorously treated preoperatively. The babies should be managed during induction as if the stomach were full, because of the danger of regurgitation of gastric contents. The neonate is intubated awake, and controlled ventilation may be maintained *without* the use of relaxants because the abdomen is very lax anyway. Postoperatively, hypoventilation and a reduced coughing mechanism may cause sputum retention and respiratory failure. Extubation takes place only when the baby is fully awake and moving vigorously. The condition is associated with perioperative morbidity and mortality, usually from respiratory causes such as secretion retention and hypoxia.

Bladder exstrophy

This serious congenital malformation affects approximately 1 in 20 000 babies; three times as many males as females. The mucosa of the bladder is laid open and the ureteric orifices are visible. The size of the exstrophy varies and sometimes the surface area of the mucosa is the same as that of a normal bladder. There is complete epispadias. As the mucosa of the bladder continues to be exposed, it becomes hyperaemic, friable and infected. Hydroureteronephrosis may develop because of oedema and, later, fibrosis which affect the ureteric orifices, causing obstruction to urine outflow.

Definitive surgical treatment is usually undertaken in the neonate before infection and secondary ureteric problems arise and while the bladder is still thin walled and flexible. The open bladder exstrophy, if left, may predispose to carcinoma. The results of closure do not necessarily indicate that full continence and a normal upper urinary tract can be expected.

The operation involves major surgery, starting with the patient prone for bilateral osteotomies of the iliac bones, after which the baby is positioned supine for formal mobilization and closure of the bladder. The pelvic osteotomies enable the pubes to be apposed and closure of the urethra to be attempted. Heavy blood loss may be expected and two good intravenous lines should be established, one of which could be central in the internal jugular vein. Hypotensive anaesthesia, so useful for this operation in older children, is rarely necessary in the neonate. Full monitoring should include oesophageal stethoscope and blood pressure cuff. Care should be taken to prevent heat loss during the long operation, particularly at the stage of turning from the prone to supine positions. The tracheal tube and intravenous lines should be very well secured to prevent accidental dislodgement during turning of the baby. While the baby is prone, pads under the pelvis and chest prevent pressure on the inferior vena cava which would increase bleeding and also decrease cardiac output.

Caudal analgesia may be used as an adjunct to anaesthesia for bladder exstrophy.

Anaesthesia for neuroradiology and neurosurgery

The principles of anaesthesia for neuroradiological investigation and neuro-surgery in neonates do not differ greatly from those in adults. All patients need very careful neurological assessment preoperatively.

Cerebral blood flow

Cerebral blood flow is normally regulated automatically to match cerebral metabolism. Decreased oxygenation of arterial blood results in an increased rate of blood flow to the brain so that tissue oxygen tension is maintained at near-normal levels. This autoregulation operates throughout a wide range of systemic blood pressure (60–180 mmHg in the adult) and even as low as 45–50 mmHg in the newborn infant. Regulation of cerebral blood flow in the preterm baby is less precise and may not function after a period of hypoxia (p. 23). Cerebral blood flow increases with increasing $Paco_2$ between 2.7 and 10.7 kPa (20 and 80 mmHg): hypocapnia tends to modify the effects of agents which increase cerebral blood flow. Damaged areas of brain, such as occur with trauma, infarction or in the region of arterio-venous malformations and tumours, lose their autoregulation so the circulation in these areas varies passively with blood pressure. If the $Paco_2$ rises and normal cerebral vessels dilate, blood is diverted from abnormal to healthy areas (intracerebral steal syndrome). The inverse intracerebral steal syndrome is seen when normally reactive cerebral vessels constrict.

The total volume of the intracranial contents cannot alter within the rigid skull of the adult, although compensatory decreases (or increases) may take place within the three constituents: brain, blood and cerebrospinal fluid (CSF). A slowly expanding space-occupying lesion will displace CSF and venous blood, so intracranial pressure (ICP) rises very slowly until no more compensation is possible. Any small increase in volume above this will cause a very large increase in ICP with severe symptoms. A neonatal skull has a capacity to expand not seen with the rigid adult skull, and increasing head circumference is the main sign of hydrocephalus, preceding symptoms of raised ICP (vomiting, irritability, seizures or severe lethargy).

All inhalation anaesthetic agents increase cerebral blood flow, as does ketamine, although intravenous induction agents, barbiturates and drugs which depress neuronal activity tend to decrease it. Halothane, like all inhalation anaesthetic agents, increases cerebral blood flow and thus intra-cranial pressure. The effect is minimal if low doses of halothane are used, and is not seen if hyperventilation is employed. This makes halothane combined with mild hyperventilation a very useful technique for neonatal neurosurgical anaesthesia. Recent work in adults suggests that isoflurane may be better because intracranial pressure is easier to control and is now being used in neonatal anaesthesia.

Anaesthesia for neuroradiology

General anaesthesia is invariably required for major neuroradiological investigations because of the need for immobility and the prolonged discomfort involved.

In addition to the problems of anaesthetizing a neonate, there are those associated with working in the x-ray department. The commonest problems are a lack of facilities for keeping the baby warm (although this can be overcome with warm coverings and a draught-free environment), lack of easy access to the patient and, often, poor lighting. There is the possibility of static electricity or electrical sparks, so cyclopropane should be avoided and, because of the risk from radiation, protective aprons must be worn by the staff. Far fewer invasive investigations have been necessary since the advent of bedside ultrasound investigations and computerized axial tomography (CT) scanning.

CT scan

Neonates may not need anaesthesia for CT scanning as restraint with a blanket will immobilize the infant for a head scan. A fit child may be sedated with chloral hydrate $30\,mg \cdot kg^{-1}$ orally 1 hour beforehand. For high-speed body and head scans, periods of apnoea with anaesthesia may be required; occasionally, intubation is also necessary for airway security in patients who are having fits or who are comatose or in respiratory failure. Contrast CT scans to show configuration of the ventricles are commonly performed using iohexol which has very few side-effects, unlike metrizamide which is epileptogenic. Investigations using nuclear magnetic resonance may also require total immobility and no metallic objects must be in the field. A relaxant technique using one of the shorter-acting drugs such as vecuronium or atracurium is ideal, and intubation should be with a PVC tube which is not markedly radio-opaque.

Lumbar air encephalography

Because of the advent of the new generation of CT scanners, lumbar air encephalography is very rarely required nowadays for children. It may still be necessary for lesions in the posterior fossa, or for confirmation of the site of obstruction to the flow of CSF if this is not obvious from the CT scan.

As for all neuroradiological and neurosurgical anaesthesia, only atropine is given for premedication. Increased steroid cover is necessary if the patient has been given dexamethasone for treatment of any intracranial problem. The patient is intubated awake using a non-kinking type of tube such as the Magill flexometallic tube, introduced with a rigid stilette. This tube must be very firmly fixed because the radiological examination requires tilting and somersaulting of the patient, during which accidental extubation may occur.

A relaxant technique with controlled ventilation is necessary for the neonate or for any patient with suspected raised intracranial pressure. The investigation takes at least 1 hour. The limbs are wrapped in foil and as much of the baby as possible is swaddled in warm coverings. The oesophageal stethoscope, ECG and blood pressure cuff should be used to monitor the patient's condition.

Respiratory signs of rising ICP will be lost with controlled ventilation so, as air is injected, careful monitoring of cardiovascular signs, such as rising pulse and blood pressure, is necessary. It is possible that an acute rise in ICP may cause coning of the brain stem, with respiratory and cardiovascular signs; the pulse rate will slow and a spontaneously breathing patient will become apnoeic. Immediate steps must be taken to relieve the ICP, and osmotic diuretics such as mannitol $2\,g\cdot kg^{-1}$ and an urgent ventricular tap may be necessary.

The anaesthetic T-piece is an ideal circuit for use in the x-ray department, as a long lead for fresh gas flow and a long expiratory limb do not alter the function of the circuit but may help the anaesthetist during the moving of the patient.

After reversal of any neuromuscular block, the patient is extubated when fully awake and returned as soon as possible to the recovery area where postoperative neurological assessment can begin.

Myelography

Myelography is performed for investigation of spinal cord injuries at birth, for cord compressions and for dysraphic lesions of the cord.

Diastematomyelia is a fissure or cleft of the spinal cord in the lumbar region, caused by transfixion of the neural tissue by a bony septum. This prevents normal ascent of the cord in the vertebral canal as the child grows and, because the cord is tethered in the lumbar region, there will be progressive neurological damage. Cutaneous haemangiomata, a lipoma or a tuft of hair may overlie the site of the spinal defect.

During the x-ray examination there is a need for many changes in position of the patient, including marked flexion of the head, and a flexible reinforced tracheal tube is therefore recommended. If the investigation includes the cervical spine, a radiolucent tube must be used; a plain Portex tube is suitable.

Premedication is with atropine, and awake intubation is carried out after preoxygenation. Intubation difficulties are occasionally encountered, as lesions of the cervical spine which need investigation may be associated with conditions such as the Klippel–Feil syndrome (p. 255).

Cisternal air myelograms are rarely performed nowadays and there are several reports in the literature of air embolism occurring during this procedure. Metrizamide, the radio-opaque contrast medium used for myelography, causes seizures if it is allowed to track up into the head. The contrast medium is given only during screening and about 5 ml is used for a neonate. The threshold for seizures is markedly reduced if the patient receives phenothiazines, so these should be avoided.

Vital signs should be monitored using an oesophageal stethoscope, ECG and blood pressure cuff. The most satisfactory anaesthetic technique involves a relaxant, controlled ventilation with oxygen, nitrous oxide and incremental halothane (0.25-0.5%). Hypotension may occur during tilting of the patient.

Great care should be taken to prevent contrast medium from draining into the head, so a head-up posture is necessary postoperatively. It is perhaps wisest to give phenobarbitone $2\,mg \cdot kg^{-1}$ i.m. after the investigation, as a precaution against seizures.

Angiography

Carotid angiograms are performed for suspected vascular malformations and arteriovenous malformations and tumours (rare in the neonatal period). Arteriovenous malformations may present with cardiac failure, and a bruit over the head will be audible. Fits will need to be controlled with specific agents such as phenobarbitone, diazepam or phenytoin.

Premedication is with atropine, and awake intubation is carried out after preoxygenation. Ventilation, which needs to be controlled for neonatal anaesthesia, is also an advantage for cerebral arteriography. A flexible reinforced tracheal tube is used. If the patient is ventilated to a Pa_{CO_2} of $4\,kPa$ (30 mmHg), normal vessels are constricted, which improves the definition of abnormal vessels. The dose of contrast medium must not exceed $4\,ml \cdot kg^{-1}$ body weight. Allergic reactions to contrast medium are relatively common and cause death in 1 in 40 000 cases. The contrast is hypertonic and causes a biphasic problem for the circulation: initial volume overload, followed by dehydration after an osmotic diuresis. Contrast media may also interfere with the clotting mechanism in which platelets are consumed. It is possible for a body to lose 10 per cent of the circulating blood volume during a carotid angiogram, and fluid overload is possible as the result of excessive flushing of the artery with saline. Digital angiography with subtraction may need prolonged apnoea during the exposure.

Some arteriovenous malformations such as aneurysm of the vein of Galen may be controlled by an embolization procedure. Emboli of small pieces of lyophylized dura or Silastic beads are flushed into the feeding artery if this can be localized. The procedure is more likely to be prolonged than an investigation, so extra care must be taken with heat maintenance and monitoring of vital signs.

Anaesthesia for neurosurgery

Neurosurgery in the neonatal period usually involves operations for developmental anomalies in the spine and cranium, for hydrocephalus or for extradural and subdural haematomas. Most operations for tumours, craniosynostosis or vascular lesions tend not to fall into this age group.

Myelomeningocele

Myelomeningocele occurs in 1-4 infants per 1000 live births, although encephalocele is much less common (1 in 5000). The measurement of α-fetoprotein (AFP) concentrations in the amniotic fluid has made possible the antenatal recognition of severe open neural tube anomalies and possible termination of the pregnancy. The maternal serum AFP may also be elevated in pregnancy when the fetus has an open neural tube anomaly (see p. 43).

After 1952, when it became possible to relieve hydrocephalus by shunt operations, a period of aggressive surgery for myelomeningocele followed in which closure of the back lesion was one of the most common emergency neonatal operations. Because of the very large numbers of badly deformed children who survived as a result of this policy, many centres now try to restrict surgical treatment at birth to those babies whose handicap later in life will be minimal. Back closure is carried out in these babies within 24–36 hours of life because to delay increases the chances of wound infection and meningitis. Some untreated babies survive, however, and in these back closure must be considered at some stage on humanitarian grounds.

Of babies with myelomeningocele or encephalocele, 80 per cent develop hydrocephalus with the Arnold–Chiari malformation (downward displacement of the pons and medulla and protrusion of the cerebellar vermis through the foramen magnum) and aqueduct stenosis. Occasionally, patients with the Arnold–Chiari malformation develop stridor as hydrocephalus progresses. This is possibly caused by traction on the vagus nerve in the posterior cranial fossa. Usually the stridor disappears after insertion of a shunt or following occipital craniectomy.

Occipital encephalocele is very commonly associated with other abnormalities such as Klippel–Feil syndrome (webbing of the neck and cervical vertebral synostosis), micrognathia and cleft palate. Such patients may be very difficult to intubate. If the neural damage is very extensive and possibly involving autonomic functions in the midbrain, surgery is usually withheld.

Surgery involves excision of the sac and preservation of the neural elements, then closure of the defect with fascial flaps and skin coverage. In the past, a very large defect needed a rotation flap of skin for cover.

Preoperatively the lesion is covered with sterile gauze, blood is crossmatched, and atropine and vitamin K (1 mg) are given as premedication. Awake intubation is performed using a plain or flexometallic tracheal tube with the patient on his side to minimize damage to the myelomeningocele or encephalocele. An assistant presses the shoulders back and supports the head in an optimum position for laryngoscopy. An alternative is to support the baby's back on a 'head ring' to protect the lesion from pressure while the baby is intubated in the usual supine position.

For surgery, the infant is positioned prone, usually with pads supporting the chest and pelvis so that the abdomen remains free from external pressure and inferior vena caval obstruction is avoided. Any venous obstruction will greatly increase bleeding from the wound. When the patient is in the prone position, care must be taken to protect the eyes—which should be taped shut after chloramphenicol eye ointment has been inserted. In certain conditions such as gross hydrocephalus or hypertelorism, the eyes may be very difficult to close and tarsorrhaphy is occasionally necessary.

Anaesthesia is usually maintained with oxygen, nitrous oxide and halo-thane up to 0.5% with controlled ventilation. Controlled ventilation is espe-cially necessary for neonates operated on in the prone position with pressure on the chest. Relaxants may be used if the surgeon does not need to use a nerve stimulator to confirm the position of nerve roots. The vital signs are monitored using an oesophageal stethoscope, ECG, blood pressure cuff and rectal temperature probe.

Maintenance of body temperature, which is so important in paediatric anaesthesia, is very difficult indeed in neurosurgery. Surgeons should be discouraged from using cold, wet drapes. The limbs and trunk must be wrapped in foil and as much contact as possible obtained between the baby and the heating pad. It is possible to put the support pads beneath the heating pad rather than between it and the baby. With most cases of occipital encephalocele some temperature fall during surgery is inevitable.

A further difficulty is encountered over the measurement of blood loss, as this is mixed with unknown quantities of CSF and saline used for irri-gation. The need for transfusion is assessed not only by estimation of blood loss but also by changes in the patient's vital signs, including the state of the peripheral circulation, pulse rate and blood pressure. As a rule, blood is needed for encephalocele but not for myelomeningocele. In infants the suboccipital bone is very vascular. Surgery for occipital encephalocele in-volves a risk of air embolism because the suboccipital bones are exposed. Careful monitoring with an oesophageal stethoscope and ECG should give warning of this potentially disastrous complication. The surgeons may also be in a position to warn the anaesthetist. Venous distension, to discourage the passage of the air into the heart, is then possible by applying pressure to the reservoir bag of the anaesthetic T-piece. Early warning of air embol-ism using a capnometer is now feasible in the newborn, using a neonatal cuvette (Hewlett-Packard).

For spinal surgery in cases of diastematomyelia the general anaesthesia principles described for excision of myelomeningocele also apply. Blood loss may be expected to exceed 10 per cent of the blood volume and this must be replaced. Careful positioning of the chest and pelvis on pads will minimize venous bleeding from the edges of vertebrae.

Occasionally lesions of the skin or subcutaneous tissues are haemangiom-atous, so an increased blood loss is to be expected. If the lesion is greater than 4 cm in diameter, the need for transfusion is inevitable.

Hydrocephalus

A large proportion of neurosurgery in the neonate is carried out for hydro-cephalus. The abnormal accumulation of CSF within the head is usually obstructive due to blockage of the fluid pathway. Communicating hydro-cephalus with an open CSF pathway into the subarachnoid space may occur after meningitis. Non-communicating hydrocephalus is due to ob-struction of the fluid pathway proximal to the subarachnoid space, such as aqueduct stenosis, or Arnold–Chiari syndrome.

Hydrocephalus is very commonly associated with myelomeningocele. The combined defect is present in 3 per 1000 live births. The excess CSF causes rapid dilatation of the ventricles, destroying the brain and producing enlargement of the cranium. The earliest sign is one of increasing head circumference, which is routinely measured in all babies following operation for myelomeningocele. Bulging fontanelle, the 'setting sun' sign of the eyes and increased spasticity of the limbs are all later signs. Papilloedema is rare because of the capacity for the infant skull to enlarge. About 10 per cent of these children will grow up to be very retarded, both physically and mentally.

Surgical treatment involves the use of a low-pressure valve draining CSF from the ventricle to the right atrium, to the pleural cavity or to the peritoneum for cases of non-communicating hydrocephalus. For communicating hydrocephalus a shunt is inserted from the lumbar subarachnoid space to the peritoneum. If the CSF is infected, surgery must be delayed because the valve will become colonized.

The most important neonatal sign of raised intracranial pressure is the tendency to apnoeic attacks: patients may need to be intubated, ventilated and a ventricular tap performed. Cardiovascular signs such as bradycardia are also indicative of raised ICP.

Preterm babies frequently develop hydrocephalus following intraventricular cerebral haemorrhage in the early days of life. Because the CSF protein is high a ventriculoperitoneal shunt may not work well, frequently becoming blocked. These small babies are better managed with intermittent tapping of the ventricle or insertion of a percutaneous Teflon cannula until the CSF protein, and thus the viscosity, is back to normal. Many of these patients are a poor risk, having residual respiratory problems such as apnoeic attacks or residual oxygen dependency and reduced lung compliance from bronchopulmonary dysplasia.

Premedication is with atropine and, after preoxygenation, awake intubation is performed with a flexible tube. Difficulties with intubation associated with a very large head may be avoided if the patient's trunk is placed on a pillow so that the head is in neutral position. Controlled ventilation is established, preferably using a relaxant/nitrous oxide/oxygen technique and the baby is monitored with oesophageal stethoscope, ECG and blood pressure cuff. Because of the relatively very large head with its disproportionate radiating surface, temperature maintenance may be difficult.

Cardiovascular instability may occur at any time and is related to changes in ICP, especially hypotension at the time of CSF tap if the ICP and systemic blood pressure were previously raised. It is necessary to ventilate the patient with 100% oxygen at this stage. The shunt most commonly used nowadays is the ventriculoperitoneal shunt. If ventriculoatrial shunts are employed, they are usually inserted under x-ray control so that the distal catheter is seen to lie in the right atrium. The ECG may also be used as a guide to positioning the atrial end of the shunt. The shunt tubing is filled with hypertonic saline and attached to the left arm ECG lead. As the tip approaches the right atrium the P-waves grow taller, and when in the correct position the P-waves become small again and biphasic. At the moment that the internal jugular vein is opened for insertion of the catheter, positive pressure on the reservoir bag of the T-piece will raise the venous pressure and prevent air embolism. Many neurosurgeons infiltrate the surgical field with lignocaine 0.5%. The maximum dose of $3\,mg\cdot kg^{-1}$ should not be exceeded.

The patient should be wide awake before extubation and be returned to the intensive care unit for neurological assessment postoperatively. Although blood is always cross-matched for this operation, it is very rarely used. Phenobarbitone $1\,mg\cdot kg^{-1}$ i.m. 6-hourly and codeine phosphate $1\,mg\cdot kg^{-1}$ i.m. 6-hourly are prescribed for sedation postoperatively, but this should very rarely be needed in the neonatal period.

Other conditions

Other neurosurgical conditions which may require surgery in the neonate include intracranial haematomas and craniosynostosis (premature fusion of the cranial sutures, leading to deformities and mental retardation). Massive blood loss may be a feature of these operations, although anaesthesia follows the general pattern of that for neurosurgery in the neonate. Blood loss may be particularly large with craniectomy for craniosynostosis, and direct measurement of arterial pressure is useful so that the systolic blood pressure can be reduced to the range $50\text{-}60\,mmHg$ using an increased halothane concentration and controlled ventilation. Induced hypotension with trimetaphan or sodium nitroprusside is not necessary in the neonate. After craniectomy, babies may lose at least 10 per cent of the blood volume into a drain or into the head bandages.

Surgery in the sitting position is very rare indeed in the neonatal period, although it is widely used for posterior fossa exploration and cervical surgery in the older child. However, the neonatal anaesthetist must be aware of the dangers of air embolism in any neurosurgical procedure where the head may be higher than the trunk.

Congenital lobar emphysema

Although rare, this condition may present as a cause of serious respiratory distress in the newborn period. The emphysematous lobe, which is commonly the left upper, right upper or right middle lobe, compresses the normal lung tissue and may displace the mediastinum (Fig. 4.13).

The aetiology was unknown in over half the cases reported in the literature. The condition can be caused by extrinsic bronchial obstruction from lymph nodes or abnormal vessels as in the absent pulmonary valve syndrome, or intrinsic obstruction associated with bronchial stenosis or cartilaginous deficiency. It can present from birth to 6 months or so of age, and the differential diagnosis includes congenital lung cyst, pneumothorax, diaphragmatic hernia and bronchial obstruction with compensatory emphysema as with inhaled foreign body. The presence of bronchial and vascular markings should help to differentiate the first two of these conditions from lobar emphysema.

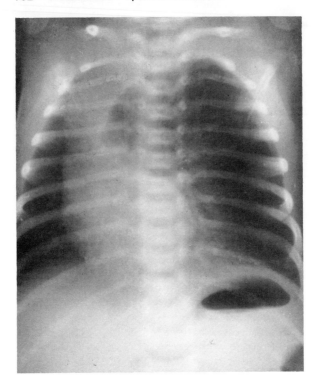

Fig. 4.13   Congenital lobar emphysema. X-ray showing mediastinal displacement to the right.

Associated anomalies

The condition is frequently associated with congenital heart disease, particularly ventricular septal defect or patent ductus arteriosus. The relationship to absent pulmonary valve syndrome has been mentioned above.

Anaesthetic management

These children may present either for bronchoscopy or for lobectomy, although bronchoscopy is not usually indicated and is dangerous in the presence of intrapleural tension problems. The only safe way of performing bronchoscopy is with spontaneous ventilation, and the bronchoscope should be passed under fairly deep anaesthesia, usually with halothane. The laryngeal inlet and upper trachea can be sprayed with lignocaine to a maximum dose of $4\,mg{\cdot}kg^{-1}$. If the surgeon decides to proceed to lobectomy, the bronchoscope should be removed and a tracheal tube inserted.

The air in the emphysematous lobe may be under tension, and the presence of nitrous oxide can increase its volume significantly.

Care should be taken with controlled ventilation because of the risk of making the emphysematous lobe even more distended or producing pneumothorax; only gentle ventilation is applied. However, once the chest is opened it is essential that controlled ventilation be performed, and this is best carried out with full muscle relaxation. Cullum, English and Branthwaite (1973) have described a technique for bronchial intubation in this condition but this is not usually required. It may be necessary to leave the tracheal tube in place postoperatively, but if it is to be removed, this should not be done until the patient is fully awake.

Postoperative care

The infant should be nursed in an oxygen-enriched environment using a head box, and a postoperative chest x-ray should be taken to confirm adequate expansion of the remaining areas of lung.

Since this condition is sometimes associated with generalized chondromalacia of the bronchial walls, it is not unusual for further lobes to become emphysematous fairly soon after the operation. New alveoli continue to develop until about 7 years of age, so the long-term outlook in terms of respiratory function may not be as poor as it at first appears.

Anaesthesia for cardiac surgery

The incidence of major congenital heart disease is estimated at 6–8 per 1000 live births. Without treatment, approximately 50 per cent of these children will die in the first year of life, one-third of the deaths occurring in the first 3 months of life. Neonates with congenital heart disease may present as emergencies because of the effects of the cardiac anomaly itself, because of the effects of prematurity or because of the presence of other major congenital abnormalities. Of the coincident defects, renal abnormalities are the most common, although cleft palate, tracheo-oesophageal fistula, abdominal malformations and other defects also occur.

Ventricular septal defect is the commonest congenital cardiac anomaly, with an incidence of 2 per 1000 live births, although at least three-quarters of these defects will close spontaneously. Patent ductus arteriosus, pulmonary stenosis and atrial septal defect have incidences of 0.5–0.7 per 1000 live births. Transposition of the great arteries, although the commonest cardiac anomaly to cause cyanosis in the newborn, is an even rarer lesion, having

Table 4.3 Open heart operations in infancy, 1971–1984, The Hospital for Sick Children, London

Age (months)	Number	Deaths
0–1	144	68 (47%)
1–6	366	87 (24%)
6–12	269	40 (15%)
Total	779	195 (25%)

a similar incidence to aortic stenosis, coarctation of the aorta and Fallot's tetralogy (0.3 per 1000 live births). Total anomalous pulmonary venous drainage, although having an incidence of only 0.1 per 1000 live births, is an extremely serious lesion in the newborn, often requiring emergency surgery because of severe hypoxia and congestive cardiac failure.

Although open heart operations in the first month of life are still associated with a higher overall mortality than in older infants (Table 4.3) and children, two points must be borne in mind. First, these operations are carried out on sick babies who would all certainly die without treatment. Secondly, many of the babies have complex, multiple lesions. If these are excluded, the mortality of the remainder is seen to be considerably lower (Table 4.4).

Table 4.4   Neonatal open heart operations, 1971–1984, The Hospital for Sick Children, London

	Number	Deaths
Simple lesions (VSD, PS, TGA)	56	18 (32%)
Complex lesions (TAPVD, truncus arteriosus, pulmonary atresia, complex AS, VSD, TGA, etc.)	88	50 (57%)
Total	144	68 (47%)

AS, aortic stenosis; PS, pulmonary stenosis; TAPVD, total anomalous pulmonary venous drainage; TGA, transposition of the great arteries; VSD, ventricular septal defect.

Preoperative management

Severe congenital cardiac anomalies in the newborn can be classified into three main categories.

1. Those which cause cardiac failure: ventricular septal defect, patent ductus arteriosus, aortic stenosis, coarctation of the aorta.
2. Those which cause cyanosis: pulmonary atresia, Fallot's tetralogy (rarely cyanosed in the neonatal period), tricuspid atresia and single ventricle with pulmonary stenosis.
3. Those which cause failure and cyanosis: transposition of the great arteries, truncus arteriosus, total anomalous pulmonary venous drainage.

Babies in cardiac failure usually develop severe hypoxaemia and acidosis, often complicated by hypoglycaemia or hypocalcaemia. Immediate assessment should include measurement of blood sugar, calcium and electrolyte levels, and arterial blood gas and acid–base analysis. Dextrose 50% should be given intravenously: $(0.2\,ml\cdot kg^{-1})$ if the blood sugar falls below $2\,mmol\cdot l^{-1}$ in a full-term neonate or $1.5\,mmol\cdot l^{-1}$ in a premature neonate. If the serum calcium is less than $2.0\,mmol\cdot l^{-1}$, intravenous 20% calcium gluconate should be given $(1\,ml\cdot kg^{-1})$. ECG and body temperature should be monitored, and the baby nursed in a suitably warm environment.

Neonates who are sick enough to require urgent surgery usually also require full intensive therapy on admission, with monitoring of direct arterial and central venous pressure. They require ventilatory support if they are in respiratory failure, inotropic support if cardiac output is low, diuretics if overhydrated and intravenous fluids if dry. Intensive support for several days may be beneficial before cardiopulmonary bypass, and could include total parenteral nutrition to improve myocardial glycogen stores.

Diagnostic procedures

Detailed investigations are required to make the diagnosis in most neonates with suspected congenital heart disease. Two-dimensional echocardiography can, together with the clinical x-ray and ECG findings, be all that is required to manage the patient in many cases, including coarctation, aortic stenosis, patent ductus arteriosus and total anomalous pulmonary venous drainage. In other cases echocardiography helps enormously in planning the catheterization. These procedures are usually carried out without general anaesthesia, and sedation is often unnecessary in the newborn baby. After the first few days of life, a sedative intramuscular injection of pethidine compound up to $0.05\,\text{ml·kg}^{-1}$ body weight is usually given half an hour prior to catheterization (1 ml pethidine compound contains 25 mg pethidine, 6.25 mg promethazine, 6.25 mg chlorpromazine). This is half the dose used in older infants. Should any additional sedation be required during the investigation, diazepam $0.1\,\text{mg·kg}^{-1}$ may be injected through the cardiac catheter. If general anaesthesia is considered essential, tracheal intubation should be performed and a nitrous oxide/oxygen mixture administered using full muscle relaxation and controlled ventilation of the lungs. It is essential to monitor inspired oxygen concentration, as it is impossible to calculate shunts if the oxygen saturation of the venous blood is too high.

The newborn baby, if premature, is especially susceptible to heat loss, and steps should be taken to prevent hypothermia. The temperature of the room should not be less than 24°C, the baby should be swathed in warm clothing and, if possible, be placed on a radiolucent heating pad. Wrapping the head and limbs in aluminium foil also helps to reduce heat loss.

In small infants, excessive amounts of blood can be removed during diagnostic sampling unless oximetry is carried out in a sterilized cuvette from which the sample can be returned to the patient. The blood volume in the neonate is approximately $85\,\text{ml·kg}^{-1}$ body weight, and loss of more than 10 per cent of this usually requires replacement. Blood should be cross-matched at the start of the procedure.

Other hazards of cardiac catheterization are rare. They include dysrhythmias from manipulation of the catheter, hypotension and occasional perforation of the heart or intramyocardial injection of contrast. Systemic hypotension may lead to increase in any right-to-left shunting and to intense hypoxia. Hypoxaemia itself may increase pulmonary vascular resistance and thus create a vicious circle of events.

The injection of contrast medium may lead to transient flushing of the skin from histamine release, and more importantly may cause an increase in pulmonary vascular resistance with fall in cardiac output, especially in patients with pulmonary hypertension. The new non-ionic contrast medium causes less of these problems; 10–$20\,ml\cdot kg^{-1}$ of isotonic fluid is given into the catheter to help offset the diuretic effect of the contrast medium.

Mortality associated with cardiac catheterization in the first month of life is probably around 5 per cent but it is difficult to separate the hazards of the investigation from those of the cardiac lesion itself.

Open heart procedures

General principles

Open heart surgery in infancy has developed greatly in the last 20 years, with falling mortality (Fig. 4.14). This is due to advances in equipment and techniques as well as to improved preoperative diagnosis. Better oxygenators are now available, of both the bubble and the membrane type, with 'priming volume' reduced to 750–1000 ml. Improved intracardiac cannulae

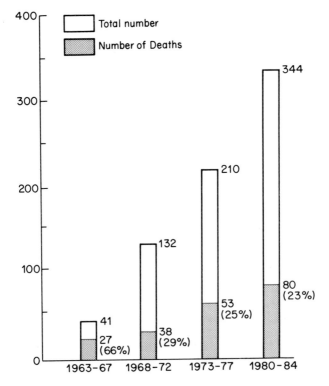

Fig. 4.14 Open heart surgery in the first year of life at The Hospital for Sick Children, London, for 5-year periods between 1963 and 1984.

and suckers cause less red cell damage, and the use of blood filters has reduced platelet–fibrin aggregation with its risk of embolization. The technique of surface cooling to 26–28°C prior to sternotomy is still used in the newborn and in older sick infants, although indications for its use vary between centres. The technique produces more even cooling, particularly of the peripheral muscle bed.

The use of profound hypothermia by blood stream cooling on bypass to temperatures of 18–20°C allows the surgeon to carry out the intracardiac repair on a bloodless motionless heart during periods of up to 60 minutes' circulatory arrest and reduces the time on bypass. Some surgeons start bypass with very cold perfusate, disregarding the conventionally accepted maximum temperature gradients between patient and perfusate (15°C). The use of this rapid cooling technique is thought to improve myocardial protection.

Perfusion technique in neonates

Until recently, fresh heparinized blood was chosen to prime the bypass for neonatal surgery because of the risk of coagulation disorders following the use of stored blood and because of the metabolic alkalosis which follows the transfusion of citrated blood. Fresh blood may be difficult to obtain, especially in an emergency, but the freshest stored blood obtainable should be used. Blood which is more than 4 days old should not be accepted unless undue delay in obtaining fresher blood threatens the patient's life.

Haemodilution should not lower the haematocrit below 30 per cent because the newborn neonate has difficulty in excreting a large fluid load. Haemodilution does, however, improve the flow characteristics of the perfusate, especially at low temperatures, and improves postperfusion urine flow; 20 mg heparin, 3 ml of 20% calcium chloride and 80 mmol sodium bicarbonate are added to each unit of blood used in the prime. Mannitol $(0.5\,g{\cdot}kg^{-1})$ may be added to improve urine output, and methylprednisolone sodium succinate (Solu–Medrone) $(30\,mg{\cdot}kg^{-1})$ to stabilize membranes. Some also add albumin to increase the oncotic pressure of the prime. Bypass flow rate is calculated at $2.4\,l{\cdot}m^{-2}{\cdot}min^{-1}$, although lower flows are often used during hypothermia.

Technique of surface cooling

The commonest method of producing surface cooling involves the use of icebags placed around the child's body, either with or without a hypothermia blanket. A specially designed hypothermia chamber has, however, been described for neonatal use.

In the commonly used technique small ice-filled plastic bags are packed around and under the body (Fig. 4.15). Care should be taken to avoid placing icebags directly over the precordium because of the risk of ventricular fibrillation, or on the extremities of limbs or in the area of the kidneys as this may reduce renal blood flow. The bags should be moved occasionally to prevent thermal damage to the skin from the ice.

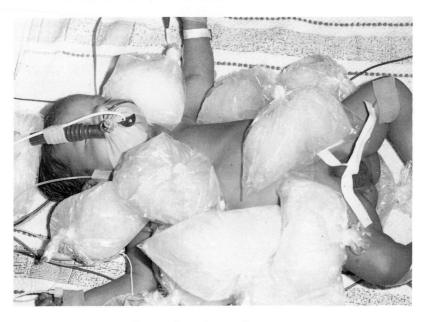

Fig. 4.15   The position of icebags for surface cooling.

While cooling is taking place, the ECG and the nasopharyngeal and oesophageal temperatures should be monitored, and arterial and central venous lines, if not already in place, should be inserted. Blood pressure should be monitored indirectly, for example with a Doppler flowmeter, until direct arterial pressure monitoring is established. Shivering and vaso-constriction should be prevented by full muscle relaxation together possibly with the addition of small doses of chlorpromazine ($0.5\,mg\cdot kg^{-1}$). As the metabolic rate slows with falling temperature, carbon dioxide production decreases, so 2.5-5% carbon dioxide should be added to the inspired gas mixture once the nasopharyngeal temperature reaches 34°C. This improves cerebral perfusion and helps prevent intense vasoconstriction. Blood gases and serum potassium should be checked regularly during cooling. Supple-ments of potassium are frequently required at this stage, as potassium may move into the cells. Arterial carbon dioxide tension (corrected for the low temperature of the blood sample) should be kept above 6 kPa (45 mmHg) and serum potassium should not be allowed to fall below $3\,mmol\cdot l^{-1}$.

Active cooling is discontinued once the nasopharyngeal temperature has reached 26-28°C. Icebags are removed, the infant is carefully dried and surgery commenced. Any sudden movements of the baby's position at this stage can cause ventricular fibrillation. Temperature usually drifts down 2°C further.

Anaesthetic management

Premedication

Neonates are given atropine ($0.02 \, \text{mg} \cdot \text{kg}^{-1}$), either alone or with pethidine compound, in reduced dosage ($0.05 \, \text{ml} \cdot \text{kg}^{-1}$) 1 hour preoperatively.

Before bypass

ECG, precordial heart beat and blood pressure should be monitored before induction of anaesthesia. The sickest babies and those in the first week or two of life may be intubated awake without difficulty, and some may already have required intubation before reaching the operating theatre. In older neonates, especially if vigorous, it may be wiser to intubate under light general anaesthesia and muscle relaxation. Halothane is potentially dangerous at this stage because of the risk of hypotension and is best avoided. It is particularly dangerous in infants with left ventricular outflow tract obstruction, where hypotension and ventricular fibrillation occur very readily and where the nitrous oxide/oxygen/muscle relaxant technique is safer. A tracheal tube of 2.5 or 3.0 mm internal diameter is passed, and either the oral or the nasal route can be used. The former is usually easier and quicker, and less likely to cause hypoxia, but a nasal tube can be secured more satisfactorily for postoperative care. It is important to make sure there is air entry to both lungs after intubation, as it is quite easy to intubate either main bronchus because of the relatively short trachea.

Arterial, central venous and peripheral venous lines can usually be inserted percutaneously. It is wise to establish a venous line as soon as possible so that resuscitative drugs can be given if required. The arterial line is preferably inserted into a radial artery and the central venous line into the internal jugular or subclavian vein by the techniques described on p. 114 et seq. In the presence of a left superior vena cava it is wise to cannulate a left-sided central vein, as pressure measurements from the right side will not warn of significant changes on the left side unless there is a good intercommunicating vein.

Major complications of cannulation of the radial artery are rare in children—provided a fine (24 s.w.g. for neonates) cannula is used—possibly because the arterial wall is healthier or because there is a better collateral blood supply. Internal jugular and subclavian vein cannulation are not free from hazard, particularly from puncture of the carotid artery with haematoma formation or from pneumothorax. The advantages are generally felt to outweigh the risks involved, which may be minimized if the tip of the needle is kept well above the thoracic inlet. It is seldom possible to advance a percutaneous cannula centrally from the antecubital fossa in infants. If venous or arterial cannulation fails, it may be necessary to cut down onto a limb vessel. Oesophageal and nasopharyngeal or rectal temperatures should also be monitored, the former reflecting blood temperature and the latter core temperature. Intermittent positive pressure ventilation (IPPV) is continued with nitrous oxide/oxygen as the basic anaesthetic, and pancuronium $0.1-0.15\,mg\cdot kg^{-1}$ for muscle relaxation. Inspired oxygen concentration should be adjusted according to the arterial oxygen tension, and inspired gas should be warmed and humidified. Narcotic supplements such as morphine (up to $0.5\,mg\cdot kg^{-1}$ after test dose) or fentanyl (up to $10\,\mu g\cdot kg^{-1}$) may be used if the cardiovascular system is stable. A supply of emergency drugs should be immediately available, including 8.4% sodium bicarbonate and 20% calcium chloride. A urinary catheter is inserted and urine output recorded regularly. Heparin $3\,mg\cdot kg^{-1}$ is given prior to insertion of the aortic cannula, and it is wise to check the level of heparinization by ensuring that the activated coagulation time (ACT) is greater than 350 seconds. Additional muscle relaxant should be given at least 10 minutes before commencement of bypass to allow time for it to be fixed at the neuromuscular end-plate, and an incremental dose of narcotic may be required at this stage.

During bypass

It is not necessary to ventilate the lungs during bypass, and opinions vary as to what gas mixture they should contain at this time. Some fill them with inert gas such as helium, but many leave them gently distended with oxygen or air at about $5\,cmH_2O$. Heparinization should be checked every 30 minutes using the ACT, but since relatively large amounts of heparin are added to the perfusate during priming, incremental doses of heparin are seldom required.

Myocardial function is preserved during bypass by the use of ice-cold cardioplegic solution injected into the aortic root and hence to the coronary arteries during aortic cross-clamping. The composition of the cardioplegic solution varies from centre to centre, but the common constituents are potassium, magnesium and procaine. The solution is infused until the myocardial temperature has dropped to 10°C. Because the aorta is clamped and the solution is aspirated to waste via the coronary sinus, little of it enters the perfusate. Cardioplegic infusion is repeated from time to time (usually every 30 minutes) to ensure that the myocardial temperature remains below 20°C and that the heart does not commence beating.

Perfusion pressure during bypass is usually kept at 50–70 mmHg. If it rises above this, it may be necessary to infuse sodium nitroprusside. The rate of this infusion must be carefully controlled, especially during periods of reduced bypass flow, in order to avoid the risk of cyanide toxicity.

Potassium levels should be checked during perfusion, and the addition of $1\,mmol\cdot kg^{-1}$ to the prime is recommended by some.

Rewarming is commenced as the intracardiac repair is completed, and this should be performed gradually, with a gradient of not more than 10°C between the temperature of the water in the heat exchanger and the blood. The skin is also rewarmed using a heating blanket, such as described on p. 96. The use of vasodilator such as sodium nitroprusside at this stage significantly improves the evenness of rewarming. Oesophageal temperature rises faster than nasopharyngeal temperature, and bypass should not be discontinued until the latter has reached 37°C and there is good peripheral circulation. Blood gases and serum potassium level should be checked immediately before coming off bypass, and left atrial (or right atrial after right heart surgery) pressure should be raised to a satisfactory level. This is usually around 10 mmHg for patients with transposition of the great arteries (TGA) but may be as high as 15 mmHg in neonates with total anomalous pulmonary venous drainage. The left atrial pressure line, if required, can be inserted by the surgeon before bypass is discontinued.

The postperfusion period

It is wise to ventilate the lungs with 100% oxygen until the haemodynamic state is stable and a satisfactory arterial oxygen tension has been obtained, after which a nitrous oxide/oxygen mixture can be recommenced. Colloidal fluid should be infused to keep the left atrial pressure at a satisfactory level. If the haematocrit is below 40 per cent, whole blood is given which should be filtered and warmed. If the haematocrit is above 40 per cent, freshly thawed plasma is preferable. If urine output is below $1 \, ml \cdot kg^{-1}$, either mannitol ($0.5 \, g \cdot kg^{-1}$) or frusemide ($1 \, mg \cdot kg^{-1}$) may be required. Potassium supplements are needed less frequently than for adults. Should blood pressure be low despite adequate filling pressure, it may be necessary to commence inotropic support with dopamine, isoprenaline or, occasionally, adrenaline. Dopamine $5-10 \, \mu g \cdot kg^{-1} \cdot min^{-1}$ is the drug of first choice, although isoprenaline may be added if the cardiac rate is below 100. These pressor agents should be administered by syringe pump or a similar controlled infusion device. If $3 \, mg \cdot kg^{-1}$ is mixed with 50 ml of 5% dextrose in a syringe, the dial setting of the pump in $ml \cdot h^{-1}$ will equal the rate in $\mu g \cdot kg^{-1} \cdot min^{-1}$.

If severe hypotension occurs or if cerebral oedema is anticipated, methylprednisolone sodium succinate may be given in a dose of $30 \, mg \cdot kg^{-1}$.

Heparin reversal is achieved in the usual way with protamine. The conventional dose of heparin ($3 \, mg \cdot kg^{-1}$) results in a blood level in the patient before bypass of $35-40 \, mg \cdot l^{-1}$. The heparin level in the bypass prime may be considerably higher than this, and since priming volume usually exceeds blood volume in the neonate the heparin level will rise towards the prime level after bypass has begun. This factor must be taken into account when calculating the reversal dose of protamine, which may be considerably greater in relation to heparin administered than for older children. Adequacy of reversal can be confirmed by the ACT.

Closed heart procedures

The main closed heart operations performed in the neonatal period are left-to-right shunts, closure of patent ductus arteriosus (PDA) and resection of coarctation of the aorta. The Blalock–Hanlon procedure to increase interatrial mixing of blood has largely been replaced by the balloon atrial septostomy, but is still performed occasionally in some complex congenital heart disease. Shunt operations are still required in a number of neonates.

The increasing use of open heart surgery has made banding of the pulmonary artery to reduce pulmonary blood flow a rarely performed operation (p. 174).

Pulmonary systemic shunts

The Blalock–Taussig (subclavian to pulmonary artery) shunt is performed on the opposite side to the aortic arch. Occasionally the shunt is established using synthetic material (Gortex). The less common Waterston (ascending aorta to pulmonary artery) shunt is carried out through a right thoracotomy. Although these shunts are seldom required for tetralogy of Fallot in the neonatal period, they may be used in conditions such as pulmonary atresia with intact ventricular septum. Oral prostaglandins are sometimes used preoperatively to stimulate growth of the pulmonary arteries.

Cyanosis and polycythaemia are common preoperatively. Hypoxia may be temporarily increased during surgery because of partial occlusion of the pulmonary artery. It is wise to ventilate with 100% oxygen during this period. Blood loss should be replaced with plasma because of the high haematocrit. Intra-arterial blood pressure monitoring is usually required for shunts in the neonatal period. Blood pressure should be measured on the arm opposite to the operative side if a Blalock–Taussig shunt is to be performed, as the pulse will be lost on the operative side. Systemic blood pressure should not be allowed to fall below 80 mmHg because of the risk that the shunt may clot. Heparin ($1 \, mg \cdot kg^{-1}$) will be required when synthetic material such as Gortex is used.

Postoperative pulmonary oedema may develop if the shunt is too large. This is more common after a Waterston shunt. Other shunts such as Potts and Glenn shunts are virtually never used nowadays.

Closure of patent ductus arteriosus (PDA)

In approximately 20 per cent of cases a PDA causes persistent chest infection and cardiac failure due to significant left-to-right shunting. These are high-risk cases despite preoperative digoxin, diuretics and antibiotics, and many are already ventilated. The operation is performed through a left thoracotomy and no particular problems should be encountered apart from those of the sick neonate in general. Postoperative respiratory failure is common, however, and IPPV may be required for some days. Fluid therapy should be restricted.

The presence of a patent ductus arteriosus may be life-saving in neonates who have a severe obstructive lesion in the pulmonary circulation, as in pulmonary stenosis or atresia. Perfusion of the lungs in these cases depends on blood passing from right to left via an atrial or ventricular septal defect, and then via the ductus arteriosus to the pulmonary artery. Closure of the ductus will cause severe hypoxaemia and precipitate the need for surgical intervention. It is possible to keep the ductus open with an intravenous infusion of prostaglandin E_1 in this situation, but this should be done only as a temporary measure while preparations are being made for urgent shunt operation. Occasionally the ductus arteriosus provides the main communication between the pulmonary and systemic circulations in transpositions in the great arteries, but oxygenation is achieved more satisfactorily in this condition by mixing pulmonary and systemic blood at atrial level. Balloon atrial septostomy should be performed as soon as possible in all cases of TGA. In coarctation of the aorta the ductus may be carrying much of the blood supply to the lower part of the body. In total anomalous pulmonary venous drainage, the presence of a patent ductus may act as a vent for the congested pulmonary vascular bed. In both these cases, however, urgent surgical correction of the cardiac anomaly is required.

Ligation of the PDA is sometimes required in premature babies with severe hyaline membrane disease. Pulmonary vascular resistance may fall from its initial high level, causing left-to-right shunting through the duct and cardiac failure. If the duct is not ligated at this stage, it may be difficult to wean the baby from controlled to spontaneous ventilation and eventually pulmonary vascular disease and bronchopulmonary dysplasia will develop.

Coarctation of the aorta

The infantile type of coarctation is commonly preductal, with much of the blood supply to the lower part of the body coming through the patent ductus. Cyanosis is common, due to the high incidence of pulmonary oedema in this condition, and in the worst cases there may be associated hypoplasia of the aortic arch or left ventricle. Other anomalies, such as PDA or ventricular septal defect (VSD), may be present. Respiratory and cardiac failure may ensue, with hypoxia and acidosis. Preoperative prostaglandin infusions and dialysis are occasionally used to preserve renal function.

Halothane should be avoided as it is very poorly tolerated. The operation is performed through a left thoracotomy, and controlled ventilation with pancuronium is the technique of choice, with 50% nitrous oxide/50% oxygen if tolerated, although even this sometimes causes hypotension, when the use of oxygen and fentanyl should be considered. As the operation usually performed is subclavian angioplasty, the arterial line must be in the right arm.

Intra-arterial pressure monitoring is mandatory, and resuscitation drugs should be immediately available. Acidosis should be corrected before the clamps are applied, and 10–20 ml of blood should be given before they are removed, as even minor degrees of hypovolaemia may cause hypotension. It may be necessary for the surgeons to reclamp the aorta several times before the clamp is finally removed. Postoperative respiratory support for at least 48 hours is essential.

Blalock-Hanlon procedure

This operation was designed to improve interatrial mixing of blood in TGA by the creation of an atrial septal defect. In neonates it is now performed only in cases of complicated TGA. The common method is to expose the right pulmonary artery and veins via a right thoracotomy, and place a clamp on the right and left atrial wall near the interatrial groove so as to include part of the septum in the clamp. The atrium is opened and a portion of septum excised. The clamp is then partially opened, allowing the septum to slip out of it, then quickly reapplied. The snares previously applied to the pulmonary vessels are then released and the atrial incision is closed. Alternatively, the operation can be performed after inflow occlusion. Whichever technique is used, it is wise to ventilate the lungs with 100% oxygen for 3 minutes before the clamps are applied, and during closure of the atrium. Major blood loss may occur, and myocardial stimulant drugs should be available. Intra-arterial blood pressure monitoring is mandatory and blood gas and acid-base state should be checked immediately before and after the period of clamping. Controlled ventilation may be required for several days after this procedure.

Pulmonary artery banding

This procedure, which reduces pulmonary blood flow in patients with left-to-right shunts, is nowadays seldom performed in uncomplicated VSD because the risks of total correction have been reduced to a low level. It is, however, used in complex lesions which are not suitable for early correction, such as a univentricular heart with high pulmonary blood flow, multiple VSD and occasionally VSD with coarctation.

The pulmonary artery is usually approached through a left thoractomy, although it may be reached from the right. A thick ligature is passed round the artery, and when this is tightened the systemic arterial pressure rises and the distal pulmonary artery pressure falls. If the band is applied too tightly, oxygen tension will fall dramatically because of inadequate pulmonary blood flow, so intra-arterial pressure monitoring and sampling facilities are mandatory.

Controlled ventilation may be required for several days after this procedure because of the severe disruption of haemodynamics which occurs.

Postoperative care

There is a high incidence of postoperative respiratory failure following open heart surgery in the newborn. All neonates are ventilated via a nasotracheal tube for a few hours following open heart surgery, and usually at least until the following morning. The techniques of intubation and ventilation are described elsewhere in this book (p. 209 et seq.).

Controlled ventilation may also be required after closed heart surgery, particularly banding of the pulmonary artery, creation of shunts or the Blalock-Hanlon procedure where respiratory support may be needed for several days. During transfer from the operating theatre to the intensive therapy unit the baby should be ventilated with oxygen, and it is wise to monitor precordial heart beat, blood pressure and ECG. Portable battery-operated machines are now available. Chest drains should be clamped for the shortest possible time, to minimize the risk of tamponade.

In the intensive therapy unit arterial pressure, right atrial pressure (and sometimes left atrial pressure), heart rate, core and peripheral temperatures should all be monitored continuously after open heart surgery. Urine output and osmolality should be recorded and blood balance should be charted every 15 minutes. Blood gas and electrolyte measurements should be performed and coagulation status checked. A chest x-ray should be taken as soon as possible to ensure full lung expansion and to check the position of the tracheal tube in relation to the carina. Blood volume should be maintained according to left atrial pressure and the haematocrit kept between 30 and 40 per cent. Tracheal suction following the injection of a small volume of saline down the tracheal tube should be performed every 15 minutes. Careful attention must be paid to the humidification of the inspired gas.

Infants may be sedated with morphine ($0.2\,mg\cdot kg^{-1}$ 2- to 3-hourly), fentanyl infusion ($4\,\mu g\cdot kg^{-1}\cdot h^{-1}$) or diazepam ($0.2\,mg\cdot kg^{-1}$ i.v. 2- to 3-hourly) as long as controlled ventilation is being used, but care must be taken with sedation during weaning to spontaneous ventilation. The place of positive end-expiratory pressure (PEEP), intermittent mandatory ventilation (IMV) and continuous positive airway pressure (CPAP) is discussed on p. 222.

Pulmonary hypertensive crisis

A reactive pulmonary vasculature is a feature of neonatal physiology, but it is seen particularly after correction of VSD, TAPVD, TGA with VSD and truncus arteriosus, in the first few weeks of life. A greater reactivity of the precapillary arteriolar region is caused by a persistent fetal type of muscularity of the arterioles or an actual increase in the amount of smooth muscle in the media of these vessels. If an increase in pulmonary vascular resistance occurs and fetal channels have been closed surgically so that right-to-left shunting cannot take place, then a low cardiac output state ensues. The systemic pressure falls as both ventricles fail together in infants, the peripheral temperature falls and the patient becomes hypoxic. At this stage the condition becomes self-reinforcing because hypoxia causes further pulmonary vasoconstriction.

The pulmonary hypertensive crisis—which is likely to be fatal—can only be suspected unless the pulmonary artery or right ventricular pressure is monitored, when the cause of the problem may be identified. This is now routine for this type of patient: a catheter is placed in the right atrium using a Seldinger technique via the right internal jugular vein and the catheter is then threaded into the pulmonary artery by the surgeon after the surgical correction but before cardiopulmonary bypass is discontinued.

Prophylaxis is better than treatment for a pulmonary hypertensive crisis, so the patients are paralysed, sedated and ventilated postoperatively for 12-24 hours with high Pa_{O_2} and avoiding catecholamines such as adrenaline which have alpha-predominant activity. If the pulmonary artery pressure does rise, a crisis may be averted by immediate hand ventilation with 100% oxygen and an increase in the sedation (e.g. a bolus of fentanyl 5-10 μg·kg^{-1} i.v.). A fully established rise in pulmonary artery pressure with a low cardiac output may be treated with tolazoline in the same

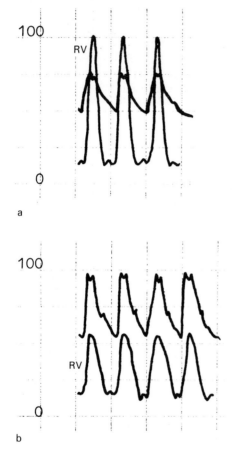

Fig. 4.16 (a) Pulmonary hypertensive crisis with right ventricular pressure (RV) greater than systemic. (b) After tolazoline: normal right ventricular pressure.

way as transitional circulation is treated, by a bolus of 1-2 mg·kg^{-1} followed by an infusion of 1-2 mg·kg^{-1}·h^{-1}. The tolazoline is weaned slowly after cardiovascular stability has been achieved for 24 hours. Paralysis and mechanical ventilation are withdrawn after a further 12-24 hours (Fig. 4.16).

Anaesthesia and respiratory obstruction

The anatomical differences between the upper airway of the neonate and that of the adult are described on p. 16. The fact that neonates are obligatory nose breathers makes them particularly susceptible to respiratory distress should blockage of the nasal airway occur. This is probably more important for caucasian babies than for negroes, in whom nasal resistance is lower. A nasogastric tube may also cause respiratory difficulty, particularly if too large or if placed in the larger nostril.

The neonatal trachea is a relatively soft structure, and dynamic compression can easily occur. Extrathoracic obstruction tends to cause inspiratory stridor, whilst intrathoracic obstruction favours dynamic compression with stridor mainly during expiration. 'Fixed' lesions of the airway such as tracheal stenosis, where little change in diameter can occur with respiration, may produce a picture of combined inspiratory and expiratory stridor.

Immediate assessment of severity

Upper airway obstruction, if severe and prolonged, may cause serious hypoxia, which can easily be fatal, or may lead to cerebral ischaemia and resultant mental retardation. The fact that a high proportion of infants with Pierre Robin syndrome are found later to have mental retardation may be due to hypoxia subsequent to severe and prolonged episodes of airway obstruction. The immediate assessment of the severity of the obstruction must be based on a rapid and thorough appraisal of the clinical signs and recent history. The amount of stridor is not on its own the most significant feature because stridor diminishes as the infant tires, so the moribund child may be almost silent.

Increase in respiratory frequency is a reliable sign of respiratory failure, rates over 60 per minute giving cause for concern. Any baby able to take a feed without undue distress is unlikely to require urgent treatment although other signs may show that immediate action is necessary to relieve the obstruction. These signs may include severe intercostal and subcostal recession, paradoxical movement of the chest and abdomen, with abdominal protrusion on inspiration, tracheal tug, sweating, cyanosis, peripheral hypoperfusion, head retraction and general restlessness. Because the compliance of the rib cage is high, intercostal recession is particularly marked. Arterial blood gases tend initially to be well maintained although hypercarbia, hypoxia and metabolic acidosis develop in sequence, as respiratory failure ensues. It is important to remember that the higher alveolar ventilation of the infant—two to three times that of the adult—results in lower ranges of carbon dioxide content in arterial blood and that levels above 5.3 kPa (40 mmHg) are abnormally elevated for an infant. However, such levels are initially well tolerated, and an elevated Pa_{CO_2} is not necessarily an indication for active intervention.

Cardiovascular deterioration occurs early in severe respiratory obstruction, with initial tachycardia, pallor or cyanosis progressing to bradycardia and cardiac arrest. Cardiac arrest is particularly likely to result in brain damage if it has been preceded by a period of severe hypoxaemia, which is usually the case in respiratory obstruction.

Clinical examination usually gives a clue to the site and possible cause of obstruction. There may be an obvious external abnormality such as malformation of the nares, micrognathia, cleft palate or swelling around the neck and face.

Causes of respiratory obstruction

The main causes of respiratory obstruction in the neonate are shown in Table 4.5. In many of these there is some underlying pathology—congenital or acquired—to which an acute or subacute obstructive episode may be added. In addition, however, obstructive apnoea may occur during sleep in the absence of apparent underlying disease, particularly in preterm infants.

Although obstructive apnoeic episodes are usually shorter in duration than central apnoeas, they are frequently associated with hypoxia. Several theories have been put forward to explain the mechanism behind these episodes, including laryngeal hyperexcitability and pharyngeal inco-ordination. Neck flexion appears to make the airways more susceptible to collapse.

Table 4.5 Causes of respiratory obstruction in the neonate

Site	No pre-existing anomaly	Pre-existing anomaly
Nose	Nasal congestion Nasogastric tube	Congenital absence Choanal atresia
Pharynx	Sleep apnoea Burns	Macroglossia (e.g. Beckwith syndrome) Cretinism Pierre Robin syndrome Treacher-Collins syndrome Cystic hygroma
Larynx	Acute laryngospasm Acquired vocal cord palsy Acquired subglottic stenosis	Atresia Laryngomalacia Congenital webs, cysts, haemangiomata Secondary to raised intracranial pressure Congenital vocal cord palsy Congenital subglottic stenosis
Trachea	Foreign body Acquired tracheal stenosis	Tracheomalacia, often associated with oesophageal atresia Congenital tracheal stenosis Extrinsic pressure: cyst, tumour, vascular ring

Nasal

Nasal obstruction may be fatal, as the neonate is an obligatory nose breather. Extreme respiratory distress with cyanosis is characteristically relieved when the infant cries, thus using its mouth for breathing.

Choanal atresia

Choanal atresia is ruled out by passing a soft rubber catheter through each nostril. If this condition is complete, obstruction by bony or membranous walls will cause severe respiratory distress in the newborn. In cases of severe airway obstruction the airway may have to established before accurate diagnosis is made.

An oral airway is inserted and fastened by tapes to the baby's cheeks until he comes to the anaesthetic room. Transnasal or transpalatal puncture and dilatation is usually performed at the age of 1–2 days.

Premedication is with atropine, and intubation is performed awake after preoxygenation through the oral airway. A 3 mm (internal diameter) preformed or Oxford tube is used and a small throat pack inserted. The T-piece will come down over the patient's chest. Ventilation is controlled using a relaxant technique with all the precautions necessary for neonatal anaesthesia and surgery. After the nasal punctures are completed, the surgeon inserts short plastic tubes which remain in place in the nose for 6 weeks. The operation usually takes 20–30 minutes. The patient is extubated fully awake after removal of the throat pack and careful suctioning of the pharynx. Pulmonary aspiration of regurgitated stomach contents is very

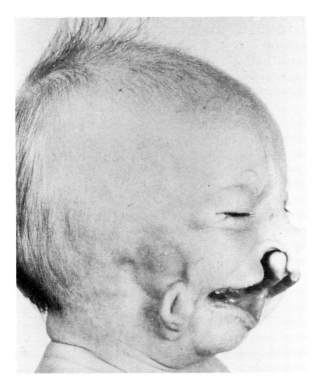

Fig. 4.17 The Treacher-Collins syndrome.

likely to occur after this operation: careful nursing observation must start at once in the postoperative ward.

Atresia may be unilateral or bilateral, and may also be associated with other congenital abnormalities such as Apert's or Treacher-Collins syndrome (Fig. 4.17).

Pharyngeal

Recent evidence has shown that pharyngeal obstruction may be an important cause of apnoea in some preterm infants, possibly due to pharyngeal or laryngeal dysfunction. It has been shown that transmural pressures greater than those normally seen during peak inspiratory flow are required to keep airways patent, suggesting that a neuromuscular mechanism is required to maintain airway patency in some infants. Neck flexion increases the opening pressure, making the airways more liable to collapse. Hyper-excitability of the laryngeal adductors has also been demonstrated in prematures, aggravated by hyperthermia.

Pierre Robin syndrome (Fig. 4.18)

This syndrome consists of cleft palate, underdevelopment of the mandible, micrognathia and a relatively large tongue (macroglossia) which may cause

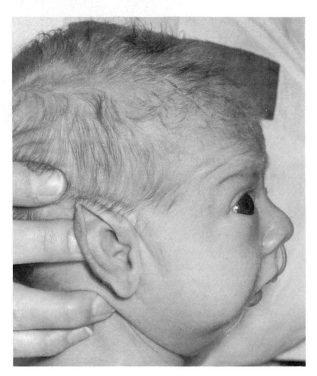

Fig. 4.18   The Pierre Robin syndrome.

pharyngeal obstruction, particularly in the supine position. Severe cases provide a challenge to airway management in the first few months of life. The infant is sometimes nursed in the prone position, but even in this position fatalities do occur. More recently the use of a nasopharyngeal airway has been suggested, but a prolonged period of tracheal intubation or even tracheostomy may be required. Suturing the tongue forward onto the mandible may relieve the respiratory obstruction in some cases but is not often practised.

Cystic hygroma

This cystic lymphangioma presents at birth as a multiloculated cystic swelling in the neck (Fig. 4.19) or, rarely, in the axilla. The swelling is soft and fluctuant, and although it is benign it frequently invades neighbouring tissues and may recur. It may not be possible to perform complete surgical removal, especially if the tumour is large or extends around the trachea or brachial plexus. Involvement of the base of the tongue and oropharynx is

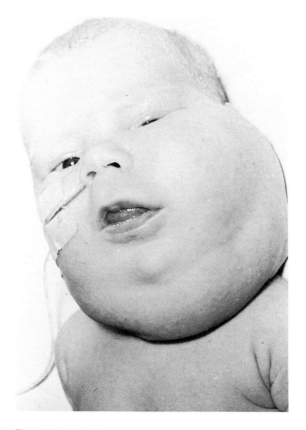

Fig. 4.19 Cystic hygroma.

common and may cause respiratory difficulties. Intrathoracic extension of this tumour is rare.

Anaesthetic management   The intraoral extension of this multilocular cystic tumour may make identification of the larynx difficult and, more importantly, may make inflation of the lungs impossible in the apnoeic patient. It is therefore essential to maintain spontaneous breathing until intubation has been performed. In the worst cases the only way to identify the larynx may be to observe the movement of air in and out of the lungs, which usually causes a number of frothy bubbles to appear between two lobules of the hygroma. Surgical removal of the tumour may be difficult as it crosses tissue planes, and blood should be available for transfusion. The child should not be extubated until fully awake, and in the worst cases tracheostomy may be necessary.

Postoperative care.   Because of the danger of bleeding into the operative site causing respiratory obstruction in the early postoperative period, these children must be observed very closely. Even the aperture of a tracheostomy tube may become obstructed by recurrent swelling in the neck.

Laryngeal

Laryngomalacia is the commonest cause of stridor at birth, and is probably due to immaturity of the laryngeal muscles and cartilages. It may occur in association with other congenital defects such as subglottic stenosis. The laxity of the supraglottic larynx allows it to be drawn into the glottis during inspiration, causing the characteristic inspiratory stridor. The condition is seldom life-threatening although it may cause feeding problems, and repeated respiratory infections are common. The diagnosis is made by direct laryngoscopy, and induction of anaesthesia may worsen the stridor. The long-term prognosis is usually good, although in some cases symptoms of persisting respiratory obstruction may remain into childhood.

Vocal cord palsy may be unilateral or bilateral, resulting from birth trauma, surgical damage to the recurrent laryngeal nerve, secondary to raised intracranial pressure, or the Arnold–Chiari syndrome, and rarely from tumours in the neck or thorax. Partial paralysis may leave the adductors relatively unopposed, creating severe stridor. In some but not all cases the stridor gradually resolves over a period of several months, during which time intubation or even tracheostomy may be required. Diagnosis is made at direct laryngoscopy, with spontaneous breathing to allow vocal cord movement to be properly assessed.

Congenital webs and cysts may arise anywhere in the larynx. The most common are situated in the glottic or subglottic area, and lateral x-ray of the neck or xerogram usually demonstrates the lesion clearly. Laryngeal haemangiomata should be suspected in any child with significant cutaneous haemangiomata, especially over the neck or anterior chest wall. They seldom give rise to airway problems at birth; stridor tends to develop within the first 3 months of life. Crying, struggling or partial airway obstruction will increase the size of the tumour by venous engorgement. Direct laryngoscopy confirms the diagnosis, and treatment is by suction diathermy or laser resection. Tracheostomy is often required.

Congenital subglottic stenosis is a relatively rare cause of airway obstruction, found more frequently in association with tracheo-oesophageal fistula or Down's syndrome. Acquired stenosis, on the other hand, still occurs more frequently than it should, and is due either to the pressure of too large a tracheal tube or to trauma from the shoulder of a tapered tube such

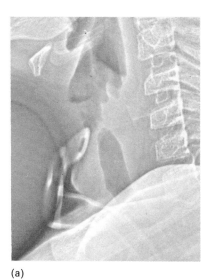
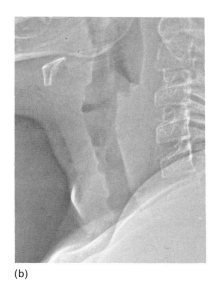

(a)   (b)

Fig. 4.20 Xerograms showing (a) complete respiratory obstruction due to subglottic stenosis, and (b) the same child after relief of the obstruction by laryngotracheoplasty. (Courtesy of J. N. G. Evans)

as the Cole pattern. Since the subglottic area, which is the narrowest part of the neonate's upper airway, is the site of the complete cartilaginous cricoid ring, there is no room for expansion, and 1 mm of oedema or fibrosis will narrow the airway by as much as 65 per cent. Stridor usually occurs within a few hours of extubation, and mild cases may respond to humidity, oxygen, intravenous dexamethasone ($0.25\,mg\cdot kg^{-1}$ followed by $0.1\,mg\cdot kg^{-1}$ 6-hourly for 24 hours), and possibly nebulized racemic adrenaline. More severe cases require a period of reintubation with a small tube, and the worst cases may require tracheostomy and eventual laryngotracheoplasty (Fig. 4.20).

Tracheal

Vascular anomalies of the aortic arch may cause compression of the trachea and oesophagus. A vascular ring is most commonly due to persistent right and left aortic arches, but can also be caused by a right-sided aortic arch and left patent ductus arteriosus, or by aberrant right subclavian, innominate or left common carotid arteries (Fig. 4.21). The trachea and oesophagus are enclosed within the vascular ring, and pressure on the trachea causes the main clinical problem, airway obstruction. This obstruction usually develops within the first few weeks after birth, is exacerbated by feeding and may become very severe. The clinical picture is that of intrathoracic respiratory obstruction, with a croaking cry, brassy cough, signs of hyperinflation of the chest, expiratory wheezes and rhonchi. Respiratory infections are common, and the diagnosis should be considered in cases of

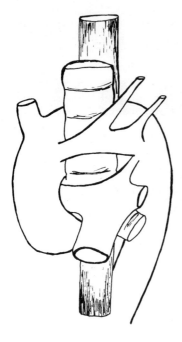

Fig. 4.21   Double aortic arch.

repeated chest infection. In severe cases the infant may adopt the hyperextended posture of opisthotonus, and sudden death from respiratory obstruction may occur. Associated cardiac anomalies may be present, particularly ventricular septal defect or bicuspid aortic valve.

Diagnosis should be confirmed as soon as possible, either by endoscopy or by barium or propyliodone (Dionosil) swallow (Fig. 4.22). These investigations should be carried out only when a skilled anaesthetist can be standing by with full resuscitation equipment. Laryngoscopy and tracheal intubation may be necessary in order to suck out any aspirated propyliodone and to relieve hypoxia.

Treatment is surgical, and incomplete division of the ring has been reported. Because the airway obstruction is low in the trachea it may occasionally be necessary to use a long tracheal tube passed into the right main

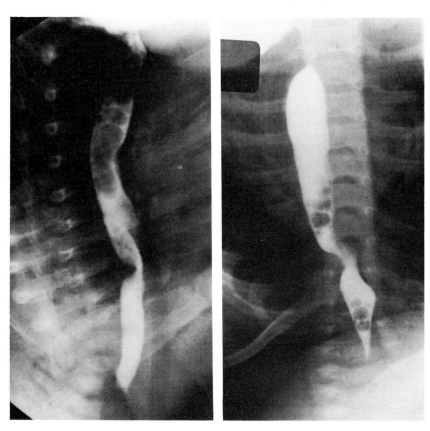

Fig. 4.22 Barium swallow, showing oesophageal compression caused by double aortic arch which was also producing severe stridor from tracheal obstruction. (Reproduced, with permission, from Hatch, 1985)

bronchus, with a side hole cut 1.5–2 cm from the tip to allow ventilation of the left lung. Care should be taken not to pass too large a tube through the obstructed area because of the risk of oedema causing postoperative stridor, and it is better to keep the tube above the lesion if possible. Surgical manipulation may cause complete airway obstruction, and severe haemorrhage may occur.

Symptoms of airway obstruction may be slow to improve postoperatively, as the trachea has often been severely distorted and some degree of tracheomalacia and tracheal stenosis is almost always present. The infant should be nursed in a humidified head box with some oxygen enrichment, and may be helped by dexamethasone (0.25–0.5 mg·kg^{-1}). In severe cases, continuous positive airway pressure, using either a nasal prong or a small tracheal tube, may be necessary. Tracheostomy may have to be considered, although the low position of the obstruction often makes this unsatisfactory. The possibility of incomplete resection of the vascular ring should be considered if postoperative respiratory obstruction persists, as in some cases a ligamentum arteriosum may be responsible for continuing symptoms.

Other rare tracheal anomalies include tracheomalacia, tracheal stenosis and external compression by cysts or tumours. Inhalation of a foreign body is also unusual in the neonatal period.

Management of respiratory obstruction

Intubation, laryngoscopy, bronchoscopy or tracheostomy may be necessary for the management of these cases. Nasal obstruction may be relieved by the insertion of an oral airway which must be strapped in place, as it will otherwise be rejected by the baby. Babies with gross nasal deformities, although rare, may need an urgent tracheostomy.

Bronchoscopy and laryngoscopy should never be undertaken lightly—especially in the neonate. Bronchoscopy is never indicated merely for removal of secretions. It should not be performed in the presence of tracheal infection or subglottic stenosis, as oedema and stridor will be intensified.

Laryngoscopy

Some of the conditions for which laryngoscopy is performed can progress to partial or complete respiratory obstruction under anaesthesia; this applies particularly to patients with micrognathia, large tongues, rigid jaws, and pharyngeal or glottic cysts or tumours. A selection of laryngoscopes and tracheal tubes of various lengths must be on hand and a surgeon must be ready to perform a tracheostomy if that becomes urgently necessary. Great care must be taken to maintain the infant's body temperature during induction of anaesthesia and surgery, and ECG and precordial stethoscope should be employed. Premedication consists only of atropine, and this should always be given because local topical analgesia is essential and only works well if adequate drying of secretions has been achieved. In spite of the advantages generally cited for controlled ventilation in neonatal anaesthesia, these are usually outweighed by the advantages of spontaneous ventilation in anaesthesia for laryngoscopy. Spontaneous ventilation is mandatory in respiratory obstruction unless the anaesthetist is certain he will be able to inflate the lungs of the paralysed patient. In children with laryngeal papillomata or cystic hygroma the movements which occur around the glottis during spontaneous breathing, with possible bubbles of saliva, may provide the only means of identification of the laryngeal inlet.

Induction of anaesthesia for laryngoscopy is usually performed with oxygen and halothane via a well-fitting face mask. The application of constant distending pressure by controlling the gas leak from the open-ended T-piece reservoir bag is sometimes extremely useful during induction in cases of respiratory obstruction, and may even lead to the complete disappearance of stridor. It is essential therefore that the mask used is one which can make a good seal with the face: the Rendell–Baker mask is not ideal for this purpose, and one with an inflatable rim is preferable despite its larger dead space. It may be impracticable to cannulate a vein before induction of anaesthesia but a vein should be cannulated as soon as possible after induction. Topical lignocaine (3–5 mg·kg^{-1}) is sprayed into the larynx and trachea when the patient is fairly deeply anaesthetized, and at this time the anaesthetist can make a first assessment of the larynx. The commonly used proprietary lignocaine (Xylocaine) spray delivers 10 mg aliquots. If microlaryngoscopy is to be performed it is wise to intubate the trachea first, in order to assess the diameter of the larynx and upper trachea, and to provide a secure airway while the microscope is set up. A small nasotracheal tube is convenient for this purpose. This is usually withdrawn into the nasopharynx during the microlaryngoscopy, and oxygen and halothane are insufflated through it. Spontaneous ventilation allows the surgeon to observe the movements of the larynx during the procedure, and this is essential in the diagnosis of prolapsing larynx, laryngomalacia, cleft larynx and vocal cord palsy.

The Sanders injector cannot be used during laryngoscopy in infants because it cannot be easily fitted to the microlaryngoscope blade and there is often difficulty in aiming the jet directly down the larynx. There is also a risk of seeding papillomata further down the airway. Intratracheal jets have been used in older children, but are dangerous if the cords close, and should not be used in neonates.

Controlled ventilation through a small nasotracheal tube will be required for the occasional patient in respiratory failure.

Bronchoscopy

Anaesthetic techniques for bronchoscopy depend on the apparatus available. Paediatric bronchoscope systems such as the Storz (Fig. 4.23) are

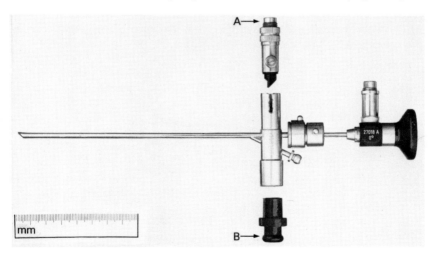

Fig. 4.23   The Storz bronchoscope, showing (A) the light carrier and (B) the attachment for the anaesthetic T-piece.

supposed to be 'ventilating' bronchoscopes, but it is very unwise to give relaxants to the patient during such an endoscopy unless one is sure that it is possible to inflate the lungs adequately through the bronchoscope. Assisted or spontaneous ventilation is possible using an anaesthetic T-piece on the side-arm of the infant bronchoscope. The smaller sized bronchoscopes have very little gap within the bronchoscope when the telescope is in place and ventilation is difficult in these circumstances. Manual ventilation is not possible during suction and insertion of the telescope, during which time a paralysed patient will become increasingly hypoxic. Bronchoscopy is performed under general anaesthesia with full local anaesthesia to the respiratory tract as described above, with oxygen and halothane delivered to the side-arm of the bronchoscope, ventilation being spontaneous or gently controlled.

Monitoring must include ECG and precordial stethoscope; if a hand is placed over the epigastrium, each breath can be felt, and the thumb on the apex can feel each heart beat. It is useful to attach two precordial stethoscopes—one on the left for breath and heart sounds, and the right only for breath sounds. This allows monitoring of respiration to both lungs independently and is especially useful when the bronchoscope is down one or other main bronchus.

The Sanders jet, which uses the Venturi principle, is seldom used for infant bronchoscopy because most endoscopists prefer the superior optical characteristics of modern fibreoptic telescopic bronchoscopes. These bronchoscopes are expensive, however, and not available in all centres. Bronchoscopy for inhaled foreign body, for example, may require the use of the Negus bronchoscope (Fig. 4.24), and when this is used, ventilation with the Venturi is preferable to spontaneous breathing. Ideally, the anaesthetic technique should allow the surgeon to change from one type of bronchoscope to another. Chest wall movements should be carefully monitored whichever technique is used. Pneumothorax is a theoretical complication of the Venturi jet, but hypoxia from inadequate ventilation is probably a more likely hazard.

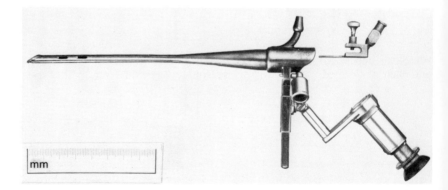

Fig. 4.24 The Negus suckling bronchoscope with Venturi attachment.

Standard pipeline pressures may be used safely if the Venturi needle in infants does not exceed 10 s.w.g. Anaesthesia can be maintained if the entrained gas includes oxygen and halothane to the side-arm of the Negus-type bronchoscope.

Pneumothorax is a complication of bronchoscopy whichever anaesthetic technique is used. Blood gas analysis has shown that ventilation with a Sanders type of Venturi is satisfactory unless the patient has severe chronic respiratory disease with markedly reduced lung compliance.

Most laryngotracheal lesions are diagnosed by laryngoscopy or bronchoscopy. The characteristic small, floppy glottis and epiglottis of laryngomalacia and vocal cord palsies will be observed. Tracheomalacia is seen during spontaneous respiration. Pulsatile swellings may be vascular in origin, although such pulsation may be transmitted and is not therefore diagnostic of a vascular origin. If the compression is caused by an aberrant subclavian artery making a vascular ring, the pressure of the tip of the bronchoscope may produce changes in the character of the radial pulses. This condition usually requires a cine swallow with contrast medium, using the image intensifier to visualize the obstruction and so make for a definitive diagnosis.

After the examination, the patient should be placed in the lateral position, the lower side being the side of any bleeding from trauma or biopsies. The patient must be observed until he is fully awake, as stridor and respiratory distress may not reappear until then.

Bronchoscopy may precipitate complete respiratory obstruction in very marginal cases by minimal oedema caused by the instrumentation. Bronchoscopy is not necessary and may be dangerous in the diagnosis of subglottic stenosis. Postoperatively the baby is nursed using a head box with humidified air or air and oxygen mixture, and should have nothing by mouth until 3 hours after the lignocaine spray to the glottis. Dexamethasone should be given (p. 183) for laryngeal oedema if stridor reappears.

Tracheostomy

This is very rarely an emergency procedure. With the advent of long-term nasotracheal intubation, tracheostomy is never required nowadays merely for respiratory support in the neonatal period. The indications for tracheostomy vary from centre to centre, but it is generally accepted that for ventilator-dependent patients tracheostomy may be delayed for many weeks and then performed, not for airway reasons but because handling, nursing and stimulating a growing baby are easier with a tracheostomy. Tracheostomy is most commonly performed for conditions of the upper airway for which tracheal intubation is unsuitable, such as subglottic stenosis, severe tracheomalacia or vocal cord palsy.

Many patients who require tracheostomy already have a tracheal tube in place. Premedication is with atropine, and preoxygenation is followed by intubation if a tube is not already in place. A very small tube may be necessary in cases of subglottic stenosis. A relaxant technique with controlled ventilation may be used. The patient is positioned with a sandbag behind the neck to extend the head maximally and to throw the trachea into prominence. Monitoring must include ECG and oesophageal stethoscope. Infant tracheostomy is a specialized and difficult operation. Cartilage must never be excised because of the risk of subsequent tracheal collapse and stenosis, nor must the incision be too high in the trachea because of the risk of subglottic stenosis. The surgeon usually makes a vertical incision through the second and third tracheal rings. If it is made lower than this, there is a risk of bronchial intubation or tube dislodgement. Some surgeons insert two stay sutures which remain in place for 7 days until the tube is changed for the first time. The uncuffed tracheostomy tube is chosen, usually one size larger than the tracheal tube in place, and then a check is made that all connections are available and that they fit. The Great Ormond

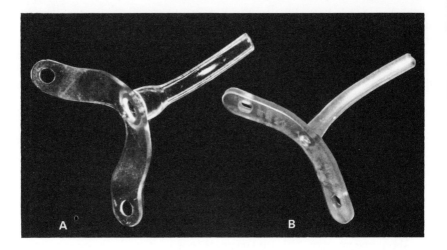

Fig. 4.25   Neonatal tracheostomy tubes: A, Great Ormond Street pattern; B, Portex.

Street (Aberdeen) non-cuffed plastic tracheostomy tube (3.5–7 mm plain) is very satisfactory, although at the moment no British Standard connections are available for them (Fig. 4.25). The patient is ventilated with 100% oxygen before the tracheal incision is made and the tracheal tube withdrawn only enough for the tracheostomy tube to be inserted. Anaesthesia is continued through the tracheostomy with a sterile connector. The tube must fit with a small air leak around it and be fixed tightly round the neck with tapes. Postoperatively a chest x-ray is taken to check the position of the tip of the tube.

The complications of tracheostomy are more severe than those of tracheal intubation. Accidental dislodgement in the first week before a track is established can be disastrous, although less so if stay sutures are employed. Severe infection, tracheal granuloma and vascular erosion are reported complications.

A tracheostomy mask with humidified air is used to prevent crusting of secretions in the tube. Eventually the epithelium in the trachea becomes stratified and humidification is usually discontinued after about 3 weeks.

References and further reading

Surgical emergencies

Andrassy, R. J. and Mahour, G. H. (1979). Gastrointestinal anomalies associated with esophageal atresia or tracheo-esophageal fistula. *Archives of Surgery* **114**, 1125.

Bohn, D. J., James, I. G., Filler, R. M., Ein, S. H., Wesson, D. E., Shandling, B., Stephens, C. and Barker, G. A. (1984). The relationship between Pao_2 and ventilation parameters in predicting survival in congenital diaphragmatic hernia. *Journal of Pediatric Surgery* **19**, 666.

Collins, D. L., Pomerance, J. J., Travis, K. W., Turner, S. W. and Papperbaum, S. J. (1977). A new approach to congenital posterolateral diaphragmatic hernia. *Journal of Pediatric Surgery* **12**, 149.

Cozzi, F. and Wilkinson, A. W. (1975). Low birth weight babies with oesophageal atresia or tracheo-oesophageal fistula. *Archives of Disease in Childhood* **50**, 791.

Dibbins, A. W. (1976). Neonatal diaphragmatic hernia: a physiological challenge. *American Journal of Surgery* **131**, 408.

Ganderer, M. W. L., Jassani, M. N. and Izant, R. J. Jr (1984). Ultrasonographic antenatal diagnosis: will it change the spectrum of neonatal surgery? *Journal of Pediatric Surgery* **19**, 404.

Girven, D. P., Webster, D. M. and Shandling, B. (1974). The treatment of omphalocele and gastroschisis. *Surgery, Gynecology and Obstetrics* **139**, 222.

Grant, D. M. and Thompson, G. E. (1978). Diagnosis of congenital tracheo-esophageal fistula in the adolescent and adult. *Anesthesiology* **49**, 139.

Greenwood, R. D. and Rosenthal, A. (1976). Cardiovascular malformations associated with tracheo-esophageal fistula and esophageal atresia. *Pediatrics* **57**, 87.

Grossfield, J. L. and Ballantine, T. V. (1978). Esophageal atresia and tracheo-esophageal fistula: effect of delayed thoracotomy on survival. *Surgery* **84**, 394.

Inkster, J. (1976). Paediatric anaesthesia and intensive care. In: *Recent Advances in Anaesthesia and Analgesia, 12.* Ed. by C. Langton Hewer and R. S. Atkinson. Churchill Livingstone, Edinburgh and London.

James, I. G. (1985). Emergencies in paediatric anaesthesia. In: *Paediatric Anaesthesia. Clinics in Anaesthesiology* **3**, no. 3.

Kliegman, R. M. and Fanaroff, A. A. (1984). Necrotizing enterocolitis. *New England Journal of Medicine* **310**, 1093.

Levin, D. L. (1978). Morphological analysis of the pulmonary vascular bed in congenital left-sided diaphragmatic hernia. *Journal of Pediatrics* **92**, 805.

de Lorimer, A. A., Tierney, D. F. and Parker, H. R. (1967). Hypoplastic lungs in fetal lambs with surgically produced congenital diaphragmatic hernia. *Surgery* **62**, 12.

McGown, R. G. (1982). Caudal analgesia in children. *Anaesthesia* **37**, 806.

Marshall, A. and Sumner, E. (1982). Improved prognosis in congenital diaphragmatic hernia: experience of 62 cases over a 2 year period. *Journal of the Royal Society of Medicine* **75**, 607.

Nixon, H. H. (1978). *Surgical Conditions in Paediatrics*. Butterworths, London.

Olivet, R. T., Rupp, W. M., Telander, R. I. and Kaye, M. P. (1978). Hemodynamics of congenital diaphragmatic hernia in lambs. *Journal of Pediatric Surgery* **13**, 231.

Rickham, P. P., Lister, J. and Irving, I. M. (Eds) (1978). *Neonatal Surgery*, 2nd edn. Butterworths, London.

Salem, M. R., Wong, A. Y., Lin, Y. H., Firor, H. V. and Bennett, E. J. (1973). Prevention of gastric distension during anesthesia for newborns with tracheo-esophageal fistula. *Anesthesiology* **38**, 82.

Sears, B. E., Carlin, J. and Tunell, W. P. (1978). Severe congenital subglottic stenosis in association with congenital duodenal obstruction. *Anesthesiology* **49**, 214.

Sivasubramanian, K. N. (1979). Techniques of selective intubation of the left bronchus in newborn infants. *Journal of Pediatrics* **94**, 479.

Spielman, F. T., Seeds, J. W. and Corke, B. C. (1984). Anaesthesia for fetal surgery. *Anaesthesia* **39**, 756.

Sumner, E. and Frank, J. D. (1981). The effect of tolazoline on the treatment of congenital diaphragmatic hernia. *Archives of Disease in Childhood* **56**, 350.

Thomas, D. F. M. and Atwell, J. (1976). The embryology and surgical management of gastroschisis. *British Journal of Surgery* **63**, 893.

Waterston, D. J., Bonham Carter, R. E. and Aberdeen, E. (1962). Oesophageal atresia: tracheo-oesophageal fistula: a study of survival in 218 infants. *Lancet* **1**, 819.

Anaesthesia for neuroradiology and neurosurgery

Creighton, R. E. (1982). Paediatric neuroanaesthesia. In: *Some Aspects of Paediatric Anaesthesia*, p. 199. Ed. by D. J. Steward. Excerpta Medica, Amsterdam.

Creighton, R. E., Relton, J. E. S. and Meridy, H. W. (1974). Anesthesia for occipital encephalocoele. *Canadian Anaesthetists Society Journal* **21**, 403.

Fitch, W. and McDowall, D. G. (1971). Anaesthesia for neuroradiological investigations. *Proceedings of the Royal Society of Medicine* **64**, 75.

Lassen, N. A. and Christensen, M. S. (1976). Physiology of cerebral blood flow. *British Journal of Anaesthesia* **48**, 719.

Leading article (1977). Screening for neural tube defects. *Lancet* **1**, 1345.

Michenfelder, J. D., Gronert, G. A. and Rehder, K. (1969). Neuroanesthesia. *Anesthesiology* **30**, 65.

Anaesthesia for cardiac and thoracic surgery

Abbott, T. R. (1977). Oxygen uptake following deep hypothermia. *Anaesthesia* **32**, 524.

Bailey, L. L., Takeuchi, Y., Williams, W. G., Trusler, G. A. and Mustard, W. T. (1976). Surgical management of congenital cardiovascular anomalies with the use of profound hypothermia and circulatory arrest. Analysis of 180 consecutive cases. *Journal of Thoracic and Cardiovascular Surgery* **71**, 485.

Barratt-Boyes, B. G., Simpson, M. and Neutze, J. M. (1971). Intracardiac surgery in neonates and infants using deep hypothermia with surface cooling and limited cardiopulmonary bypass. *Circulation* **43**, 44.

Battersby, E. F., Hatch, D. J. and Towey, R. M. (1977). The effects of prolonged nasotracheal intubation in children. A study in infants and young children after cardiopulmonary bypass. *Anaesthesia* **32**, 154.

Buckberg, G. D. (1979). A proposed solution to the cardioplegic controversy. *Journal of Thoracic and Cardiovascular Surgery* **77**, 803.

Cooper, D. K. C. (1979). Study of the factors contributing to the mortality associated with open heart surgery in infants. *Thorax* **34**, 138.

Cullum, A. R., English, I. C. W. and Branthwaite, M. A. (1973). Endobronchial intubation in infancy. *Anaesthesia* **28**, 66.

Driscoll, D. J., Gillette, P. C. and McNamara, D. G. (1980). The use of dopamine in children. *Journal of Pediatrics* **92**, 309.

Ebert, P. A. (1978). Aspects of myocardial protection. *Annals of Thoracic Surgery* **26**, 495.

Elliott, R. B., Starling, M. B. and Neutze, J. M. (1975). Medical manipulation of the ductus arteriosus. *Lancet* **1**, 140.

English, I. C. W., Frew, R. M., Piggott, J. F. and Zaki, M. (1964). Percutaneous catheterisation of the internal jugular vein. *Anaesthesia* **24**, 521.

Glover, W. J. (1977). Management of cardiac surgery in the neonate. *British Journal of Anaesthesia* **49**, 59.

Hatch, D. J., Cogswell, J. J., Taylor, B. W., Battersby, E. F., Glover, W. J. and Kerr, A. A. (1973). Continuous positive airway pressure after open heart operations in infancy. *Lancet* **2**, 469.

Johnston, A. E., Radde, I. C., Steward, D. J. and Taylor, J. (1974). Acid–base and electrolyte changes in infants undergoing profound hypothermia for surgical correction of congenital heart defects. *Canadian Anaesthetists Society Journal* **21**, 23.

Keith, J. D., Rowe, R. D. and Vlad, P. (Eds) (1978). *Heart Disease in Infancy and Childhood*, 3rd edn. Macmillan, New York.

Kirklin, J. W. (1973). *Advances in Cardiovascular Surgery*. Grune & Stratton, New York.

Leading article (1975). Congenital heart disease: incidence and aetiology. *Lancet* **2**, 692.

Lippmann, M., Nelson, R. J., Emmanouilides, G. C., Diskin, J. and Thiebault, D. W. (1976). Ligation of patent ductus arteriosus in premature infants. *British Journal of Anaesthesia* **48**, 365.

Martin, J. T. (1976). Case history number 93: congenital lobar emphysema. *Anesthesia and Analgesia* **55,** 869.

Pang, L. M. and Mellins, R. B. (1975). Neonatal cardiorespiratory physiology. *Anesthesiology* **43,** 171.

Pick, M. J., Hatch, D. J. and Kerr, A. A. (1976). The effects of positive end expiratory pressure on lung mechanics and arterial oxygenation after open heart surgery in young children. *British Journal of Anaesthesia* **48,** 983.

Robinson, S. and Gregory, G. A. (1980). Fentanyl-air/oxygen anaesthesia for PDA ligation in infants less than 1500 grams. *Anesthesia and Analgesia* **59,** 556.

Stark, J. (1980). Current status of cardiac surgery in early infancy. In: *Proceedings of the 8th European Congress of Cardiology*, Paris, 22nd–26th June 1980, p. 253. Karger, Basel.

Stranger, P., Heymann, M. A., Tarnoff, H., Hoffmann, J. I. E. and Rudolph, A. M. (1974). Complications of cardiac catheterization of neonates, infants and children—a three-year study. *Circulation* **50,** 595.

Subramanian, S., Wagner, H., Vlad, P. and Lambert, E. (1971). Surface-induced deep hypothermia in cardiac surgery. *Journal of Pediatric Surgery* **6,** 612.

Vidne, B. A. and Subramanian, S. (1976). Surface-induced profound hypothermia in infant cardiac operations: a new system. *Annals of Thoracic Surgery* **22,** 572.

Wakusawa, R., Shibata, S. and Okada, K. (1977). Simple deep hypothermia for open heart surgery in infancy. *Canadian Anaesthetists Society Journal* **24,** 491.

Anaesthesia for airway obstruction

Hatch, D. J. (1985). Acute upper airway obstruction in children. In: *Recent Advances in Anaesthesia and Analgesia*—15, p. 133. Ed. by R. S. Atkinson and A. P. Adams. Churchill Livingstone, Edinburgh.

Maze, A. and Bloch, E. (1979). Stridor in pediatric patients. *Anesthesiology* **50,** 132.

Miyasaka, K., Sloan, I. A. and Froese, A. B. (1980). Evaluation of jet injector Sanders' technique for bronchoscopy in paediatric patients. *Canadian Anaesthetists Society Journal* **27,** 117.

5

Postoperative care

Introduction

Neonatal intensive care, where the neonatal paediatrician, anaesthetist, surgeon and nurses all work together as part of a multidisciplinary team, is a large and expanding subject which we have not attempted to cover in this book. We have, however, tried to bring together in this chapter those aspects of postoperative care which are essential to the safe practice of neonatal anaesthesia, some of which have been touched on in previous chapters.

Postoperative respiratory failure

Aetiology

Respiratory failure may occur as a result of medical, surgical, neurological, metabolic or renal disease, and supportive therapy must be accompanied by the appropriate treatment of the underlying disease.

The neonate has limited reserves of lung function. Oxygen consumption per unit of body weight is approximately twice that of the adult, and any increase may lead to inadequate tissue oxygenation. The increase in oxygen consumption which occurs in response to cold has been described on p. 24 et seq., and the importance of taking every precaution to avoid heat loss from a neonate has been stressed. The baby should be covered with warm Gamgee or similar material as soon as the operation has finished, and returned to an incubator or placed under a heat canopy as soon as possible. The incubator should be preheated and left switched on close to the operating theatre. Even inside an incubator the temperature can be hostile to the naked neonate, especially if premature, so the baby is covered with a heat shield and the head with a bonnet.

Severe hypoxaemia may result from increase in the work of breathing, reduction in ventilation/perfusion ratio in the lungs, pulmonary venous congestion or oedema, or from intrapulmonary or intracardiac right-to-left shunting. Increased interstitial fluid in the neonatal lung is a very common occurrence in the perioperative period associated with inappropriate ADH secretion and relative fluid overload. Failure of oxygen transport may also cause tissue hypoxia, as in hypovolaemia, cardiac failure, hypotension, red

195

cell haemolysis or reduced 2,3-DPG content of blood. Hypoxaemia may occur secondary to hypoventilation in cases of postanaesthetic depression, intracranial haemorrhage, raised intracranial pressure or neurological degenerative conditions such as Werdnig–Hoffmann's disease.

Intrapulmonary shunting may occur when the already small functional residual capacity (FRC) is reduced. This is more likely to happen after intrathoracic operations or after major intra-abdominal surgery where the diaphragm may be forced upwards by pressure from below. Severe disturbances in lung function may follow cardiac surgery in the newborn because of reduced compliance and lung volume and increased resistance, with consequent increase in the work of breathing. In other babies, pre-existing respiratory problems—such as surfactant deficiency causing alveolar instability in hyaline membrane disease (HMD), pulmonary hypoplasia in cases of congenital diaphragmatic hernia, meconium aspiration or lung soiling in oesophageal atresia—may be the main factor contributing to postoperative respiratory failure. Apnoeic attacks associated with a low postconceptual age are exacerbated by general anaesthesia, increasing in severity and frequency. Many patients ventilated in the early neonatal period have some degree of residual bronchopulmonary dysplasia with reduced lung compliance and oxygen dependency. Other postoperative respiratory problems are related to large airway pathology such as laryngeal oedema, vocal cord palsy or tracheomalacia.

Assessment

It is clear that the above factors contribute to postoperative respiratory therapy being required relatively frequently in the neonate. In a recent series of admissions to the neonatal surgical intensive care unit at Great Ormond Street, 28 per cent of babies required intermittent positive pressure ventilation (IPPV) after *non-cardiac* surgical operations (Table 5.1).

The criteria for IPPV after neonatal surgery vary from centre to centre. Most people agree that a period of IPPV is desirable after open heart surgery in neonates, and almost always after closed heart surgery because, if this is required in the first month of life, it suggests that the baby is

Table 5.1 Admissions (excluding myelomeningocele) to the neonatal surgical units, 1979–1983, The Hospital for Sick Children, London

Diagnosis	No.	Ventilated	Deaths
Abdominal surgery:			
General	893	107 (12%)	61 (7%)
Exomphalos	69	15 (22%)	15 (22%)
Gastroschisis	44	41 (93%)	5 (11%)
Necrotizing enterocolitis	94	90 (96%)	16 (17%)
Tracheo-oesophageal fistula/atresia	200	64 (32%)	21 (11%)
Diaphragmatic hernia	168	112 (67%)	45 (27%)
Miscellaneous	148	21 (14%)	23 (16%)
Total	1616	450 (28%)	186 (12%)

extremely sick. Opinions vary widely, however, about the place of IPPV after non-cardiac surgery in the neonate. A few advocate elective ventilation after almost all operations whilst others confine this approach to high-risk groups of neonates such as those with congenital diaphragmatic hernia, gastroschisis or oesophageal atresia, especially if the oesophageal anastomosis is tight. The approach generally adopted by the authors is to decide each case on clinical grounds, but where there is any doubt as to the adequacy of respiratory function, respiratory support is undertaken.

Although a well-conducted general anaesthetic should have little effect itself on postoperative lung function in the neonate, each case must be carefully assessed at the end of surgery. A decision not to ventilate postoperatively should be postponed until it is clear that adequate spontaneous ventilation has returned, and that the baby stays well oxygenated when breathing room air. If there is any doubt about the adequacy of respiration—whether because of hypothermia, residual narcosis, incomplete reversal of muscle relaxants or any other factor—some form of respiratory support should be instituted. The demand for respiratory support is increasing in paediatrics as morbidity falls and expertise grows, with increasing survival rates of premature babies (Fig. 5.1).

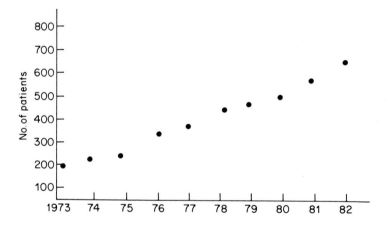

Fig. 5.1   Increase in the numbers of patients requiring mechanical ventilation over the 10 years 1973–1982 at The Hospital for Sick Children, London.

Clinical and radiological assessment

Whatever ventilatory policy is adopted, clinical assessment supported by blood gas and acid-base analysis is central to good respiratory care. Small babies have a fixed tidal volume, so attempts to increase alveolar ventilation cause an increase in respiratory rate. Thus, increasing respiratory frequency and pulse rate are early clinical signs of respiratory difficulty, often accompanied by some evidence of increase in the work of breathing, such as flaring of the alae nasi and suprasternal, intercostal and subcostal recessions. Grunting respiration is a sign that the baby is increasing the distending pressure within his lungs in an attempt to maintain the FRC in states of reduced lung compliance. A respiratory frequency above 60 breaths per minute suggests fairly severe respiratory distress. The degree of spontaneous activity, including crying and ability to accept a feed, should be carefully recorded, and responsiveness to simple manoeuvres such as the taking of blood pressure should be noted. Restlessness should be regarded as a sign of hypoxia unless proved otherwise. Periodic respiration is not uncommon in the newborn, especially if premature, and has been discussed on p. 14. Apnoeic spells lasting longer than 10 seconds, sometimes accompanied by bradycardia or cyanosis, are probably pathological, so increasing duration or frequency of attacks may be an indication for constant distending pressure in the form of CPAP. Because of the close relationship between respiratory and cardiovascular failure, respiratory assessment must always include observation of pulse rate. The state of the peripheral circulation is assessed by the quality of the peripheral pulses and temperature of the skin.

Respiratory failure exists if two or more of the following are present: retractions, respiratory rate above 70, cyanosis or intractable apnoea.

Repeated clinical assessment, preferably by the same person, is essential in deciding whether a baby is improving or deteriorating; babies should not be allowed to accumulate secretions or to become exhausted, as they may suddenly decompensate and stop breathing. Any sudden deterioration should raise the possibility of pneumothorax or hypoglycaemia. A chest x-ray may exclude or confirm the presence of cardiomegaly, collapsed areas of lung, pneumothorax or collection of fluid. Elevation of one side of the diaphragm by two vertebral spaces after thoracic surgery suggests the possibility of phrenic nerve damage, although fluoroscopy is necessary for complete diagnosis and to assess the degree of paradoxical movement.

Blood gas analysis

Arterial blood gas and acid-base estimations provide essential support to, but do not replace, clinical judgement. Babies who, after surgery, are not maintaining an arterial oxygen tension between 6.7 and 10.7 kPa (50-80 mmHg) when breathing oxygen-enriched mixtures or whose arterial carbon dioxide tension is rising above 6.7 kPa (50 mmHg) are likely to require ventilatory assistance, although sometimes IPPV is indicated on purely clinical grounds, even in the presence of relatively normal blood gases, or if gas exchange deteriorates in spite of a trial of CPAP with, for example, a nasal prong.

In the newborn, repeated arterial blood samples may be obtained by catheterization of an umbilical artery. Electrodes are also available which can be inserted into the artery to provide continuous measurement of oxygen tension (Pao_2) or oxygen saturation. Both techniques have their advocates, and blood samples for independent blood gas analysis can be withdrawn by either method. The umbilical and lower limb arteries will contain a lower arterial oxygen tension than upper limb arteries if there is significant right-to-left shunting through a patent ductus arteriosus. This difference is a very useful warning of the magnitude of a shunt caused by increasing pulmonary vascular resistance. The umbilical artery is available for use only for the first day or two of life and there is an increased risk of thromboembolism if the catheter is left in place for more than 72 hours. Many clinical situations can be managed by repeated sampling from peripheral arteries or from samples of 'arterialized' capillary blood. The oxygen tension of samples taken during crying is of little value and it is always wise to record the inspired oxygen concentration at the time of sampling for reference purposes. Femoral artery puncture carries the risk of prejudicing the blood flow to the lower limb and also the possibility of causing a septic arthritis of the hip. If repeated samples are required or if mechanical ventilation is necessary, a 22 or 24 s.w.g. cannula should be placed percutaneously in a radial artery. This artery is best identified by shining a cold light source through the wrist from the dorsal side, although a pre-existing haematoma will obscure the artery.

The continuous measurement of transcutaneous oxygen and carbon dioxide tensions is now practicable due to improvements in the design of heated skin electrodes. These non-invasive electrodes show how easily hypoxia can occur with such manoeuvres as handling, feeding and tracheal suction and are especially useful in preterm babies at risk from retinopathy of prematurity. Not only are repeated samples of arterial blood difficult to obtain from such babies, but levels of Pao_2 above and below what are considered safe will be missed without continuous measurement. There is a reasonable correlation between cutaneous and arterial gas levels when the peripheral circulation is good, although they may not be maintained if the peripheral circulation fails, during periods of hypotension or in patients with generalized cutaneous dilatation as may occur with tolazoline therapy. Absolute levels of Pao_2 may not always be exactly matched, but these electrodes are reliable in showing trends. The amount of heat energy required to heat the area of skin beneath the electrode is a rough guide to the adequacy of the peripheral circulation and hence the cardiac output. The electrodes are moved every 4 hours for a term baby to prevent blistering of the skin, but every 2 hours for a very small baby.

Cutaneous CO_2 monitoring, also using heated electrodes, is less reliable even under normal conditions, but during haemorrhagic shock and other low cardiac output states there is an increase in tissue CO_2 giving higher $TcPco_2$ values than the $Paco_2$. This difference relates indirectly to the haemodynamic status and may be a guide to cardiac output.

Oximeters which accurately measure oxygen saturation in the skin regardless of its pigmentation or thickness are useful, especially in preterm babies in whom oxygen therapy is expected to give less than 100 per cent saturation (equivalent to Pao_2 9.3–10.7 kPa (70–80 mmHg)).

Acute respiratory failure is a clinical diagnosis, supported by radiological and blood gas data, but there are occasions—particularly in chronic lung disease and in the management of patients on longer term IPPV—when a more objective assessment of resistance, compliance and lung volume is useful. For this reason, methods of measurement of these parameters are described briefly below.

Lung mechanics

Resistance

Airways resistance alone may be measured with a whole body plethysmograph. In this technique, which has been modified for babies, the subject breathes quietly from a heated circuit containing a pneumotachograph whilst enclosed in an air-tight chamber. Airways resistance is calculated from the simultaneous measurement of flow from the pneumotachograph and of pressure changes within the chamber. The inspired gas must be heated to 37°C and humidified to prevent these pressure changes being affected by differences between inspired and expired gas volumes. Measurement of the resistance of the airways plus lung tissue, known as *total pulmonary resistance*, may be obtained using the simultaneous measurement of flow and oesophageal pressure (Fig. 5.2). The former signal can be

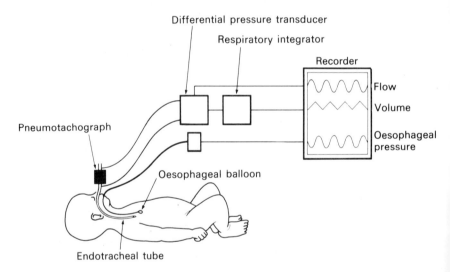

Fig. 5.2 System for assessing respiratory function in babies. (Reproduced, with permission, from Hatch, 1975)

obtained from a pneumotachograph and the latter from a thin-walled oesophageal balloon (Fig. 5.3).

Oesophageal balloons for use in the newborn must be carefully made, and each one's static and dynamic accuracy should be checked. The volume of air to be used in a balloon should be determined from the *in vitro* pressure/volume curve; the best results are obtained with balloons of 30–50 mm length, and with a diameter of 7.5 mm and a wall thickness of 0.045–

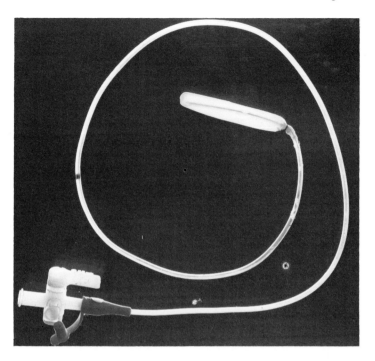

Fig. 5.3   Oesophageal balloon.

0.075 mm mounted on a 6 or 8 FG catheter and connected to a suitable pressure transducer. The balloon should be inserted into the lower oeso-phagus and its position checked by ensuring that mouth pressure changes and oesophageal pressure changes recorded simultaneously are identical when the subject attempts to breathe against an occluded airway. In sick infants with gross chest wall distortion, measurements of oesophageal pres-sure are inaccurate and should not be used. Passive total expiratory resistance can also be measured from the time constant of a relaxed expir-ation following brief airway occlusions. Pulmonary resistance is usually measured at the midpoint of inspiration and expiration.

Compliance

Compliance, or lung stiffness, is measured by volume change per unit pres-sure change. An estimation of compliance may be obtained using the pneu-motachograph and oesophageal balloon system described above if the basic assumption is made that there is no air flow at end-tidal points (Fig. 5.4). Dynamic compliance measurements obtained in this way will be erroneous when resistance is high or during rapid rates of breathing, and in these circumstances static measurements give more reliable information about the elastic properties of the lungs. The classic method of measuring static com-pliance by inflating the lungs with known volumes of air from a calibrated

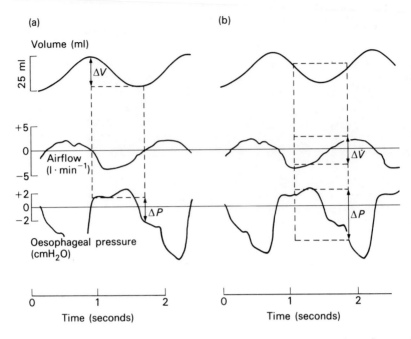

Fig. 5.4 Calculation of (a) dynamic compliance, $\triangle V/\triangle P$, at points of zero flow, and (b) total pulmonary resistance, $\triangle P/\triangle \dot{V}$, at points of mid volume.

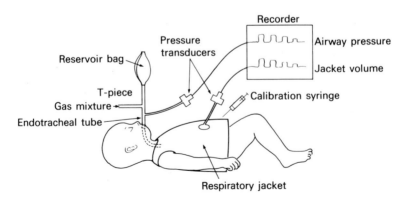

Fig. 5.5 Measurement of static compliance using the respiratory jacket. (Courtesy of B. W. Taylor)

syringe is of limited clinical use because it requires general anaesthesia, muscle relaxation and a non-leaking airway. The use of a respiratory jacket to measure thoracic volume change overcomes these difficulties. The thin-walled rubber jacket covers the chest and abdomen and is inflated to 3 cmH₂O. During quiet breathing, small pressure changes occur in the jacket and these can be calibrated by the injection of known volumes of air from a side-arm syringe. Static compliance is measured by recording changes in thoracic volume when stepwise changes in pressure are applied to the airway. These pressure changes can be applied in apnoeic patients by holding the reservoir bag of a T-piece circuit at a constant pressure for 2 or 3 seconds at the end of each inflation and then allowing the pressure to drop to atmospheric (Fig. 5.5). In spontaneously breathing patients the stepwise pressure change can be produced from a large pressurized reservoir drum. The technique can be used via a tracheal tube or with a face mask or a weighted spirometer. An alternative approach is to use the intermittent occlusion technique during tidal breathing.

Lung volumes

Since compliance and resistance (or, more commonly, its reciprocal conductance) are volume-dependent it is helpful to know the lung volume at which these measurements are made. Values of compliance divided by lung volume are referred to as 'specific compliance'. Lung volume measurements are also valuable in their own right because abnormalities, either reductions or increases, may be of clinical significance. There are two main techniques for the measurement of lung volume.

1. Dilution techniques.   These rely on the dilution of known quantities of an inert gas with the air contained in the lungs. They do not measure any air in the chest which is not in communication with the major air passages. The volume obtained by these measurements is known as the functional residual capacity (FRC). The principal techniques used are the closed circuit helium method and the open circuit nitrogen washout method, both of which have been adapted for use in young children.

2. Whole body plethysmography (Fig. 5.6).   Lung volume is calculated from changes in pressure recorded simultaneously at the mouth and within the plethysmograph when the subject attempts to breathe against a temporary obstruction. The measurement obtained is usually referred to as thoracic gas volume (TGV). Accuracy of the measurement can be improved, particularly in infants with severe airway obstruction or airway closure, by performing airway occlusions at lung volumes above FRC.

Management

In the postoperative or intensive care unit, all newborns are nursed in the neutral thermal environment in an incubator. The benefit of swaddling infants has been described in Chapter 1; this applies even in incubators

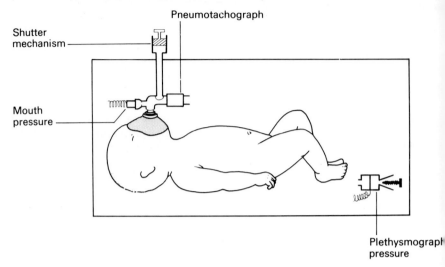

Fig. 5.6 Infant whole body plethysmography.

because, in the UK, the maximum permitted incubator temperature is 36°C. Incubator temperatures can vary considerably around the set point and their performance can be improved by the use of servo-controlled devices. These depend, however, on the skin probe remaining properly attached to the baby, not getting wet and not being covered by anything. Overhead radiant heaters improve access to the baby and can also be servo-controlled, but they increase evaporative water loss. The open type of incubator (e.g. Dräger Babytherm; Fig. 5.7) with an overhead heater of a servo type is more satisfactory for access by the medical and nursing staff and by equipment for phototherapy and portable x-rays. It is suitable for larger newborns whose management after complex surgery involves mechanical ventilation, chest drains, arterial and venous lines and a urinary catheter. Very small babies usually need to be in an enclosed type of incubator (e.g. Vickers; Fig. 5.8) because they require a high neutral thermal environment. A heat shield within the incubator or a sheet of 'bubble mat' (Sancell) over the baby is additional protection. Servo-control mechanisms theoretically may deprive the physician of the clinical information derived from changes in the infant's skin temperature, but in practice the difference between core and peripheral temperatures is still a good guide to cardiac output—the normal difference being 2°C.

Modern intensive care incubators incorporate alarm systems for temperature of the air and the baby, optional monitors for oxygen concentration and weighing scales so that the baby can be weighed while remaining inside the incubator.

Apnoeic episodes in susceptible infants should be anticipated by nursing the baby using an apnoea alarm. Apnoea mattresses are available which work on the principle that respiratory movements are transmitted to a segmented, air-filled mattress and air movement from one segment to an-

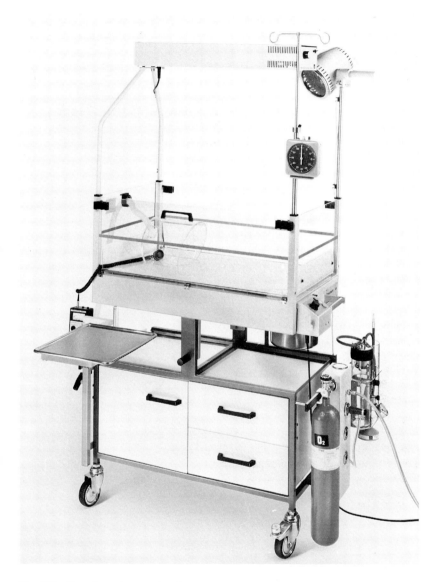

Fig. 5.7 Open intensive care incubator with overhead heater. (Dräger Babytherm)

other is detected. These mattresses are successful, although they give many false negative and positive alarms. They may detect struggling as a respiratory movement as well as failing to detect apnoea of up to 10 seconds, especially if the alarm is detecting the heart beat because the baby is incorrectly placed. Transthoracic impedance types of monitor using ECG leads

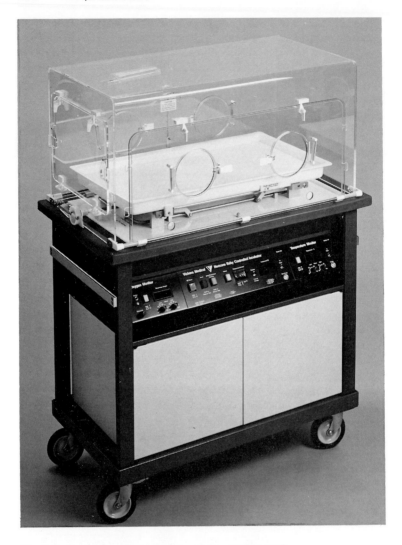

Fig. 5.8   Enclosed intensive care incubator. (Vickers Ltd)

are also successful, but the electrodes may fall off. A third type of apnoea alarm detects changes in the curvature of the abdominal wall.

ECG monitoring with a rate counter, soft bleep and alarm system is essential for all sick babies.

Other intensive care monitoring includes core and peripheral temperatures, arterial pressure either directly with an arterial line or indirectly using an automatic blood-pressure measuring device and central venous pressure.

Oxygen therapy

An increased inspired oxygen concentration is necessary for many babies postoperatively—after thoracotomy or major abdominal surgery, after large blood transfusions or if respiratory distress is present. An oxygen headbox is necessary to achieve accurate and steady concentrations of oxygen over 25% in an incubator (Fig. 5.9). The concentration should be measured using an independent oxygen analyser of the fuel cell sensor type. The resultant Pa_{O_2} or Tc P_{O_2} should be measured. The gases should be fully humidified to about 34°C (at least 95 per cent saturated) using a heated water-bath

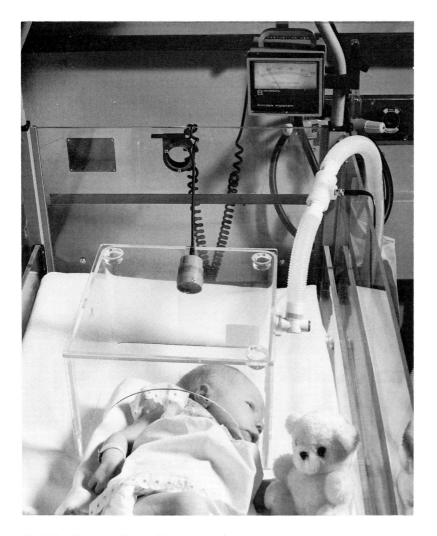

Fig. 5.9   Plastic head box with oxygen analyser.

type of humidifier at a flow of 6 l·min^{-1} to prevent accumulation of carbon dioxide within the headbox. A servo-controlled type of humidifier (e.g. Bennett Cascade Mark II) which meets all electrical safety requirements is satisfactory if the temperature probe is close to the baby but not within the incubator. One disadvantage with this type of humidifier is that if the gas flow is increased from a previously steady state, the baby will be exposed to gas hotter than is desirable. The contents of the bowl are usually maintained at a temperature which is 'self-pasteurizing', but the bowl should be exchanged for a sterile one every 24–48 hours. If cold oxygen is used, there will be stimulation of the trigeminal area of the face and an undesirable increase in metabolic oxygen demand.

Ultrasonic nebulizers are not commonly used for the newborn because they produce a very fine cold mist which may overhydrate the baby. They tend to be more expensive and are more difficult to sterilize between cases. If such a humidifier is used a water gain of at least 2 ml·kg^{-1}·h^{-1} should be included in the fluid balance.

High inspired oxygen concentrations are used as necessary to give as normal a Pao_2 as possible, although not if the low Pao_2 is caused by a fixed intracardiac right-to-left shunt as in transposition of the great arteries (TGA) or pulmonary valve atresia.

Infants of less than 36 weeks' gestational age are at risk from retinopathy of prematurity (cicatricial retrolental fibroplasia) caused by the vasoconstrictive effects in the preterm retinal vessels of high Pao_2. The safe level of Pao_2 and duration of effect are unknown but it is wisest to aim for a value between 9.3 and 10.7 kPa (70–80 mmHg). Other factors such as blood flow, the level of adult haemoglobin, temperature, haematocrit and metabolic activity must operate because the condition is reported in patients who have never received an increased inspired oxygen concentration and also in patients with cyanotic congenital heart disease. A retinal examination should be undertaken by an ophthalmologist before discharge from hospital for all preterm patients who have received oxygen therapy.

Bronchopulmonary dysplasia (BPD)

BPD (ventilator lung) is a progressive fibrocystic destruction of the lung architecture associated with intubation, oxygen therapy and mechanical ventilation, and occurs especially in preterm newborns with surfactant deficiency or pulmonary hypoplasia. It can be diagnosed with confidence if the chest x-ray changes of cystic infiltration and streaky fibrosis are seen (Fig. 5.10). High inspired oxygen concentrations are implicated in the production of this lung damage, but BPD is probably caused by several factors such as high ventilatory pressures, high inspired oxygen concentrations, poor mucociliary function and chronic infection. Prolonged alveolar concentrations in excess of 60% oxygen are causal, although the relative importance of each of the factors is unknown. With BPD, as destruction of lung architecture progresses there is a need for increasing inspired oxygen concentrations and airway pressures, causing a vicious cycle which may end in death or cor pulmonale unless the factors causing the BPD can be

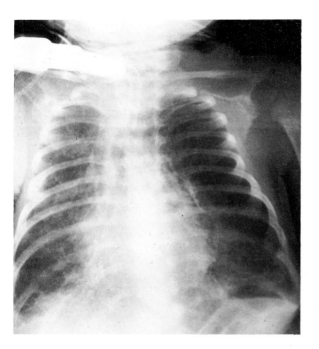

Fig. 5.10 Bronchopulmonary dysplasia. X-ray showing grossly overinflated lungs and evidence of severe parenchymal damage.

minimized. It is possible that all small babies sustain some degree of lung damage however they are ventilated, even with modern infant ventilators. Recovery tends to be rather slow, but, because of the great capacity of the infant lung to regenerate, the condition is not usually fatal. The administration of vitamin E may help to protect against oxygen toxicity. A high pulmonary blood flow, for example, with a patent ductus arteriosus increases the risk of BPD.

Nasotracheal intubation

If the infant is to be intubated postoperatively for IPPV or CPAP, it is better to change the tube from an orotracheal to a nasotracheal one for what may be prolonged respiratory support. Nasal tubes are preferred for long-term intubation because the fixation is more secure, there is greater comfort for the patient and ease of nursing, which includes improved mouth care, and also allows the infant to suck. The oral fixation which may be associated with dental, palatal and tracheal damage is certainly unsuitable for prolonged intubation after the immediate neonatal period. Prolonged nasotracheal intubation for respiratory support is now a well-accepted technique for all age groups in paediatric practice.

A technique of fixation using a Tunstall connector and an Oxford swivel (Figs. 5.11 and 5.12) has been in use at the Hospital for Sick Children,

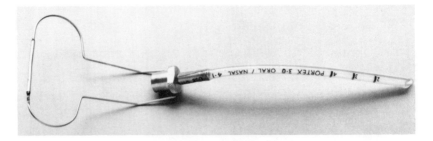

Fig. 5.11   Plain Portex tube with Tunstall connector.

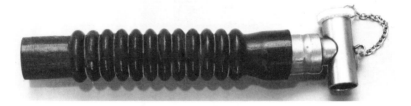

Fig. 5.12   Catheter mount with Oxford swivel connector.

London, for 15 years with great success. The tube should be radio-opaque, have clear centimetre graduations and a Murphy 'eye' to overcome inadvertent obstruction of the bevel of the tube by the side wall of the trachea. Shouldered tubes of the Cole type are not used because they have significantly greater resistance to gas flow caused by turbulence at the shoulder and are associated with an incidence of laryngeal damage.

   With the oral tracheal tube still in place and an assistant ventilating the baby, an uncut 3 mm (or 2.5 mm) plain PVC (tissue tested) nasotracheal tube is lubricated and passed through the nares as far as the glottis. This is done using a laryngoscope. The tracheal tube is cut to the desired length so that its tip lies midway between the glottis and the carina—an extra 3 cm on the length of the tube. A Tunstall connection or similar device is fixed into the nasal tube and, as the oral tube is removed by the assistant, the nasal one is inserted through the glottis using intubating forceps and then secured as shown in Fig. 5.13. Auscultation should reveal bilateral air entry and a check chest x-ray should show the tip of the tracheal tube lying in the midpoint of the trachea. The correct size of tracheal tube is that which allows normal controlled ventilation with the application of constant distending pressure if this is required, but which also allows a slight air leak at an airway pressure of 25–30 cmH$_2$O (Table 5.2). The leak must be present at all times and checked daily. If the leak disappears (subglottic oedema), this is an indication for the tracheal tube to be changed to one a size smaller (not smaller than 2.5 mm internal diameter). It is our practice to change the tube from one nostril to the other every 10 days to preserve the symmetry

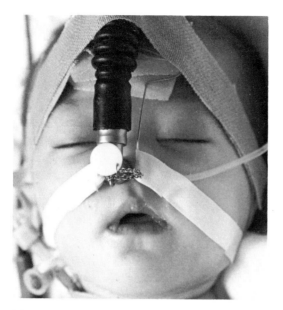

(a)

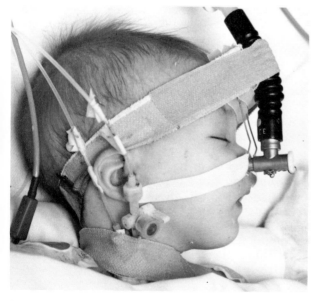

(b)

Fig. 5.13   Nasotracheal intubation using the Tunstall connector with secondary fixation to the forehead.

Table 5.2   Nasal tracheal tube sizes for newborns

Patient's weight (kg)	Tube size (i.d.) (mm)	Tube length (cm)
0.7–1.0	2.5	8.5– 9.0
1.0–1.5	2.5	9.0– 9.5
1.5–2.0	3.0	9.5–10.0
2.0–2.5	3.0	10.0–10.5
2.5–3.0	3.0	10.5–11.0

of the nostrils and to prevent pressure sores. After this length of time, the plastic of the tube hardens as plasticizers are leached out. Small rings of Stomadhesive around the tube prevent pressure of the tube and connector on the nares.

Earlier changing of the tube may be necessary in patients with low cardiac output or cyanotic congenital heart disease, as ulceration occurs more commonly in these patients.

With meticulous care it is possible to use tracheal tubes for respiratory support for prolonged periods with a very low complication rate.

All the complications of prolonged tracheal intubation are avoidable.

1. *Dislodgement* by accident is prevented by firm fixation of the tube which is of the correct length. Secondary fixation of a short catheter-mount to the forehead prevents traction on the ventilator tubing being directly transmitted to the tracheal tube. Such an accident need not be a disaster in a good intensive care unit if the problem is recognized promptly. Dislodgement is less likely to occur if the patient is maintained in a lightly sedated state.

2. *Blockage* of the tube by inspissated secretions is prevented by humidification of the inspired gases to full saturation at a temperature approaching that of the body (35–44 mg of water vapour per litre gas flow at $37°C = 80–100\%$ relative humidity). Most commercial humidifiers do not come up to these standards, and some of the water vapour condenses in the patient tubing. We thus find it necessary to instill 0.5 ml physiological saline down the tracheal tube every 30 minutes, followed by suction with a sterile soft rubber catheter. Suctioning is potentially hazardous, as it may introduce infection; disposable gloves should be worn and a sterile technique used. It may also cause dangerous hypoxia because ventilation is discontinued and intrapulmonary oxygen concentration is reduced to a degree proportional to the length of time suctioning takes place and the negative pressure is applied, and is greater than with an equal length of time of apnoea. Suction pressure should be limited to 100–150 mmHg and suction time to 15 seconds with suction taking place only on withdrawal of the catheter. Techniques do exist whereby suctioning can take place while IPPV continues and negative pressure is minimized in the airways if the diameter of the suction catheter does not exceed 70 per cent of the tracheal tube diameter—this is difficult when small tubes are used. Suction can also cause traumatic lesions of the tracheal mucosa, but these are minimized if soft catheters with an end hole (not whistle-tip) are used. The nursing staff should always know the exact length of the tracheal tube and ensure that

the suction catheter passed is longer than this, otherwise secretions at the tracheal end of the tube may not be reached.

3. *Subglottic stenosis* is potentially the most serious long-term complication; it is entirely avoidable by ensuring that the tube is never too tight in the subglottic cricoid ring of cartilage so that there is a demonstrable air leak between the tube and the mucosa at all times. Pressure on the mucosa causes necrosis and ulceration which eventually heals with fibrous stricture. When the trachea is intubated for infective lesions in older infants, such as laryngotracheobronchitis, or acute epiglottitis, exactly the same criteria are used for sizing the tracheal tube, although usually a tube considerably smaller than normal is needed to achieve the mandatory leak. In our series of 5000 babies and children with prolonged intubation over the past 10 years there has been no case of subglottic stenosis.

4. *Post-extubation stridor* occurs rarely and is most commonly seen after short intubations (24-36 hours) or in patients with Down's syndrome. Very rarely does the condition require reintubation, but usually responds to dexamethasone $0.25\,mg\cdot kg^{-1}$ i.v. followed by $0.1\,mg\cdot kg^{-1}$ i.m. 6-hourly for 12 hours. If a baby does need to be reintubated for laryngeal oedema a tube 0.5 mm smaller should be used.

5. *Nasal ulcers* may occur even with careful techniques. These heal normally if the tube is changed to the other nostril.

Suctioning and instillations of saline take the place of natural expulsion of secretions by mucociliary activity and coughing. Intubated patients should also receive chest physiotherapy 2- to 4-hourly as a prophylactic measure, and all the techniques of physiotherapy—vibration, percussion, manual lung expansion—are applicable to the neonate, although care must be taken in patients whose cardiac function is poor, as a fall in Pao_2 may cause a further fall in cardiac output. An electric toothbrush may be used for vibration of consolidated lobes, and manual ventilation with air or oxygen with a few sustained breaths of $25\,cmH_2O$ pressure will expand alveoli collapsed by suction or atelectasis associated with secretions.

There is no place for bronchoscopy for removal of secretions or for treatment of lobar collapse. These conditions are more safely dealt with by intubation and physiotherapy.

Because of the *very* low morbidity of tracheal intubation in all sizes of neonates it is our practice to institute mechanical ventilation only after the patient has been intubated. This is not necessarily the practice in other centres where babies are ventilated with tightly fitting face masks or through a nasal prong. This is possible only if pulmonary compliance is near normal and ventilating pressures are low. Securing the airway with a tube has the additional advantage of allowing full tracheal toilet.

Tracheostomy

Tracheostomy is usually preferred when an artificial airway is required for more than a few weeks. It is our practice to resort to tracheostomy if, after 4-6 weeks of intubation, there is no sign that this can be discontinued in the foreseeable future. Tracheostomy is more convenient for the nursing staff and enables the patient to become more mobile and more easily stimulated. There is a lower resistance to gas flow and occasionally after tracheostomy, a patient previously dependent on mechanical ventilation will begin to be weaned from full respiratory support.

Mechanical ventilation

Most mechanical ventilators which can deliver a low flow rate are suitable for paediatric use, and success often depends more on the skill and judgement of the medical and nursing staff than on the characteristics of a particular machine. Major criteria for the choice of ventilator must include reliability, an efficient humidifier, accurate control of inspired oxygen concentration, a reliable and effective alarm system and ease of sterilization both during and after its use. All parts of the patient circuit, including those within the machine, should be autoclavable and sets of patient-tubing be available to change every 48 hours. For infected patients a bacteriological filter for expired gases minimizes dispersion of bacteria to the atmosphere of the intensive care unit. The Siemens Servo range is suitable for newborns but the most satisfactory are the new generation of infant ventilators based on the T-occluding principle with facilities designed to minimize the factors causing BPD. *The art of mechanical ventilation and the design of specialized infant ventilators have the same basic aim—that of minimizing this lung damage.*

Examples of these machines include Bourn BP 200, Bear Cub, 2001, Vickers Neovent, Dräger Babylog, and these are generally suitable for infants up to 10 kg body weight (Fig. 5.14). These pressure-generating machines cope with small leaks in the circuitry, but not with situations of changing compliance. Tidal volume becomes a function of the *preset* peak inspiratory pressure and the pulmonary compliance (Fig. 5.15). Thus the tidal volume is the variable and, although not usually directly monitored, it must be indirectly assessed by frequent arterial $Paco_2$ estimations or the use of a transcutaneous CO_2 electrode. Peak inspiratory pressure is easy to control and square wave ventilation with effective pressures is easy to produce. The Siemens Servo 900 range is also suitable for small babies (Fig. 5.16). The minute volume is preset so that peak pressure is a variable depending on lung compliance.

Modern infant ventilators have a variety of facilities which help to minimize bronchopulmonary dysplasia, as discussed below.

Alveolar ventilation tends to be optimal when patients are ventilated at rates lower than their spontaneous breathing rate and the Pao_2 may increase if the ventilator rate is reduced. Initially the rate is set at 30, but the machines have the facility for higher rates (e.g. up to 150 per minute) to be used as a means of reducing damaging peak pressures. The rate must be related to the inspiratory/expiratory time ratio; otherwise, insufficient time is available for expiration if the respiratory rate is too high.

Very high frequency IPPV using oscillations up to 20 Hz is still largely experimental but would be used for the same purpose of preventing baro-

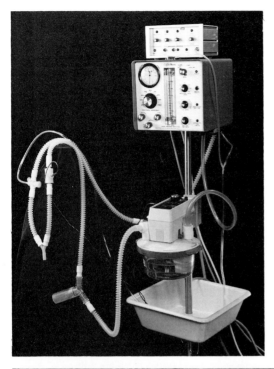

(a)

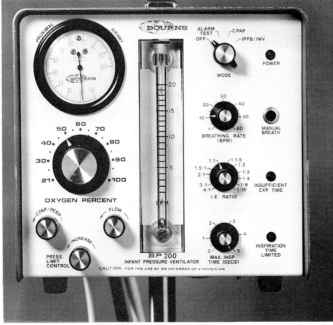

(b)

Fig. 5.14   Bourn BP 200 infant ventilator.

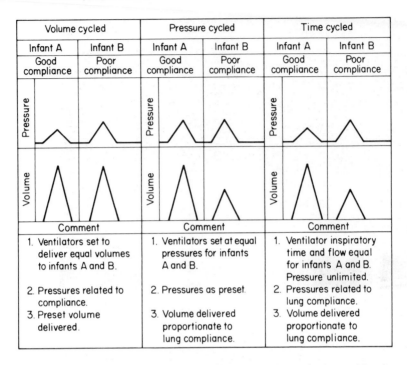

Volume cycled		Pressure cycled		Time cycled	
Infant A	Infant B	Infant A	Infant B	Infant A	Infant B
Good compliance	Poor compliance	Good compliance	Poor compliance	Good compliance	Poor compliance

Comment	Comment	Comment
1. Ventilators set to deliver equal volumes to infants A and B.	1. Ventilators set at equal pressures for infants A and B.	1. Ventilator inspiratory time and flow equal for infants A and B. Pressure unlimited.
2. Pressures related to compliance.	2. Pressures as preset.	2. Pressures related to lung compliance.
3. Preset volume delivered.	3. Volume delivered proportionate to lung compliance.	3. Volume delivered proportionate to lung compliance.

Fig. 5.15 The effect of pulmonary compliance on pressure and volume with volume-, pressure- and time-cycled ventilators. (Reproduced, with permission from Goldsmith and Karotkin 1981)

trauma to the lungs. Such oscillation must work by enhancing gas diffusion rather than bulk delivery of gases to the alveoli.

The mean airway pressure (MAP), which is the mean pressure transmitted to the airway over a series of respiratory cycles, has a direct relationship to gas exchange. MAP is represented by the area under the curve of inspiratory and expiratory pressure (Fig. 5.17). Machines should have the facility for increasing MAP by the techniques of: (1) increasing inspiratory flow rate to give a square wave pattern, (2) increasing peak inspiratory pressure, (3) reversing inspiratory to expiratory time (I/E) ratio and (4) increasing positive end-expiratory pressure.

1. *A square wave form* is probably better for small babies with stiff lungs, especially those with RDS, and is a way of increasing MAP without resorting to increasing peak pressure.

2. *Peak pressure* may need to be increased to improve gas exchange, but levels greater than 25–30 cmH$_2$O are implicated in producing lung damage.

3. *Reversal of I/E ratio* from 1:1 to 2:1 increases MAP and is useful in improving gas exchange with the stiff lungs of RDS. The facility for changing I/E ratio must be available, but it does not have universal application as Pao_2 may fall, as may cardiac output by a decrease in venous return (Table 5.3). Very little of the mean increased intrapulmonary pressure is

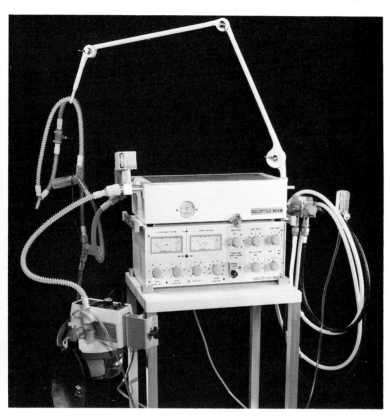

Fig. 5.16 Siemens Servo 900B ventilator.

transferred to the mediastinum, when the lungs are stiff, so little effect on
the cardiac output is to be expected. As the lungs improve, the mean
intrathoracic pressure must be reduced. Alterations in I/E ratio may allow
the inspired oxygen concentration to be reduced to potentially less dangerous levels. The optimal I/E ratio is unpredictable, the optimal being found
by blood gas analysis; 1:1 is the usual starting figure for infants. During a
recovery phase of respiratory disease a reversed I/E ratio should be returned
to normal, avoiding air trapping as compliance improves.

4. A ventilator must have the facility for *application of PEEP* (this is the
accepted term for constant distending pressure applied during controlled
ventilation). The ability of a constant distending pressure to improve arterial oxygenation at a given inspired oxygen concentration depends on the
relationship between functional residual capacity (FRC) and the closing
volume (CV) in the lungs. When CV exceeds FRC, airway closure occurs
during tidal breathing (as in young children). This increases both right-to-
left intrapulmonary shunting and the alveolar–arterial oxygen gradient (A–
aDO_2). The effect is greater in pathological states of the lung associated with

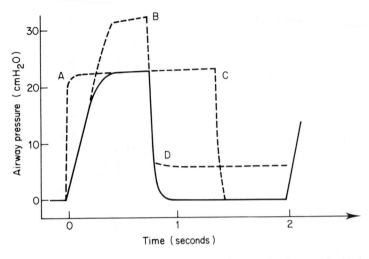

Fig. 5.17   Increases in mean airway pressure (area under the graph) with A, square wave form; B, increasing peak airway pressure; C, reversed I/E ratio; and D, constant distending pressure. (Reproduced, with permission from Goldsmith and Karotkin 1981)

fluid retention. With the application of a constant distending pressure, alveoli in the mid-region of the lungs open (those in the dependent parts of the lungs are already maximally taking part in ventilation), thus increasing FRC in relation to CV, decreasing intrapulmonary shunting, and decreasing $A-aDO_2$ (so-called alveolar recruitment). Early application of constant distending pressure to neonatal lungs affected by hyaline membrane disease improves gas exchange and may decrease the severity of the disease by reducing surfactant consumption. The net effect of PEEP on oxygen delivery to the tissues is variable and depends on a balance of factors, including possible reduction of the cardiac output in hypovolaemic patients or after cardiac surgery. Levels of PEEP up to 8–10 cmH2O are used in an

Table 5.3   The effect of reversal of the I/E ratio on oxygenation

	Hyaline membrane disease (age 1 day)		Bronchopulmonary dysplasia (age 4 months)	
Time	15.00	16.00	11.45	12.57
I/E	1 : 2	2 : 1	1 : 2	2 : 1
F_{IO_2}	1.0	1.0	0.55	0.55
Frequency	36	36	30	30
pH	7.05	7.25	7.33	7.27
P_{aCO_2}	9.3 kPa (70 mmHg)	5.1 kPa (38 mmHg)	5.9 kPa (44 mmHg)	6.5 kPa (49 mmHg)
Base excess	−15.9	−12	−3.5	−6.3
P_{aO_2}	2.0 kPa (15 mmHg)	8.0 kPa (60 mmHg)	14 kPa (105 mmHg)	7.2 kPa (54 mmHg)

attempt to lower the required inspired oxygen concentration. It is suggested that PEEP settings may parallel Fio_2 requirements so that an infant on 80% oxygen for pulmonary reasons needs $8 cmH_2O$ PEEP, 90% $9 cmH_2O$, and 100% $10 cmH_2O$ PEEP. Overinflation of areas in the lung already fully inflated will increase pulmonary vascular resistance by compression of the capillary bed. An increase in PVR over systemic will cause hypoxaemia, which may explain why Pao_2 may fall with the application of PEEP. PEEP is usually contraindicated in patients with low pulmonary blood flow (e.g. pulmonary atresia) or if the blood flow is borderline (e.g. after the Fontan operation) or with hypovolaemia or low cardiac output. Higher levels of PEEP increase the risk of alveolar rupture and tension pneumothorax.

The level of PEEP is maintained until the Fio_2 is less than 60 per cent and at this stage the pressure is gradually reduced to a level of $4-5 cmH_2O$ so that weaning from the ventilator may begin.

Intermittent mandatory ventilation (IMV)

Neonatal ventilators should now be fitted with integral CPAP mechanisms to facilitate the weaning process, and indeed most use IMV (see below). This mode involves mandatory lung inflations provided by the ventilator at preset tidal volumes, in between which the patient breathes spontaneously at constant distending pressure. As the patient improves, it is possible to decrease gradually the number of mandatory breaths until ventilatory support is completely withdrawn. The patient is then breathing from a CPAP circuit. This method of weaning is a great advance, allowing as it does a gradual transition from mechanical ventilation to spontaneous breathing and is very convenient, but it may not decrease the actual time of weaning. An IMV system ideally has a continuous fresh gas flow so no extra work of breathing is involved. The long response time of the ventilator and tubing and the large inspired volume necessary make the demand type (e.g. Servo 900B or C) unsuitable for infants. It is possible to convert such a system into a continuous flow type by providing a parallel fresh gas flow to the inspiratory circuit using a one-way valve and a reservoir bag (Fig. 5.18).

Principles of mechanical ventilation

There is no rigid technique for applying mechanical ventilation to infants and no wide agreement as to which technique is the most effective. Ventilator settings based on body weight or surface area are of little practical help because they take no account of reduced pulmonary compliance nor of the internal compliance of the tubing and humidifier unit.

With pressure preset infant ventilators, the peak pressure is set at $25 cmH_2O$ for patients with stiff lungs, but a setting of 15 is more appropriate if the compliance is normal. The rate is set at 25–30 per minute and an initial I/E ratio of 1:1 with inspiratory time at 1 second and PEEP at $4-5 cmH_2O$ with inspired oxygen concentration set at the level necessary before IPPV was started. It is an advantage to display the pressure trace to see what has been achieved in terms of wave form and I/E ratio.

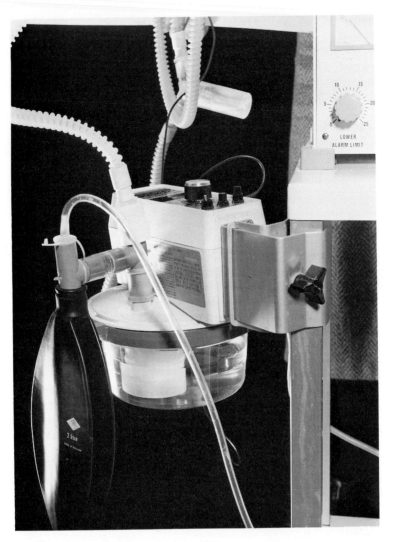

Fig. 5.18 IMV valve for use with the Siemens Servo 900B or C ventilators to provide a continuous fresh gas flow.

A preset tidal volume of $8-10\,ml\cdot kg^{-1}$ is set for flow-generating, volume-preset machines such as the Servo range.

Observation of chest movement and auscultation of lung fields give a good guide to the adequacy of ventilation, but direct measurement of arterial P_{CO_2} and P_{O_2} is absolutely essential to the establishment and maintenance of patients on respiratory support. All patients should have an arterial line for blood gas analysis during institution of mechanical ventilation. All other non-invasive monitoring such as end-tidal CO_2, transcutaneous O_2 and CO_2 electrodes must be regularly calibrated against the results of arterial blood gas analysis.

If there is potential for normal oxygenation, Fio_2 should be maintained at a level to give a Pao_2 of approximately 13.3 kPa (100 mmHg). Preterm babies are at risk from retinopathy of prematurity before full vascularization of the retina has taken place. The fetal retina is normally supplied by blood of low Pao_2 so 8-10.7 kPa (60-80 mmHg) is the optimal Pao_2 for the preterm baby.

A $Paco_2$ of 4.7-5.1 kPa (35-38 mmHg) is satisfactory if this is easily achieved with reasonable peak inflation pressures. Greater hyperventilation is used only in an attempt to overcome transitional circulation in the neonate or a pulmonary hypertensive crisis after open heart surgery or to reduce intracranial hypertension.

Ventilator settings of rate, wave form, inspiratory pause, expiratory times and distending pressure are adjusted to achieve optimal alveolar ventilation and gas exchange at *minimal* mean airway pressure and inspired oxygen concentration.

Most babies can be ventilated using simple sedatives if the blood gases and pH are normal and the patients are otherwise comfortable (Table 5.4).

Table 5.4   Suitable drugs for use in ventilated infants

Morphine	0.2 mg·kg^{-1} i.v. as necessary or *infusion* 2 ml·h^{-1} i.v. of 0.5 mg·kg^{-1} in 50 ml 5% dextrose
Diazepam	0.2 mg·kg^{-1} i.v. as necessary
Chloral hydrate	30 mg·kg^{-1} via nasogastric tube as necessary
Pancuronium	0.1 mg·kg^{-1} i.v. as necessary

Mild hyperventilation helps to reduce the drive to spontaneous ventilation in many patients in addition to the administration of small doses of sedative drugs. However, small babies with severe respiratory disease who need limitation of peak airway pressure and changes in I/E ratio and who otherwise would not be controlled require muscle relaxants to obtund damaging respiratory effort. Such patients include those with lung hypoplasia (congenital diaphragmatic hernia), transitional circulation, severe RDS and those with a low cardiac output. Pancuronium 0.1 mg·kg^{-1} i.v. may be given as necessary.

A circuit for manual ventilation, such as an anaesthetic T-piece, with a supply of pure oxygen must be available for each patient on mechanical ventilation, so that if machine failure occurs, the intensive care nurse can ventilate the patient by hand until the machine fault is rectified.

Pollitzer et al. (1981) give evidence that gas exchange is improved in paralysed patients and the risks of producing BDP are minimized.

Paralysed patients must also be sedated; an infusion of morphine is suitable.

Weaning

All therapy (which includes antibiotics, diuretics, bronchodilators and physiotherapy) of ventilated patients is aimed at achieving cardiovascular, biochemical and neurological stability. When Pa_{CO_2} is less than 6.7 kPa (50 mmHg) and Pa_{O_2} more than 10.7 kPa (80 mmHg) at an Fi_{O_2} of 0.5 with peak inflation pressures less than 25 cmH$_2$O, weaning from the ventilator may begin.

Full cardiac output is necessary to support spontaneous ventilation so that if the patient needs, for example, dopamine 6 μg·kg^{-1}·min^{-1} or less, this is not a contraindication to weaning, rather the reverse. The pH must be normal with a normal Pa_{CO_2}, as a baby will hypoventilate to the point of apnoea to compensate for a metabolic alkalosis as seen, for example, with hypokalaemia. The continuing need for high airways pressure and high Fi_{O_2} are discouraging signs.

It is important not to leave babies breathing through a tracheal tube without end-expiratory pressure, particularly those with low pulmonary compliance. Zero end-expiratory pressure allows the stiff lungs to collapse progressively so that closing volume encroaches further on the FRC with increasing right-to-left intrapulmonary shunting and hypoxaemia. As lung volume falls, airways resistance to gas flow rises, increasing the work of breathing and the oxygen consumption. This will increase any hypoxia already present. With a tracheal tube in place, the normal glottic mechanism whereby an infant can generate 2–3 cmH$_2$O end-expiratory pressure is lost. The grunting, so characteristic of infants with respiratory distress, is thought to be an attempt to overcome the cause of the distress by delaying alveolar emptying and minimizing the time during which airway closure can occur.

Sedation should not be withheld from children before weaning starts, as a well sedated baby is more likely to accept the change from controlled to spontaneous breathing than one who is restless. The non-respiratory depressant drugs such as chloral hydrate are ideal for this purpose. IMV, with gradual withdrawal of respiratory support, is most satisfactory, usually starting with 15 breaths; babies who need more than 20 IMV breaths are probably not yet ready to wean. Distending pressure helps to maintain FRC during spontaneous breathing and minimizes the work of breathing and oxygen consumption by reducing the resistance of the airways to gas flow. Ventilation is shifted to a higher point in the pressure/volume curve, thus increasing FRC and oxygenation (Fig. 5.19). The clinical signs of adequacy of respiratory function, such as low and steady respiratory rate and absence of intercostal retractions, are the most helpful guide with blood gas analysis to confirm clinical impressions. The blood gas data can be within normal limits when the work of breathing is judged to be unacceptably high.

Weaning may be a protracted affair if the lungs are infected, if there is significant cardiac failure, a high pulmonary blood flow, pulmonary vascular disease or if bronchopulmonary dysplasia has developed. The rate of reduction of IMV depends entirely on the response and clinical state of the patient. Extubation is considered when the IMV has been withdrawn and the patient has been breathing with CPAP for a length of time (usually overnight), with a low respiratory rate and minimal secretions and satisfac-

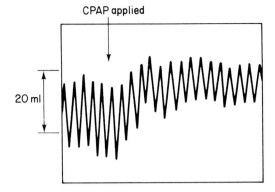

Fig. 5.19 Change in FRC when a distending pressure of 1 kPa (10 cmH₂O) is applied. (Reproduced, with permission, from Hatch, 1981)

tory levels of Pao_2 and $Paco_2$ with inspired oxygen concentration below 40%.

Constant positive airway pressure (CPAP)

Also known as constant distending pressure during spontaneous ventilation, this is now always used for weaning small patients from ventilators and also for respiratory support in some patients who do not need mechanical ventilation. CPAP may be delivered via a nasotracheal tube, one nasal prong, a face mask or a head box with a tight seal around the neck as originally described by Gregory *et al.* (1971). All methods have advantages and disadvantages, so the choice often depends on the practice in a particular centre. CPAP can be delivered from the circuit of a mechanical ventilator or from either a modified T-piece circuit as in (Fig. 5.20) or a modified Bain system which relies on a fresh gas flow of three times the patient's minute volume. On the expiratory side, a water manometer is used to read the pressure and as a safety 'blow-off' value to prevent excessive pressures developing. A reservoir bag with a controlled leak acts to smooth the level of pressure and prevents gross fluctuations within the system.

A distending pressure of 6–8 cmH₂O is suitable to begin with, although this is gradually reduced in a stepwise fashion after the inspired oxygen concentration has been reduced to 40% or lower. Patients are extubated from levels of 3 cmH₂O CPAP. The incidence of pneumothorax with high levels of CPAP is estimated to be as high as 6 per cent, and suitable equipment for relief of pneumothorax must be at hand. Transillumination of the thorax using a fibrelight lead is a useful technique for immediate diagnosis of a pneumothorax. In an emergency, a short needle should be inserted into the pleural cavity through the second intercostal space in the midclavicular line and the air aspirated. A formal chest drain should then be inserted and connected to an underwater seal.

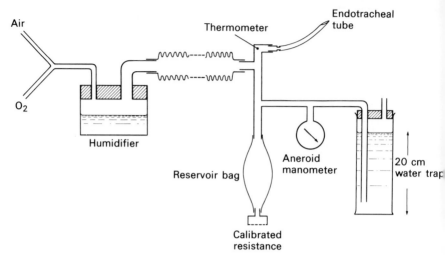

Fig. 5.20   Modified T-piece circuit used for application of CPAP. (Reproduced, with permission, from Hatch *et al.*, 1973)

Patients with poor lung compliance may be dependent on CPAP, and this may be continued after extubation using one nasal prong (Fig. 5.21). After extubation there may be temporary incompetence of the larynx and impaired ciliary function. Pulmonary atelectasis is very common, and repeated intubation may be required for physiotherapy and suction. Occasionally, temporary support with CPAP via the nasal prong is needed until the competence of the glottis is restored.

CPAP via a nasal prong is commonly used to treat moderate to severe apnoea of prematurity. The increased oxygenation and stimulation of chest wall stretch receptors reduce the intensity and frequency of the apnoeic

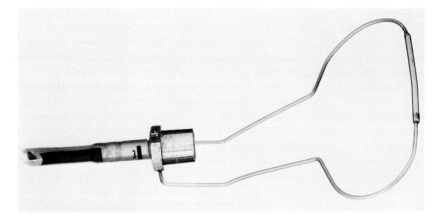

Fig. 5.21   Nasal prong for the administration of PEEP.

attacks. CPAP pressures greater than $10\,cmH_2O$ are not recommended, and unsatisfactory clinical and blood gas state (e.g. Pao_2 less than $6.7\,kPa$ ($50\,mmHg$) on 100% O_2) at this level of pressure are indications for intubation and mechanical ventilation.

Intensive care for cerebral protection

The infant brain may be subject to a variety of insults in the early days of life which may prejudice complete recovery of the baby from other major pathology. Neurological damage may be the limiting factor in successful recovery from birth asphyxia, neonatal sepsis or major surgery. Up to 40 per cent of preterm babies may have neurological handicap, although many of these are slight.

Cerebral damage may occur directly from birth asphyxia, low cardiac output states, prolonged acidosis and hypoglycaemia. Indirect damage occurs following intraventricular haemorrhage (IVH) when ventricular enlargement ensues, which is not usually seen as clinical hydrocephalus in the early stages.

Cerebral oedema following the primary insult may cause secondary damage to brain cells by a compression effect within the rigid cranium. In older children and adults this is seen as cerebral oedema with the CT scan and raised intracranial pressure (ICP) with direct monitoring of ICP which is now routine in most intensive care units. Newborns have a very flexible skull, so rises of ICP secondary to a primary insult such as hypoxia are not as great and there is no indication for direct measurement of ICP in the newborn. Papilloedema is a very late sign of increased ICP, occurring up to 48 hours after CT has shown cerebral oedema.

A cerebral insult is manifest clinically by seizures, which should be immediately brought under control as the seizures themselves may cause further cerebral damage. A lumbar puncture examination is performed for any patient with seizures. IVH is now readily diagnosed at the bedside by sonoencephalography, and this is performed routinely in preterm babies at risk from IVH. Real-time ultrasound gives a very good image of the neonatal brain. The risk factors associated with IVH are discussed on p. 24; they include prematurity, maternal bleeding, birth asphyxia, hypercarbia, metabolic acidosis and, possibly, the administration of hyperosmolar sodium bicarbonate. It is likely that the autoregulation of cerebral blood flow is inactivated by a period of hypoxia, and during this time IVH is possible. IVH is graded according to severity in order to establish a relationship between this and the degree of neurodevelopmental handicap which will be manifest later in life.

It is hoped that a series of intensive care manoeuvres to maintain oxygenation, prevent brain swelling and control seizures may reduce this incidence of handicap.

The EEG is used to detect seizures in a very sedated or paralysed baby and also to help in the diagnosis of brain death by the use of auditory evoked potentials.

The babies are mechanically ventilated and paralysed to establish normal oxygenation and a Pa_{CO_2} between 3.3 and 4 kPa (25–30 mmHg) to reduce cerebral oedema. Lower Pa_{CO_2} increases the possibility of cerebral ischaemia by vasoconstriction. Seizures are controlled by phenobarbitone 10 mg·kg^{-1} followed 6 hours later by 10 mg·kg^{-1}·24 h^{-1} in two doses, to maintain a serum barbiturate level of 50–80 μmol·l^{-1}. Phenobarbitone is a very long-acting drug in the newborn and its sedative and respiratory depressant effects may be seen for several days after the last dose. A normal cardiac output is maintained first with plasma or blood to give a normal cardiac filling pressure. If the systemic blood pressure and peripheral temperature are low then dopamine 2–5 μg·kg^{-1}·min^{-1} is indicated. A bleeding tendency is treated with fresh blood or blood products such as fresh-frozen plasma and platelet concentrate. Hydrocephalus may be treated by multiple tapping of the ventricles through the anterior fontanelle.

Maintenance fluids are restricted, and frusemide, up to 1 mg·kg^{-1} i.v. 12-hourly, is used to increase plasma osmolality (not more than 320 mmol.l^{-1}), which decreases cerebral water. Dexamethasone 0.25 mg·kg^{-1} i.v. 6-hourly may reduce cerebral oedema by stabilizing membranes and decreasing CSF production.

If seizures still persist then diazepam in doses of 0.2 mg·kg^{-1} i.v. should bring them under control. The claim that barbiturates have a particular role in cerebral protection is largely based on animal work. This is controversial, and higher doses of barbiturates may cause a fall in cardiac output and thus reduce cerebral perfusion pressure. They do, however, reduce cerebral metabolism and control seizures, dramatically reduce intracranial hypertension and generally make the central nervous system unresponsive. Barbiturates may also scavenge certain free radicals which are released after neuronal ischaemia and which may destroy mitochondrial membranes.

After 24–36 hours of stability without seizures it may be possible to withdraw respiratory support gradually, although phenobarbitone may be required for a considerable time.

Intravenous feeding

Fluid balance and intravenous feeding

The principles of intravenous therapy are discussed on p. 77, but a general guide for postoperative fluid management is to give approximately 3 ml·kg^{-1}·h^{-1} i.v. for the period in which no oral intake is possible. A suitable solution for maintenance therapy is 4% dextrose with 0.18% saline, although abnormal losses such as gastric aspirate should be replaced with physiological saline and potassium and calcium supplements administered as indicated by the serum electrolyte values. In the immediate postoperative period some fluid restriction is advisable, possibly beginning with 40 ml·kg^{-1}·day^{-1}, rising to 80 ml·kg^{-1}·day^{-1} by the sixth postoperative day. Potassium is included after the first postoperative day.

Such a regimen is inadequate in its calorific value and will not sustain growth, so it is used only for short periods of time. In some infants after major surgery or with necrotizing enterocolitis, protracted diarrhoea, extreme prematurity or renal failure, parenteral nutrition is required, sometimes for very prolonged periods. Patients with gastroschisis and exomphalos have impaired gut motility and may require total parenteral nutrition (TPN) for 6 weeks or more. Such nutrition has made a great contribution to the reduction in mortality of these conditions. Temporary malabsorption occurs, with glucose intolerance especially in sick preterm babies. Because brain growth is very rapid in the first few weeks of life, starvation at this time will interfere with development of the central nervous system. If the enteral feeding is unsatisfactory then TPN should be instituted.

Maintenance of complete intravenous feeding requires the strictest of aseptic techniques and intensive nursing care. Solutions for TPN are now prepared in a specialized aseptic department organized by the hospital pharmacy. Dosages and regimens are computer-based and involve automatic filling of containers so that the intensive care unit is provided with one or two containers of prepared sterile solutions for each patient for a 24-hour period. The nursing workload is reduced, as the container is changed only once every 24 hours and the administration rate needs no further adjustment after it has been initially set.

Solutions are pumped at a constant rate into the superior vena cava or right atrium through a long Silastic catheter, using a peristaltic or syringe pump. To minimize the risk of infection, the catheter is tunnelled subcutaneously for some distance before it enters the vein and a bacterial filter is fitted into the system as near the patient as possible. (Intralipid will not pass through bacterial filters.) The catheters are usually inserted surgically, although it is possible to pass a Silastic catheter through a 19 s.w.g. scalp vein needle in a scalp or arm vein, when it can be expected to pass centrally on a flow-guided principle. Some centres recommend that peripheral veins be used on a rotational basis and that the site of venepuncture be changed every 24 hours. With care, employing Teflon 22 or 24 s.w.g. cannulae, it is possible to maintain TPN for 4–6 weeks using peripheral veins. Many units employ an intravenous therapy team to resite peripheral infusions so that the best use is made of what veins are available. Eventually a central catheter such as Broviac or Hickman is necessary. These silicone rubber catheters have a Teflon cuff which is buried within the skin tunnel when the catheter is introduced surgically. The cuff reduces bacterial contamination from the skin and also provides an anchor to prevent accidental dislodgement of the catheter. They may stay in place for considerable lengths of time without trouble.

All fluids for newborns, including TPN, should be administered accurately with either a syringe pump or a drip-rate controller. Syringe pumps are relatively cheap with low cost disposables and will accurately deliver even very low rates ($0.1 \, ml \cdot h^{-1}$) and thus are particularly suitable for the administration of, for example, inotropic agents, but can be used for plasma, blood or TPN. Volumetric pumps are more expensive and need special administration sets which are also expensive. Simpler drip-rate controllers which use standard microburette infusion sets are very satisfactory for infusions of TPN where complete accuracy of rate is not absolutely necessary. The variability of drop size makes accurate determination of flow rate difficult. Dangers of pumps are inadvertent extravascular infusion, air embolism and fluid overload. To prevent accidental gross fluid overload no more fluid should be put in the burette than is necessary for a period of 1–2 hours.

Frequent biochemical monitoring is necessary, using microtechniques which allow tests to be performed on very small volumes of blood. Acidosis and dehydration must be corrected before commencing intravenous feeding, especially when hypertonic or fructose-containing solutions are used. Fat emulsions are contraindicated in patients with hyperlipidaemia and in the presence of poor bone marrow function. They may be used cautiously in patients with mild liver dysfunction, although daily estimations of liver transaminases should be made. Infused fat should be rapidly cleared from the circulation. If the serum becomes turbid, this suggests that too much fat is being given. The clearance of lipid may be reduced in small-for-gestational-age infants and those of less than 32 weeks' gestation. The load of Intralipid is best spread over 24 hours, which is easily achieved with an infusion pump. Fat pigment is seen in the Kupffer cells of the liver but does not seem to interfere with liver function. The inclusion of Intralipid in doses of 4 g fat·kg^{-1} body weight each day (non-irritant to veins) has meant that peripheral veins may be used for longer periods before resorting to central veins where risks of infection and serious venous thrombosis are greater.

Regimens are available which are effective in maintaining positive nitrogen balance and growth for many months. The caloric requirement is not less than 0.42 MJ·kg^{-1} (100 kcal·kg^{-1}) body weight per 24 hours.

Solutions for complete intravenous feeding include the following.

1. *Amino acid solutions*, of which several are commercially available. All solutions also contain a non-nitrogenous source of calories such as glucose, ethanol or sorbitol. The L-forms of the amino acids are more effective in maintaining positive nitrogen balance (e.g. Vamin; Table 5.5). In addition to the eight amino acids essential for adult growth, histidine, proline, alanine and cystine are essential for infant growth. Aminosol–fructose–ethanol (AFE) and Vamin contain all the amino acids for the growing infant, but the osmolality of these two solutions is very high. They are, however, the most appropriate solutions for use in infancy, but their infusion rate should not exceed AFE 48 ml·kg^{-1} and Vamin 72 ml·kg^{-1}·day^{-1} because the fructose they contain will cause metabolic acidosis. In practice, Vamin Glucose is the most satisfactory solution for use in infants.

2. *Fat emulsions.* Intralipid is the usual fat solution used (as 10 or 20%), prepared from fractionated soyabean oil and in the form of triglycerides. The fat is rapidly cleared from the plasma, even in the newborn, at a rate of up to 8 g fat·kg^{-1} body weight per 24 hours. The addition of heparin may increase the clearance rate of the fat but this is controversial. The infusion of fat is restricted to 4 g fat·kg^{-1}·day^{-1} at a rate not exceeding 0.5 g fat·kg^{-1}·h^{-1}. The solution is usually introduced at 1 g·kg^{-1}·day^{-1}, and if the serum is not turbid then the amount is increased.

Table 5.5   The constituents of Vamin Glucose

Presentation

Clear, straw-coloured solutions for intravenous use containing pure crystalline L-amino acids together with glucose and added electrolytes to the following formula:

L-Alanine	3.0 g	L-Proline	8.1 g
L-Arginine	3.3 g	L-Serine	7.5 g
L-Aspartic acid	4.1 g	L-Threonine	3.0 g
L-Cysteine/Cystine	1.4 g	L-Tryptophan	1.0 g
L-Glutamic acid	9.0 g	L-Tyrosine	0.5 g
Glycine	2.1 g	L-Valine	4.3 g
L-Histidine	2.4 g	Glucose	100.0 g
L-Isoleucine	3.9 g	Sodium	50 mmol
L-Leucine	5.3 g	Potassium	20 mmol
L-Lysine	3.9 g	Calcium	2.5 mmol
L-Methionine	1.9 g	Magnesium	1.5 mmol
L-Phenylalanine	5.5 g	Chloride	55 mmol

in each 1000 ml (pH 5.2). Sterile and pyrogen-free.

Nitrogen per litre: 9.4 g, corresponding to about 60 g of first-class protein. Caloric content per litre 2.7 MJ (650 kcal) of which 1.7 MJ (400 kcal) are provided by glucose.

(Courtesy of Kabi Vitrum Ltd.)

3. *Monosaccharides*. There is no agreement as to which source of calories is preferable. Fructose is said to be less irritant to veins and is less dependent on insulin for its further metabolism. Urinary losses of fructose are greater than glucose and the former may therefore result in a greater osmotic diuresis. Hypoglycaemia may occur during fructose infusion, so at least 50 per cent of the infused carbohydrate should be given as dextrose.

Ethyl alcohol is included in AFE as $2.5 \, g \cdot dl^{-1}$. Its toxicity is a limiting factor in infancy and its inhibitory action on antidiuretic hormone causes increased urinary losses of water and electrolytes.

Vitamins are required, although exact requirements are not well worked out. A multivitamin infusion is given in a dose of 3 ml daily with folic acid 0.5 mg daily, vitamin K 3 mg twice weekly and vitamin B_{12} 100 μg once monthly. If intravenous feeding is continued for more than 1 week, biotin 0.5 mg daily and choline chloride 150 mg daily must be given. Weekly infusions of plasma $10 \, ml \cdot kg^{-1}$ will provide the necessary trace metals (Table 5.6).

The volumes of each nutrient are increased daily, with maximum volumes being achieved on the fourth day. On the first day, one-third of the total requirements ($150 \, ml \cdot kg^{-1} \cdot 24 \, h^{-1}$) are given as 20% Intralipid, 15% glucose and Vamin Glucose, the remaining fluid being given as 4% dextrose with 0.18% saline. On the second day, the volumes are doubled and if the clinical and biochemical state of the patient is satisfactory, then full volumes are achieved after 4 days (Fig. 5.22).

Small volumes of each solution are given in a rotational system so that

Table 5.6 A regimen for complete intravenous feeding of infants (all values per kg per 24 hours)

Solution	Volume (ml)	MJ [kcal]	Amino acids (g)	Na$^+$ (mmol)	K$^+$ (mmol)	Cl$^-$ (mmol)	Ca^{2+} (mmol)	Mg^{2+} (mmol)
Vamin	50	0.14 [34]	3.5†	2.5	1.0	2.5	0.125	0.075
15% Glucose	70	0.18 [42]						
20% Intralipid	20	0.15 [36]						
MgSO$_4$ (0.5 mmol Mg^{2+}·ml^{-1})	0.3							0.150
K$_2$HPO$_4$ (1 mmol K$^+$·ml^{-1})	1.0				1.0			
10% Calcium gluconate (0.25 mmol Ca^{2+}·ml^{-1})	3.5						0.875	
Total	145.3*	0.43 [102]	3.5	2.5	2.0	2.5	1.0	0.225

* Due to osmotic diuresis total fluid volume may need to be increased using 4% dextrose in 0.18% saline.
† Caloric value included in total calories.

(From Harries, 1971)

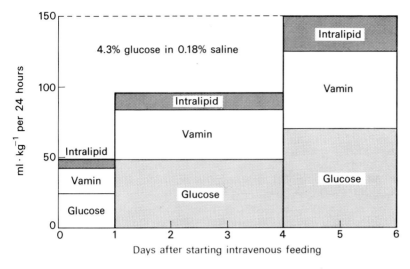

Fig. 5.22 A technique for the introduction of infusates for complete intravenous feeding in infants. (Reproduced, with permission, from Harries, 1971)

an even distribution of solutions during a 24-hour period is achieved. For example:

Vamin Glucose   30 ml for 1 hour
Dextrose 15%   30 ml for 1 hour
Intralipid   10 ml for ½ hour
0.18% Saline   30 ml for 1 hour
Vamin Glucose   30 ml for 1 hour   etc.

A series of three-way stopcocks is arranged to which the required number of drip sets can be attached.

No solutions, drugs or electrolytes may be added to Intralipid or to amino acid or carbohydrate infusions. Vitamins and electrolytes are given into the infusion chamber containing dextrose–saline, but each electrolyte solution must be given separately or precipitation may occur with mixtures. The daily requirements of Ca^{2+} and K^+ must be given in spaced doses to obviate the danger of cardiac arrhythmia with excessive concentrations.

All infusion tubing, drip sets and solutions are changed every 24 hours. If possible, limited oral feeding should be continued during total intravenous feeding, even with severe diarrhoea, to maintain a continuous 'trophic' stimulus to the small intestinal mucosa. Intraluminal substrates exert a trophic effect on the small intestinal mucosa, that effect being mediated by gastrointestinal hormones such as gastrin.

Intravenous alimentation must not be withdrawn abruptly or hypoglycaemia may develop. High levels of circulating insulin are stimulated by the infusions and the levels persist after withdrawal of the feeding. Oral feeding should be reintroduced over several days before the intravenous alimentation is withdrawn.

Complications of intravenous alimentation are very common and include septicaemia with organisms such as *Candida albicans, Staphylococcus aureus* and *Escherichia coli.* All procedures are undertaken with the strictest of aseptic precautions. Topical antibiotics combined with nystatin at the point of skin entry may reduce the incidence of infections. Central venous catheters must be removed if blood cultures are found to be positive. Small neonates are especially vulnerable to infections, and it has also been postulated that metabolic changes accompanying the correction of malnutrition may predispose the infant to infection. Marked electrolyte disturbances and severe acidosis are sometimes seen. Phlebitis and venous obstruction are common, although the incidence is reduced by including isotonic fat emulsions in the regimen (e.g. Intralipid). Catheter dislodgement may occur, with extravasation of solutions into the surrounding tissues.

As most of the amino acid solutions contain relatively high sodium concentrations and are markedly hyperosmolar, excess may cause oedema and cardiac failure.

Intravenous feeding can be expected to provide all the nutrient agents essential for normal growth in the small baby, including the essential amino acids and agents required for brain cell replication and maturation of the central nervous system. Levels of amino acids which are too low or too high may produce irreversible brain damage in young infants. High circulating levels of blood ammonia have been reported in infants fed intravenously, and this, too, is a potential source of brain injury.

References and further reading

Respiratory failure—assessment

Auld, P. A. M., Nelson, N. M., Cherry, R. B., Rudolph, A. J. and Smith, C. A. (1963). Measurement of thoracic gas volume in the newborn infant. *Journal of Clinical Investigation* **42**, 476.

Beardsmore, C. S., Helms, P., Stocks, J., Hatch, D. J. and Silverman, M. (1980). Improved esophageal balloon technique for use in infants. *Journal of Applied Physiology* **49**, 735.

Cassidy, G. (1983). Transcutaneous monitoring in the newborn infant. *Journal of Pediatrics* **10**, 837.

Chiswick, M. L. and Milner, R. D. G. (1976). Crying vital capacity. Measurement of neonatal lung function. *Archives of Disease in Childhood* **51**, 22.

Conway, M., Durbin, G. M., Ingram, D., McIntosh, N., Parker, D., Reynolds, E. O. R. and Soutter, L. P. (1976). Continuous monitoring of arterial oxygen tension using a catheter tip polarographic electrode in infants. *Pediatrics* **57**, 244.

Cook, C. D., Sutherland, J. M., Segal, S., Cherry, R. B., Mead, J., McIlroy, M. B. and Smith, C. A. (1957). Studies of respiratory physiology in the newborn infant. III. Measurements of mechanics of respiration. *Journal of Clinical Investigation* **36**, 440.

Fox, W. W., Schwart, J. G. and Shaffer, T. H. (1977). A new approach for measuring functional residual capacity (FRC) in the intubated infant. *Pediatric Research* **11**, 570.

Gerhardt, T., Bancalari, E., Cohen, H. and Maciar-Loza, M. (1977). Respiratory depression at birth—value of Apgar score and ventilatory measurements in its detection. *Journal of Pediatrics* **90**, 971.

Hatch, D. J. (1975). The measurement of pulmonary function. In: *Recent Advances in Paediatric Surgery, 3*. Ed. by A. W. Wilkinson. Churchill Livingstone, Edinburgh and London.

Helms, P. (1982). Problems with plethysmographic estimation of lung volume in infants. *Journal of Applied Physiology* **53**, 698.

Helms, P., Taylor, B. W., Milner, A. D. and Hatch, D. J. (1982). A critical assessment of a jacket plethysmograph for use in young children. *Journal of Applied Physiology* **52**, 267.

Huch, A. and Huch, R. (1977). Technical, physiological and clinical aspects of transcutaneous Po_2 measurements. In: *Non-invasive Clinical Measurement*. Ed. by D. E. M. Taylor and J. Whamond. Pitman Medical, Tunbridge Wells.

Lesouef, P. N., Lopes, J. M., Miller, N. and Bryan, A. C. (1984). Influence of chest wall distortion on esophageal pressure. *Journal of Applied Physiology* **55**, 353.

Olinsky, A., Bryan, A. C. and Bryan, M. H. (1976). A simple method of measuring total respiratory system compliance in newborn infants. *South African Medical Journal* **50**, 128.

Milner, A. D., Hull, D., Hatch, D. J. and Cogswell, J. J. (1972). A new method for measuring static compliance in infants and young children. *Clinical Science* **43**, 689.

Peabody, J. L., Willis, M. M., Gregory, G. A., Tooley, W. H. and Lucey, J. F. (1978). Limitations and advantages of transcutaneous oxygen electrodes. *Acta Anaesthesiologica Scandinavica* (Suppl.) **68**, 76.

Phelan, P. D. and Williams, H. E. (1969). Ventilatory studies in healthy infants. *Pediatric Research* **3**, 425.

Tepper, R. S., Reynaldo, D. and Taussig, L. (1984). Noninvasive determination of total respiratory system compliance in infants by the weighted spirometer method. *American Review of Respiratory Disease* **130**, 461.

Zin, W. A., Pengelly, L. O. and Milic-Emili, J. (1982). Single breath method for measurement of respiratory mechanics in anaesthetised animals. *Journal of Applied Physiology* **52**, 1266.

Respiratory failure—management

Aberdeen, E. (1965). Tracheostomy care in infants. *Proceedings of the Royal Society of Medicine* **58**, 900.

Battersby, E. F., Hatch, D. J. and Towey, R. M. (1977). The effects of prolonged naso-endotracheal intubation in children: a study in infants and young children after cardio-pulmonary bypass. *Anaesthesia* **32**, 154.

Bohn, D. J., Miyasaki, K., Marchak, B. E., Thompson, W. K., Froese, A. B. and Bryan, A. C. (1980). Ventilation by high frequency oscillation. *Journal of Applied Physiology* **48,** 710.

Boros, S. J., Matalou, S. V., Ewald, R., Leonard, A. S. and Hunt, C. E. (1977). The effect of independent variations in inspiratory:expiratory time ratio and end expiratory pressure during mechanical ventilation in hyaline membrane disease: the significance of mean airway pressure. *Journal of Pediatrics* **91,** 794.

Brünstler, I., Enders, A. and Versmold, H. T. (1982). Skin surface pCO_2 monitoring in newborn infants in shock: effect of hypotension and electrode temperature. *Journal of Pediatrics* **100,** 454.

Clark, C. E. Clayman, R. I., Roth, R. S., Sniderman, S. H., Lane, B. and Ballard, A. A. (1981). Risk factor analysis of intraventricular hemorrhage in low birth weight infants. *Journal of Pediatrics* **99,** 625.

Downes, J. J. (1974). Intermittent mandatory ventilation. *Archives of Surgery* **109,** 519.

Downes, J. J. and Raphaely, R. C. (1975). Pediatric intensive care. *Anesthesiology* **43,** 238.

Drummond, W. H., Gregory, G. A., Heymann, M. A. and Phibbs, R. A. (1981). The independent effects of hyperventilation, tolazoline, and dopamine on infants with persistent pulmonary hypertension. *Journal of Pediatrics* **98,** 603.

Fox, W. W., Gewitz, M. H. and Berman, L. S. (1977). The Pao_2 response to changes in end expiratory pressure in the newborn respiratory distress syndrome. *Critical Care Medicine* **5,** 226.

Fox, W. W., Berman, L. S., Dinwiddie, R. and Shaffer, T. H. (1977). Tracheal extubation of the neonate at $2-3\,cmH_2O$ continuous positive airway pressure (CPAP). *Pediatrics* **59,** 257.

Goldsmith, J. P. and Karotkin, E. H. (1981). Assisted ventilation of the neonate. W. B. Saunders, Philadelphia.

Gregory, G. A., Kitterman, J. A., Phibbs, R. H., Tooley, W. H. and Hamilton, W. K. (1971). Treatment of idiopathic respiratory distress syndrome with continuous positive airways pressure. *New England Journal of Medicine* **284,** 1333.

Halliday, H. L., McClure, G. and Reid, M. (1981). *Handbook of Neonatal Intensive Care.* Ballière Tindall, London.

Hatch, D. J. (1977). Anaesthesia for cardiac surgery in the first year of life. In: *Anaesthesia for Cardiac Surgery and Allied Procedures.* Ed. by M. A. Branthwaite. Blackwell Scientific, Oxford.

Hatch, D. J. (1981) Anaesthetic equipment for neonates and infants. *British Journal of Hospital Medicine* **26,** 84.

Hatch, D. J. (1985). Acute upper airway obstruction in children. In: *Recent Advances in Anaesthesia and Analgesia—15,* p. 133. Ed. by R. S. Atkinson and A. P. Adams. Churchill Livingstone, Edinburgh.

Hatch, D. J., Cogswell, J. J., Taylor, B. W., Battersby, E. F., Glover, W. J. and Kerr, A. A. (1973). Continuous positive airway pressure (CPAP) after open heart operations in infancy. *Lancet* **2,** 469.

Hayes, B. and Robinson, J. S. (1970). The assessment of methods of humidification of inspired air. *British Journal of Anaesthesia* **42**, 94.

James, L. S. and Lanman, J. T. (Eds) (1976). Symposium: Retrolental fibroplasia. *Pediatrics* **57**, Supplement, 591.

Lou, H. L., Lassen, N. A. and Friis-Hansen, B. (1977). Low cerebral blood flow in hypotensive perinatal distress. *Acta Neurologica Scandinavica* **56**, 343.

Mackersie, A. M., Hatch, D. J. and Farnsworth, G. M. (1980). Ventilatory management of neonates undergoing surgery. *British Journal of Anaesthesia* **52**, 273.

Milner, A. D. (1980). Bronchopulmonary dysplasia. *Archives of Disease in Childhood* **55**, 661.

Myers, T. F., Milsap, R. L., Krauss, A. N., Auld, P. A. M. and Reidenberg, M. M. (1980). Low-dose theophylline therapy in idiopathic apnea of prematurity. *Journal of Pediatrics* **96**, 99.

Phibbs, R. H. (1977). Oxygen therapy: a continuing hazard to the premature infant. *Anesthesiology* **47**, 486.

Pollitzer, M., Reynolds, E. O. R., Shaw, D. G. and Thomas, R. (1981). Pancuronium during mechanical ventilation speeds recovery of lungs of infants with hyaline membrane disease. *Lancet* **1**, 346.

Reynolds, E. O. R. (1974). Pressure waveform and ventilator settings for mechanical ventilation in severe hyaline membrane disease. *International Clinics in Anesthesiology* **12**, 269.

Reynolds, E. O. R. and Taghizadeh, A. (1974). Improved prognosis of infants mechanically ventilated for hyaline membrane disease. *Archives Disease in Childhood* **49**, 505.

Roberton, N. R. C. (1976). CPAP or not CPAP? *Archives of Disease in Childhood* **51**, 161.

Roberton, N. R. C. (1981). *A Manual of Neonatal Intensive Care.* Edward Arnold. London.

Schöber, J. G., Stübing, K. and Kuhwald, R. (1981). Abstracts of the International Workshop on continuous pCO_2 monitoring by skin surface sensors. *Intensive Care Medicine* **7**, 249.

Sjostrand, U. (1980). High frequency positive pressure ventilation (HFPPV): a review. *Critical Care Medicine* **8**, 345.

Speidel, B. D. and Dunn, P. M. (1976). Use of nasal CPAP to treat severe recurrent apnoea in very preterm infants. *Lancet* **2**, 658.

Stocks, J. G. (1972). The management of respiratory failure in infancy. *Anaesthesia and Intensive Care* **1**, 486.

Sumner, E. and Frank, J. D. (1981). The effect of tolazoline on the treatment of congenital diaphragmatic hernias. A report of its successful use to reverse a transitional circulation in four patients. *Archives of Disease in Childhood* **56**, 350.

Svenningsen, N. W., Blennow, G., Lindroth, M., Gäddlin, P. O. and Ahlström, H. (1982). Brain-orientated intensive care treatment in severe neonatal asphyxia. *Archives of Disease in Childhood* **57**, 176.

Thorburn, R., Lipscomb, A. P., Stewart, A., Reynolds, E. O. R., Hope, P. L. and Pape, K. (1981). Prediction of death and major handicap in very preterm infants by brain ultrasound. *Lancet* **1**, 1119.

Workshop on Bronchopulmonary Dysplasia (1979) *Journal of Pediatrics* **95,** 815.

Intravenous feeding

Baum, J. D. and Aynsley-Green, A. (1975). Intravenous feeding in children. *Clinical Trials Journal,* Suppl. 1, **114.**

Broviac, J. W., Cole, J. J. and Scribner, B. H. (1973). A silicone rubber atrial catheter for prolonged alimentation. *Surgery, Gynecology and Obstetrics* **136,** 602.

Harries, J. T. (1971). Intravenous feeding in infants. *Archives of Disease in Childhood* **46,** 855.

Harries, J. T. (1978). Aspects of intravenous feeding in childhood. In: *Advances in Parenteral Nutrition.* Ed. by Ivan Johnston. MTP Press, Lancaster.

Kiely, E. (1984). One hundred consecutive central venous catheters in children. *Zeitschrift für Kinderchirurgie* **39,** 332.

Leading article. (1977) Intravenous feeding in infancy. *British Medical Journal* **1,** 1490.

Pildes, R. S., Cornblath, M., Warren, I., Page-El, E., di Menza, S., Morrit, D. M. and Peeva, A. (1974). A prospective controlled study of neonatal hypoglycemia. *Pediatrics* **54,** 5.

6

Resuscitation of the newborn

Asphyxia at birth

Between 5 and 13 per cent of newborn infants fail to breathe immediately after delivery, and more than 50 per cent of the deaths in the first week of life occur in this group. A better understanding of the effects of acute asphyxia has been obtained as a result of experimental work in animals asphyxiated before the onset of breathing by immersion in saline. An initial period of tachypnoea and tachycardia is followed by a variable period of primary apnoea. If oxygen is administered at this stage it usually leads to the onset of regular respiration within a short period of time. If the asphyxia is allowed to continue, however, primary apnoea is followed by a series of gasping breaths which eventually stop as a severe mixed respiratory and metabolic acidosis develops (Fig. 6.1). The heart rate falls rapidly after the onset of asphyxia, then plateaus or rises slightly during the period of gasping, to fall again after the last gasp. Cardiac activity may continue for 5–10 minutes after the gasping ceases, and the period between the last gasp and cardiac arrest is known as terminal or secondary apnoea. During this period blood pressure falls. After a few minutes of terminal apnoea, brain damage will rapidly ensue unless effective resuscitation involving artificial ventilation with or without external cardiac massage is instituted. Administration of intravenous glucose and bicarbonate during resuscitation to combat the hypoglycaemia and acidosis improves the cardiac output and helps minimize the likelihood of cerebral damage.

The clinical picture in the human neonate will depend on the severity and duration of intrapartum asphyxia together with the degree of depression resulting from drugs given to the mother (Table 6.1).

If the asphyxia has been acute and of short duration, without severe acidosis or significant drug depression, a picture similar to that described above may be seen, although if the initial shallow breaths or gasps succeed in establishing alveolar ventilation regular respiration will soon start. In the presence of moderate acidosis (pH < 7.2) from prolonged intrapartum asphyxia or drug depression the gasping may not be adequate to establish effective alveolar ventilation or may be completely absent, so primary apnoea may progress into terminal apnoea. If pH is less than 7.0 at birth the baby will be limp and pale and already in terminal apnoea.

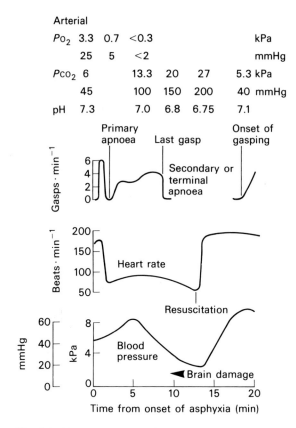

Fig. 6.1 Response to asphyxia and resuscitation by artifical ventilation in rhesus monkeys. (Redrawn, with permission, from Dawes, 1968)

Assessment

It is not always easy to decide in the newborn infant at birth whether apnoea is primary or terminal. The Apgar scoring system (Table 6.2) has been widely used as a method of assessing the infant's condition, a score of less than 4 being highly suggestive of terminal apnoea. *There is, however, a danger that resuscitation will be delayed in an attempt to assess the Apgar score correctly.* A simplified score based on heart rate at birth and the time taken for spontaneous respiratory movements to appear has been described by Chamberlain and Banks (1974) and may be just as useful. Whatever scoring system is used, it is most important to make a rapid assessment of ventilation, circulation and neurological status (Roberton and Rosen, 1982). The pressure required to inflate the lungs of an infant who has not taken a breath is often greater than for normal ventilation, so it is important to record whether initial lung expansion has taken place. The interval between birth and the first breath is usually less than 30 seconds. Observation

Table 6.1   Drugs commonly given to mothers and their effects on fetus and neonate.

Drugs given to mother	Fetal and neonatal problems
Opiates	Respiratory depression. Premature infant achieves higher brain levels, and has retarded metabolism and diminished renal excretion
Pethidine	Respiratory depression. Breakdown products are also depressant and have a maximal effect between 2 and 3 hours
Tranquillizers	Additive to analgesic depression. Some sedatives cause hypothermia and prolonged hypotonia
Diazepam	Hypothermia and apnoea. Long half-life. May diminish normal fetal heart rate variation
Ultra-short-acting barbiturates	Least depression if less than 250 mg of thiopentone is used and 4–8 minutes elapse between induction and delivery
Nitrous oxide	Minimal depression that becomes worse with time of exposure. Neonatal pulmonary excretion could cause diffusion anoxia
Halothane	May abolish fetal heart rate distress patterns in low concentrations. Diabetic infants may become hypoglycaemic
Other vapours and cyclopropane	Minimal depression in carefully controlled analgesic levels
Neuromuscular blocking drugs	Gallamine easily transferred across the placenta. All require close control. Only pancuronium not yet detected in newborn
Local anaesthetics	Fetal bradycardia with overdose, paracervical block, accidental intravenous or fetal injection
Magnesium	Hypotonia and respiratory depression if maternal plasma level high
Alcohol	Acidosis, hypoglycaemia, CNS depression if grossly excessive amounts given

(From Davenport and Valman, 1980)

of ventilatory rate, rhythm and depth helps in the assessment of drug-induced respiratory depression or airway obstruction.

Measurement of both heart rate (by auscultation rather than by palpation) and peripheral perfusion is essential in the assessment of hypoxia and low cardiac output. Bradycardia below 100 beats per minute and pale cold limbs are ominous signs which dictate immediate resuscitation. Neurological status is crudely assessed by observation of muscle tone, the presence or absence of spontaneous movements and reflex conjunctival, pharyngeal or inflation reflexes. Head's reflex (p. 14) is an encouraging sign that the baby is still in a state of primary apnoea and is often followed by the onset of regular spontaneous breathing. Boon, Milner and Hopkin (1979) showed

Table 6.2   The Apgar score

	0	1	2
Colour	White	Blue	Pink
Heart rate	0	<100	>100
Activity in response to pharyngeal suction	Nil	Grimace	Cough
Respiration	Absent	Gasping or irregular	Regular or crying lustily
Muscle tone	Limp	Reduced or normal with no active movements	Normal with active movements

that a rejection response was common, frequently causing expulsion of gas from the lungs whilst the inflation pressure was maintained.

The possibility of fetal asphyxia developing at birth should be suspected in cases of fetal distress, prematurity, difficult forceps or breech delivery, twins (especially the second twin) and rhesus incompatibility. Infants born by caesarian section are also at risk, especially if the interval between induction of anaesthesia and delivery is prolonged. The situation may be complicated by the technique of cord clamping. Early clamping is known to lead to hypovolaemia and this is associated with a higher incidence of respiratory distress syndrome (RDS). Birth asphyxia and late cord clamping are associated with a reduction in FRC, reduction in compliance, low arterial oxygen tension and high carbon dioxide tension.

Prognosis

The Apgar score is of little prognostic value, and on the whole the outlook following recovery from a period of acute asphyxia is generally accepted to be good. Even delays of as long as 20 minutes in establishing spontaneous respiration in very low birth weight babies without cardiac arrest have been shown to have little influence on the eventual outcome.

It has been shown, however, that if resuscitation is started early in terminal apnoea the infant can be expected to commence regular spontaneous respiration within a few minutes, whilst if resuscitation is delayed onset of spontaneous respiration may not occur for 20–30 minutes or even longer. Administration of glucose and correction of acidosis may shorten this time.

There appears to be a high risk of permanent brain damage in any baby in whom regular spontaneous breathing is not established within 30 minutes of a period of circulatory arrest (Table 6.3). If, however, regular spontaneous breathing, as opposed to the intermittent gasping which may occur in severe asphyxia, is established within 30 minutes the risk of cerebral damage is less.

The outlook following chronic intrapartum asphyxia is less certain. One group of babies have been identified who, following intrapartum bradycar-

Table 6.3 The prognosis for babies receiving cardiac massage for circulatory arrest within 15 minutes of birth

Time taken for regular spontaneous respiratory movements to develop after the circulation was restored	Outcome		
	Normal	Quadriplegia	Dead
≤30 min	26	0	2
>30 min	1	9	12

(From Hey, 1977b)

dia and meconium-stained liquor, develop problems of cardiorespiratory adaptation after delivery, with intractable persistence of the fetal circulation. The outlook for these babies can be improved by a combination of alkali therapy and artificial ventilation in an attempt to keep them mildly alkalotic, as this makes reversion to fetal circulation less likely. It seems reasonable to start the regimen early in this group. The presence of prolonged fetal distress or serious intrapartum haemorrhage appears to increase the risk of cerebral palsy, and as long as resuscitation is commenced within a few minutes of birth it seems that the likelihood of any eventual handicap is mainly determined by events occurring *in utero*.

Moderate or severe acidosis (pH < 7.2) may inhibit surfactant synthesis, and may be associated with an increased incidence of RDS, especially in premature babies. Hey showed that early active intervention in cyanosed babies led to a 20 per cent fall in mortality from RDS. Prevention of intrapartum asphyxia might be expected to lead to a further fall in mortality. Birth asphyxia can also cause a reduction in cardiac output, and even cardiac failure, pulmonary oedema, renal and hepatic damage, and widespread metabolic disturbances. It has also been identified as one of the causes of necrotizing enterocolitis.

Resuscitation technique

Immediately after delivery of the head, the infant's pharynx should be gently aspirated, although care must be taken not to touch the back of the pharynx as this may induce reflex apnoea or laryngospasm. Pharyngeal drainage is encouraged by placing the baby in the head-down position. If central cyanosis is present, oxygen should be administered. The baby should be dried and quickly wrapped in a warm towel at birth and placed on a flat surface, preferably under a heating canopy because neonates lose heat rapidly during resuscitation. The temperature of the delivery room should be as high as can be tolerated by the staff, for the same reason. If the infant has not begun to breathe by 30 seconds after birth, a close-fitting face mask should be applied and the lungs gently inflated two or three times with oxygen. Face mask resuscitation is effective only if used with a resuscitator capable of producing a sustained inflation pressure for more than 1 second because of inevitable leaks around the mask. Vyas, Milner and Hopkin (1983) have shown that gastric distension is unlikely to occur with pressures less than 3.5 kPa (35 cmH$_2$O).

There is still uncertainty regarding the pressures and frequencies at which the lungs should be ventilated during resuscitation. Unfortunately, what is adequate for most babies is insufficient for a few. Hey (1977b) suggested that an inflating pressure of 3 kPa (30 cmH$_2$O) maintained for a little more than 1 second appeared to be the best way of initiating aeration of the lungs, although he admitted that slightly higher pressures might be required to expand them in some babies.

Boon, Milner and Hopkin (1979) found that an opening pressure of 2 kPa (20 cmH$_2$0) was sufficient to expand the lungs in most asphyxiated babies, but Milner and Vyas (1982) point out that it may be necessary to hold the lungs inflated for up to 5 seconds to obtain an adequate FRC.

In practice, if the baby has taken a breath, resuscitation can usually be achieved using a face mask, but if there are no respiratory movements at the end of 1 minute, if the heart rate is less than 100 beats per minute at any time, if mask ventilation is not producing effective alveolar ventilation or if there is obstruction by meconium or secretions, tracheal intubation should be performed and the lungs should be inflated to not more than 3 kPa (30 cmH$_2$O) for approximately 1 second.

The first few breaths may be shallow and hard to detect but the tidal volume usually increases rapidly in the absence of drug depression or severe prolonged asphyxia so that adequate gas exchange is established within 2 minutes. It is occasionally necessary to inflate the lungs with pressures slightly greater than 3 kPa (30 cmH$_2$O) or to hold the lungs inflated for up to 5 seconds and pneumothorax is rare in these situations except in cases of pulmonary hypoplasia. If spontaneous breathing does not commence, intermittent positive pressure ventilation (IPPV) should be started at a rate of 15 times a minute. After the first inflation, care should be taken not to apply pressures higher than 3 kPa (30 cmH$_2$O) to the airway. Inflating pressures of up to 6 kPa (60 cmH$_2$O) can be achieved with high flow rates relatively easily even if a simple water manometer set at 3 kPa (30 cmH$_2$O) is incorporated into the circuit.

If adequate expansion of the lungs is not achieved, the position of the tracheal tube should be checked, as it may be in the oesophagus or in one of the bronchi. The stomach should be deflated by the passage of an intragastric tube. The most reliable sign of successful resuscitation is an increase in heart rate, which should usually exceed 100 beats per minute within 30 seconds of starting IPPV. If this does not occur, it suggests that the asphyxia is very severe and external cardiac massage should be commenced. The continued occurrence of occasional gasps after the onset of regular respiration should be viewed with suspicion, and if these continue for more than 30 minutes the possibility of intraventricular cerebral haemorrhage, hypoglycaemia or metabolic acidosis should be considered. Gasps occurring without the onset of regular respiration suggest hypoplasia of the lungs. Gross hypoplasia is frequently associated with congenital diaphragmatic hernia, and lesser degrees are seen in severe rhesus incompatibility. In Potter's syndrome, pulmonary hypoplasia is associated with renal anomalies and peculiarities of the face, including large low-set ears and prominent facial creases.

Circulatory arrest

If the heart rate does not increase to more than 100 beats per minute within 30 seconds of effective IPPV, external cardiac massage should be commenced. This can be carried out by slight pressure over the lower part of the sternum with two thumbs or fingers (Fig. 6.2). If an effective circulation is not obtained within 3–4 minutes, it may be wise to give an intracardiac injection of 2–4 mmol of sodium bicarbonate. Although the use of continuous infusions of glucose or bicarbonate has been suggested, there appears to be little evidence of their value.

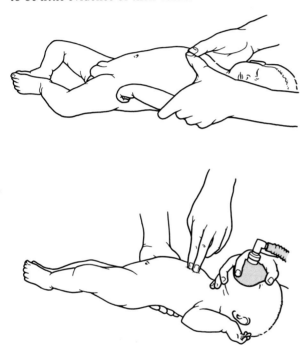

Fig. 6.2 Alternative positions of the hands for external cardiac massage in infants. (Reproduced, with permission, from Davenport and Valman, 1980)

Drug therapy

The empirical use of sodium bicarbonate has been mentioned above; if, after successful resuscitation, residual acidosis is suspected an arterial blood sample should be taken and base deficit corrected with bicarbonate according to the formula:

$$\text{dose of bicarbonate} = 0.3 \times \text{body weight} \times \text{base deficit}$$
$$\text{(mmol)} \qquad\qquad \text{(kg)}$$

It is usual to commence with a half correction.

If the mother has received pethidine or morphine (see Table 6.1) within 2 hours of delivery, a pharmacological antagonist can be given to the infant. Naloxone in an intramuscular dose of $0.005-0.01 \, mg \cdot kg^{-1}$ is suitable.

Since circulatory insufficiency immediately after birth is usually associated with severe bradycardia rather than ventricular fibrillation or asystole, myocardial stimulant drugs are seldom required.

Equipment

Equipment for cardiopulmonary resuscitation should be readily available at all times, and should be checked regularly to ensure that it is complete and reliable when required (Table 6.4).

Table 6.4   Neonatal resuscitation equipment

Self-inflating resuscitator	Needles
Tracheal tubes	Scalp vein needles
Tube connectors	Stethoscope
Laryngoscope	Scissors
Face mask	Umbilical catheters
Chest drain	Gastric tube
Suction catheters	Dextrostix
Syringes	

Drugs
Sodium bicarbonate—8.4%
Adrenaline—1 : 10 000
Calcium chloride—10 mmol in 10 ml
Naloxone (Narcan Neonatal) —0.01 $mg \cdot kg^{-1}$
Water for injection
Saline
Dextrose—50% (dilute to 12.5%)
Heparin

Resuscitators

Although ventilation of the lungs can be performed with a T-piece, a certain amount of training is required, and it cannot be used in situations where there is no oxygen. A number of self-inflating resuscitators are commercially available which overcome these difficulties (Fig. 6.3). Any assessment of these resuscitators should include an evaluation of the ease with which they can be used, whether the state of the lungs can be determined by the 'feel' of an inflating bag, the maximum inspired oxygen fraction (Fio_2) which can be achieved and the ease with which the resuscitator can be sterilized. Table 6.5 shows an evaluation of these factors for three commercially available resuscitators, together with the maximum pressure which could be achieved when inflating dummy lungs of compliance 1 and 5 $ml \cdot cmH_2O^{-1}$. It also shows the length of time during which an inflating pressure can be sustained.

Although there is evidence that excised lungs tend to rupture at autopsy

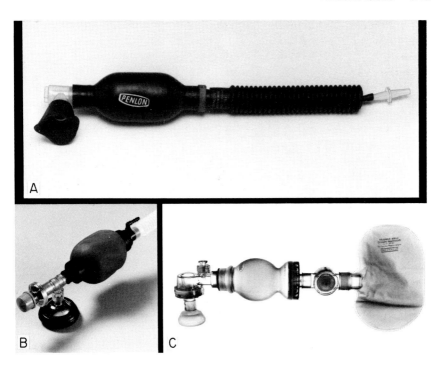

Fig. 6.3   Three neonatal resuscitators: A, Penlon; B, Vickers–Laerdal; and C, Ambu.

when inflated above 3 kPa, alveolar rupture and pneumothorax are seldom encountered in clinical practice during resuscitation, and the vigorous infant creates considerably higher transpleural pressure changes during crying. All the neonatal resuscitators assessed in Table 6.5 were capable of reaching the inflating pressures recommended by Hey when inflating a dummy lung of low compliance $(1\,ml \cdot cmH_2O^{-1})$ but some were unable to produce a sustained pressure.

The ability to produce a high F_{IO_2} is also important, and there is no evidence to suggest that a high F_{IO_2} for a short period immediately after birth produces retrolental fibroplasia. Resuscitators should also be supplied with a close-fitting face mask of appropriate size and terminate in a standard 15- to 22-mm connector to allow attachment to a standard tracheal tube adaptor.

Tracheal tubes

Cole pattern tracheal tubes are popular in neonatal resuscitation because of the ease with which they can be passed into the trachea by relatively untrained staff. The increase in diameter above the short tracheal portion of the tube makes bronchial intubation unlikely, but the tube can be dis-

Table 6.5 Assessment of the performance of three neonatal resuscitators when ventilating dummy lungs of compliance 5 ml·cmH²O⁻¹ and 1 ml·cmH²O⁻¹

Make	Maximum inspiratory pressure		Sustained pressure(s)	Maximum FiO_2	Ease of use	'Feel' of the lungs	Sterilization
	Compliance = 5	Compliance = 1					
Ambu	100	142	1.5	0.8	+ +	+ +	+ (120°C)
Penlon	76	130	0.5	0.9	+ +	+	+
Laerdal:	40	52					
With safety valve			0.5	1.0	+ +	+ +	+ +
Without safety valve	80	95	1.2	1.0	+ +	+ +	+ +

placed into the oesophagus fairly easily. The widened portion of the tube can occasionally be forced through the laryngeal inlet, causing laryngeal damage, and in this case bronchial intubation becomes a possibility. Because of the high incidence of laryngeal problems with these tubes, they cannot be recommended for prolonged airway management. It should also be remembered that the sudden change in diameter causes turbulent flow even at low flow rates, with increased resistance to breathing (Figs. 6.4 and

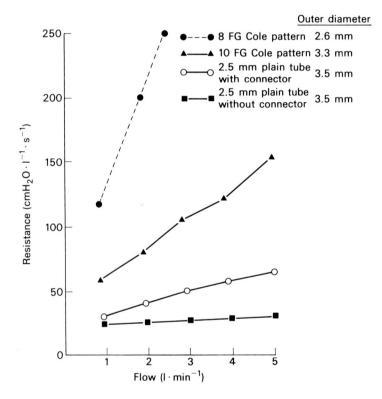

Fig. 6.4   Resistance of plain and Cole pattern tracheal tubes.

6.5). For this reason the smallest Cole pattern tubes, which may have an internal diameter of little more than 1 mm, should not be used with spontaneous breathing for more than a few minutes (Table 6.6).

Other resuscitation equipment

Resuscitation of the newborn is best performed on a firm surface of adequate height, with equipment readily available for oxygen administration, pharyngeal suction, tracheal intubation and ventilation of the lungs. These conditions are provided by a resuscitation trolley such as the Resus-

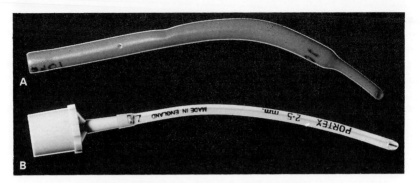

Fig. 6.5 The sudden change in diameter of a 10 FG Cole pattern tube (A) gives it a similar resistance to a 2.5 mm plain tube with connector (B).

Table 6.6 The dimensions and resistance of Cole pattern tracheal tubes without connectors

Tube	Tracheal end		Connector end		Resistance ($cmH_2O \cdot l^{-1} \cdot s^{-1}$) flow ($l \cdot min^{-1}$)		
	i.d. (mm)	o.d. (mm)	i.d. (mm)	o.d. (mm)	1	3	5
8 FG:							
Warne	1.5	2.6	2.7	4.7	135	250	—
Rusch	1.4	2.6	4.2	6.6	78	450	—
10 FG:							
Warne	1.9	3.3	3.3	5.3	54	84	120
Rusch	2.0	3.2	4.2	6.0	33	50	68
Portex 2.0 mm	2.2	3.5	3.7	5.4	35	38	52
12 FG:							
Warne	2.5	4.0	4.0	6.4	21	32	47
Rusch	2.4	4.4	4.2	7.0	19	30	44
Portex 2.5 mm	2.7	4.0	3.7	5.4	13	20	23
14 FG:							
Warne	2.8	4.3	4.5	6.6	12	20	22
Rusch	3.0	4.9	4.2	7.8	9	16	22
Portex 3.0 mm	3.0	4.7	5.1	7.0	7	12	16

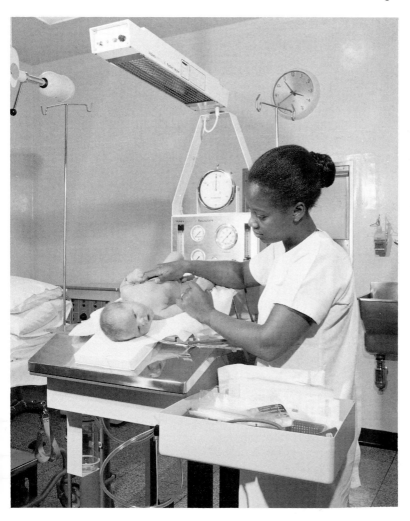

Fig. 6.6 The Vickers Resuscitaire.

citaire (Fig. 6.6), which also incorporates an overhead heating canopy to minimize heat loss. A manometer to prevent excessive airway pressures being used during ventilation is essential.

Laryngoscopes and masks are discussed on p. 88.

References and further reading

Boon, A. W., Milner, A. D. and Hopkin, I. E. (1979). Physiological responses of the newborn infant to resuscitation. *Archives of Disease in Childhood* **54,** 492.

Cave, P. and Fletcher, G. (1968). Resistance of nasotracheal tubes used in infants. *Anesthesiology* **29**, 588.

Chamberlain, G. and Banks, J. (1974). Assessment of the Apgar score. *Lancet* **2**, 1225.

Davenport, H. T. and Valman, H. B. (1980). Resuscitation of the newborn. In: *General Anaesthesia*, 4th edn. Ed. by T. C. Gray, J. F. Nunn and J. E. Utting. Butterworths, London.

Dawes, G. S. (1968). Foetal and Neonatal Physiology. Yearbook Medical, Chicago.

Godfrey, S. (1974). Growth and development of the respiratory system—functional development. In: *Scientific Foundations of Paediatrics*. Ed. by J. A. Davies and J. Dobbing. Heinemann Medical, London.

Hatch, D. J. (1978). Tracheal tubes and connectors used in neonates—dimensions and resistance to breathing. *British Journal of Anaesthesia* **50**, 959.

Hey, E. N. (1977a). The care of babies in incubators. In: *Recent Advances in Paediatrics*, 4. Ed. by D. Gairdner and D. Hull. Churchill Livingstone, Edinburgh and London.

Hey, E. N. (1977b). Resuscitation at birth. *British Journal of Anaesthesia* **49**, 25.

Hull, D. (1977). Lung expansion and ventilation during resuscitation of asphyxiated newborn infants. *Journal of Pediatrics* **75**, 47.

Milner, A. D. and Vyas, H. (1982). Lung expansion at birth. *Journal of Pediatrics* **101**, 879.

Milner, A. D., Vyas, H. and Hopkin, I. E. (1984). Efficacy of face mask resuscitation at birth. *British Medical Journal* **289**, 1563.

Roberton, N. R. C. and Rosen, M. (1982). Safer resuscitation of the newborn. *Clinics in Obstetrics and Gynaecology* **9**, 415.

Samson, H. H. (1974). Resuscitation of the newborn—an improved neonatal resuscitator. *South African Medical Journal* **48**, 628.

Yvas, H., Milner, A. D. and Hopkin, I. E. (1983). Face mask resuscitation: does it lead to gastric distension? *Archives of Disease in Childhood* **58**, 373.

Vyas, H., Milner, A. D., Hopkin, I. E. and Falconer, A. D. (1983). Role of labour in the establishment of functional residual capacity at birth. *Archives of Disease in Childhood* **58**, 512.

Weiner, P. C., Hogg, M. I. J. and Rosen, M. (1977). Effects of naloxone on pethidine-induced neonatal depression. 1. Intravenous naloxone. 2. Intramuscular naloxone. *British Medical Journal* **2**, 229.

Appendix I
Unusual medical conditions in the neonate with implications for the anaesthetist

Achondrogenesis:
    Parenti-Fraccaro type

Very short neck
Short limbs
Early death

    Langer–Saldingto type

Very large head
Short limbs
Early death

Adrenogenital syndrome

Defect in hydrocortisone synthesis—
need hydrocortisone
Virilization of the female
Electrolyte disturbances

Albright–Butler syndrome

Renal tubular acidosis
Hypokalaemia

Analbuminaemia

Very low serum albumin
Sensitive to drugs bound to albumin (e.g.
curare)

Andersen's syndrome

Mid-facial hypoplasia
Airway and intubation problems

Apert's syndrome

Hypertelorism
Craniosynostosis
May have congenital heart disease—
antibiotics necessary
Intubation difficulties

Arnold-Chiari syndrome	See p. 158
Arthrogryposis multiplex congenita	Congenital contractures Airway problems Difficult veins
Ask-Upmark kidney	Hypertension Areas of renal hypoplasia
Ataxia telangiectasia	Abnormal movements Telangiectasia of skin Defective immunity—sterile equipment and precautions Anaemia—correct preoperatively
Barter's syndrome	Metabolic alkalosis and hypokalaemia Overproduction of prostaglandin E Poor response to noradrenaline Electrolyte abnormalities
Beckwith's syndrome (Beckwith-Wiedemann)	High birth weight Macroglossia, exomphalos—airway problems Persistent hypoglycaemia—careful monitoring
Blackfan-Diamond syndrome	Congenital hypoplastic anaemia Defect in erythropoiesis Steroid therapy
Bloch-Sulzberger syndrome	Ecto- and mesodermal defects Bullous skin eruptions Microcephaly Spastic paralysis
Bonnevie-Ullrich syndrome	Similar to Turner's syndrome Redundant skin of neck Congenital heart disease
Cardiofacial syndrome	Congenital heart disease Localized facial paralysis
Carpenter's syndrome	Characteristic facies Congenital heart disease—antibiotics necessary Mandibular hypoplasia—airway problems
Cat-eye syndrome	Trisomy 22 without cleft palate

Central core disease	Hypotonia Risk of malignant hyperpyrexia Poor respiratory function
Cerebrohepatorenal syndrome (Zellweger's syndrome)	Jaundice Renal failure Cardiac failure Hypotonia
Chediak–Higashi syndrome	Immunodeficiency; recurrent infections— need to use sterile techniques Thrombocytopenia
Chotzen's syndrome	Craniosynostosis Renal abnormalities with failure Difficult intubation
Conradi–Hunerman syndrome	Chondrodysplasia Dwarfism Cataracts Difficulty with intubation Poor veins
Cri-du-chat syndrome	Odd cry Microcephaly Hypertelorism Cleft palate Cardiac anomalies
Crigler–Najjer syndrome	Congenital jaundice Glucuronyl transferase deficiency
Crouzon's disease	Craniosynostosis Hypertelorism Difficult intubation
Dandy–Walker syndrome	Hydrocephalus Posterior fossa enlargement
Diastematomyelia	See p. 157
DiGeorge's syndrome	Absent thymus and parathyroids Immunodeficiency; recurrent infections Stridor Cardiac anomalies
Down's syndrome (trisomy 21)	Hypotonia Mental retardation

	Duodenal atresia Airway problems Cardiac anomalies; often atrioventricular defects
Ebstein's anomaly	Congenital heart disease Tricuspid valve anomaly Severe dysrhythmias
Edward's syndrome (trisomy 18)	Most have heart disease Micrognathia Intubation difficulties
Ellis-van Creveld syndrome	Ectodermal defects; short extremities Congenital heart defects Poor lung function with chest abnormalities Abnormal maxilla Intubation difficulties
Epidermolysis bullosa	Bullae from minor skin trauma Some types very severe Care with face masks and intubation
Familial periodic paralysis	Weakness secondary to K^+ disturbance Care with muscle relaxants
Fanconi's anaemia	Pancytopenic anaemia Renal malformations Radial dysplasia—absent thumbs
Focal dermal hypoplasia (Goltz syndrome)	Papillomas of mucous membranes, especially of airway
Gangliosidosis, type I	Progressive neurological respiratory failure Early death
Glycogen storage disease: Types I-VIII (Cori's types):	Features include: 　Cardiac symptoms 　Hepatic symptoms: bleeding tendency 　Hypoglycaemia 　Skeletal muscles affected
I von Gierke's disease	Glucose-6-phosphatase deficiency Hypoglycaemia
II Pompe's disease	Massive cardiomegaly
III Cori's (Forbes') 　　disease	Hepatomegaly Hypotonia

Goldenhar syndrome	Mandibular hypoplasia—airway problems Congenital heart disease
Gorlin–Chaudry–Moss syndrome	Craniofacial dysostosis— difficult intubation Patent ductus arteriosus
Hallerman–Streiff syndrome	Mandibular hypoplasia Microphthalmia Glaucoma
Hermansky–Pudlak syndrome	Albinism Haemorrhagic disease
Holt–Oram syndrome	Radial dysplasia Congenital heart disease
Jervell–Lange-Nielsen syndrome (cardio-auditory)	Congenital deafness Cardiac conduction defects Sudden death
Jeune's syndrome (asphyxiating thoracic dystrophy)	Severe chest malformations— need mechanical ventilation Renal failure
Kasabach–Merritt syndrome	Haemangioma Thrombocytopenia
Kleeblattschädel	Clover leaf skull Facial abnormality Intubation difficulties
Klippel–Feil syndrome	Fusion of cervical vertebrae— difficult intubation Cleft palate
Klippel–Trenaunay–Weber syndrome	Haemangioma of whole limb Cardiac failure
Kneist syndrome	Dwarfism Cleft palate Limited joint movement
Larsen's syndrome	Congenital joint dislocations Hydrocephalus Subglottic stenosis

Leopard syndrome	Hypertelorism—intubation difficulties Congenital heart disease Pulmonary stenosis Hypospadias Kyphoscoliosis; respiratory failure later Dark spots on the skin
18-Long arm deletion	Mental retardation Cleft palate Long hands Cardiac anomalies
Maple syrup urine disease	No metabolism of leucine, isoleucine and valine Hypoglycaemia Neurological damage Acidotic episodes
Meckel's syndrome	Microcephaly, micrognathia, cleft epiglottis Heart disease Renal dysplasia
Moebius' syndrome	Paralysis of VI and VII cranial nerves Micrognathia—difficult intubation Lung damage with recurrent aspiration
Mucopolysaccharidoses: types I to VII including Hurler and Hunter syndromes (gargoylism)	Intubation difficulty Cardiorespiratory failure
Myasthenia congenita	No relaxants
Myotonia dystrophica	Weakness and myotonia Cardiac arrhythmias Respiratory failure Suxamethonium causes myotonia
Nager's syndrome	Afrofacial dysostosis Cleft palate Micrognathia Gastroschisis
Nesidioblastosis	See p. 79
Noack's syndrome	Craniosynostosis—intubation difficulties Anomalies of digits

Noonan's syndrome	Micrognathia Failure to develop Cardiac anomalies Renal dysfunction
Oppenheim's disease	Amyotonia congenita
Oral-facial-digital syndrome	Cleft palate Mandibular and maxillary hypoplasia Hydrocephalus Polycystic kidneys
Patau's syndrome (trisomy 13)	Microcephaly Micrognathia Ventricular septal defect Cleft palate Abnormal haemoglobins
Pfeiffer syndrome	Hypertelorism Craniosynostosis Syndactyly Intubation difficulties
Pierre Robin syndrome	Cleft palate Micrognathia and glossoptosis— intubation difficulties Congenital heart disease
Potter's syndrome	Renal agenesis (oligohydramnios) Typical facies—low-set ears Pulmonary hypoplasia
Prader-Willi syndrome	Hypotonia Hypoglycaemia Absent reflexes Poor respiratory effort
Prune belly syndrome	Absent abdominal musculature Poor respiratory effort Renal anomalies
Radial aplasia–thrombocytopenia	Absent radius Thrombocytopenia Cardiac defects
Respiratory distress syndrome	See p. 60
Reye's syndrome	Liver failure Encephalopathy Respiratory failure

Riley–Day syndrome
(familial dysautonomia)

Deficiency of dopamine-β-hydroxylase
Autonomic instability
Sensitivity to catecholamines
Recurrent aspiration to lungs

Ritter's disease

Toxic epidermal necrolysis
Staphylococcal infection
Very severe desquamation

Romano–Ward syndrome

Prolonged QT
Sudden heart block

Rubella syndrome

Mental retardation
Deafness
Cataract
Interstitial pneumonia
Osteolytic trabeculation in metaphyses
Cardiac anomalies, especially ventricular
septal defect

Russell–Silver syndrome

Low birth weight
Very large head
No hydrocephalus

Scimitar syndrome

Lung hypoplasia
Systemic arterial supply
Venous drainage to IVC

Short arm deletion syndromes
(rare chromosomal syndromes
4P, 18q, 21q, 22q)

Typical facies
Cleft palate
Heart disease
Poor prognosis

Smith–Lemli–Opitz syndrome

Microcephaly
Skeletal anomalies with hypotonia and
respiratory failure
Increased susceptibility to infection

Stickler syndrome

Micrognathia
Cleft palate
Retinal detachment

Sturge–Weber syndrome

Vascular naevus
Intracranial haemangioma

Tay–Sachs disease

Lipoidosis—infantile type
Mental, motor degeneration

Treacher-Collins syndrome	Micrognathia and choanal atresia—intubation difficulties Heart disease Deafness
Trisomy 22	Microcephaly Micrognathia Congenital heart disease Cleft palate
Turner's syndrome	XO females Webneck Micrognathia Congenital heart disease Renal anomaly
VATER syndrome	Vertebral anomalies Ventricular septal defect Anal atresia Tracheo-oesophageal fistula Radial dysplasia Renal anomalies
Werdnig-Hoffmann disease	Severe muscular atrophy Respiratory failure—resulting in early death
Williams syndrome (infantile hypercalcaemia syndrome	Mental retardation Coarse hair Aortic and pulmonary stenosis Characteristic facies
Wilson-Mikity syndrome	Prematurity Severe lung disease with fibrosis and cysts (aetiology unknown)
Wiskott-Aldrich syndrome	Thrombocytopenia Immunological deficiency Poor prognosis
Wolff-Parkinson-White syndrome	ECG shows prolonged QRS Paroxysmal tachycardia and other arrhythmias Effects accentuated by neostigmine
Wolman's disease	Failure to thrive Xanthomatous infiltration of heart, liver, etc.

Appendix II
Guidelines for drug dosage in paediatric anaesthetic practice

All drugs are given on the basis of body weight (kg)

Premedication

Atropine $0.02\,mg\cdot kg^{-1}$

> up to 2.5 kg   0.15 mg
> 2.5–8 kg   0.2 mg   i.m. $\frac{3}{4}$ hour preoperatively

Glycopyrrolate $0.004–0.008\,mg\cdot kg^{-1}$

Injection pethidine compound (Inj. Peth. Co.) $0.07\,ml\cdot kg^{-1}$ i.m. $\frac{3}{4}$ hour preoperatively. (Used only before open heart surgery in the neonate.)

> 1 ml contains: pethidine   25 mg
>   promethazine   6.25 mg
>   chlorpromazine   6.25 mg

For cardiac catheters, Peth. Co. up to $0.05\,ml\cdot kg^{-1}$ i.m. may be given $\frac{1}{2}$ hour before catheterization.

Anaesthetic agents   all are given intravenously unless stated otherwise

Thiopentone $2–4\,mg\cdot kg^{-1}$

Suxamethonium $1–2\,mg\cdot kg^{-1}$
                  $1\,mg\cdot kg^{-1}$ for intermittent use in neonates;
                  total dose up to 25 mg

Atracurium $0.5\,mg\cdot kg^{-1}$; dilute to $1\,mg\cdot ml^{-1}$
                  Infusion $8\mu g\cdot kg^{-1}\cdot min^{-1}$

260

Pancuronium	$0.06\,mg\cdot kg^{-1}$; dilute to $0.2\,mg\cdot ml^{-1}$
Tubocurarine	$0.2\,mg\cdot kg^{-1}$; dilute to $0.25\,mg\cdot ml^{-1}$
Vecuronium	$0.1\,mg\cdot kg^{-1}$; dilute to $0.4\,mg\cdot ml^{-1}$ Infusion $1.5\,\mu g\cdot kg^{-1}\cdot min^{-1}$

Ketamine:
| induction | $2\,mg\cdot kg^{-1}$ i.v. (or $10mg\cdot kg^{-1}$ i.m.) |
| maintenance | $1\,mg\cdot kg^{-1}$ i.v. |

Reversal

Atropine and neostigmine:
| atropine | $0.025\,mg\cdot kg^{-1}$ |
| neostigmine | $0.05\,mg\cdot kg^{-1}$ |

| Glycopyrrolate | $0.01\,mg\cdot kg^{-1}$ |

Analgesics   intraoperative—for cardiac anaesthesia only

Pethidine	$1\,mg\cdot kg^{-1}$ (maximum dose)
Morphine	$0.2\,mg\cdot kg^{-1}$; up to $1\,mg\cdot kg^{-1}$ total dose for open heart surgery
Fentanyl	Up to $10\,\mu g\cdot kg^{-1}$

Antibiotics   by i.m. or i.v. injection

Ampicillin	Up to $50\,mg\cdot kg^{-1}$	6-hourly for severe infections
Cloxacillin	$12.5\,mg\cdot kg^{-1}$	6-hourly
Erythromycin	$12.5\,mg\cdot kg^{-1}$	8-hourly
Cephalothin	$25\,mg\cdot kg^{-1}$	6-hourly
Gentamicin	$2\,mg\cdot kg^{-1}$	8-hourly
Metronidazole	$7.5\,mg\cdot kg^{-1}$	6-hourly i.v.
Penicillin	$25\,mg\cdot kg^{-1}$	6-hourly

Other drugs   by i.v. injection unless stated otherwise

| Chlorpromazine | 1 mg increments up to $0.5\,mg\cdot kg^{-1}$ |
| Dexamethasone | $0.25\,mg\cdot kg^{-1}$ i.v., then $0.1\,mg\cdot kg^{-1}$ 6-hourly i.m. for three doses
For cerebral oedema, up to $0.5\,mg\cdot kg^{-1}$ |

Digoxin	Total digitalizing dose: $0.05\,mg\cdot kg^{-1}$
	one-third stat
	one-third 4–6 hours
	one-third 8–12 hours
	Maintenance: one-tenth digitalizing dose b.i.d.
	For premature babies, total dose: $0.03\,mg\cdot kg^{-1}$

Droperidol $0.3\,mg\cdot kg^{-1}$

Frusemide $1\,mg\cdot kg^{-1}$, repeatable

Hydrocortisone $1\,mg\cdot kg^{-1}$

Indomethacin $0.2\,mg\cdot kg^{-1}$

Labetalol $0.2\,mg\cdot kg^{-1}$ increments up to $1\,mg\cdot kg^{-1}$

Lignocaine $1\,mg\cdot kg^{-1}$ (maximum dose $3\,mg\cdot kg^{-1}$)

Mannitol   Test dose: $0.5\,g\cdot kg^{-1}$

Methoxamine   Dilution to $0.5\,mg\cdot ml^{-1}$; careful increments of $0.25\,mg$ to achieve desired result

Methylpred- $30\,mg\cdot kg^{-1}$
nisolone

Naloxone $10\,\mu g\cdot kg^{-1}$

Phentolamine   Dilution to $1\,mg\cdot ml^{-1}$; increments of $0.5\,mg$ for desired result

Practolol   Dilution to $1\,mg\cdot ml^{-1}$; increments of $0.5\,mg$; maximum dose $0.5\,mg\cdot kg^{-1}$

Propranolol   Dilution to $0.1\,mg\cdot ml^{-1}$; increments of $0.05\,mg$; maximum dose $0.1\,mg\cdot kg^{-1}$

Prostacycline 4–$20\,nanog\cdot kg^{-1}$; min^{-1}

Prostaglandin E_1 $30\,\mu g\cdot kg^{-1}$ in 50 ml 5% dextrose $1\,ml\cdot h^{-1}$
or E_2

Sodium $3\,mg\cdot kg^{-1}$ in 100 ml of 5% dextrose. Do not exceed
nitroprusside 1–$1.5\,mg\cdot kg^{-1}$ total dose in 24 hours

Theophylline $6\,mg\cdot kg^{-1}$

Tolazoline 1–$2\,mg\cdot kg^{-1}$ over 3 minutes; then infuse the same dose hourly

Postoperative agents   NO ROUTINE ANALGESIA IS NECESSARY IN THE NEONATE

Codeine phosphate $1\,mg\cdot kg^{-1}$ Do NOT give i.v. because it causes a severe fall in cardiac output

Fentanyl	Infusion $100\mu g \cdot kg^{-1}$ in 50 ml 5% dextrose
	$2 \text{ ml} \cdot hr^{-1} = 4 \mu g \cdot kg^{-1} \min^{-1}$

Pethidine	$1 \text{ mg} \cdot kg^{-1}$	i.m. or i.v.	TO BE USED
Papaveretum	$0.2 \text{ mg} \cdot kg^{-1}$	i.m. or i.v.	ONLY FOR PATIENTS ON
Morphine	$0.2 \text{ mg} \cdot kg^{-1}$	i.m. or i.v.	VENTILATORS
	Infusion $\frac{1}{2} \text{ mg} \cdot kg^{-1}$ in 50 ml		
	5% dextrose run at $2 \text{ ml} \cdot h^{-1}$		

Phenobarbitone	$1\text{--}2 \text{ mg} \cdot kg^{-1}$	i.m. to control seizures (4-hourly if necessary)

Diazepam	$0.2 \text{ mg} \cdot kg^{-1}$	orally	
Triclofos elixir	$30 \text{mg} \cdot kg^{-1}$	orally	or via nasogastric tube
Syrup of chloral	$30 \text{ mg} \cdot kg^{-1}$	orally	4-hourly if necessary
Promethazine	$0.5\text{--}1 \text{ mg} \cdot kg^{-1}$	orally	

Inotropic agents — DILUTIONS ONLY ARE GIVEN. The effect of administration must be monitored. The strength may be increased if fluid restriction is necessary. Start at a rate of 5–10 microdrops per minute ($= 5\text{--}10 \text{ ml} \cdot h^{-1}$)

Adrenaline	Up to 1 mg in 100 ml of 5% dextrose (1 ml of 1:1000 contains 1 mg)
Isoprenaline	Up to 1 mg in 100 ml of 5% dextrose
Dobutamine	$6 \text{ mg} \cdot kg^{-1}$ in 100 ml 5% dextrose
	$1 \text{ ml} \cdot h^{-1} \equiv 1 \mu g \cdot kg^{-1} \cdot \min^{-1}$
Dopamine	$6 \text{ mg} \cdot kg^{-1}$ in 100 ml 5% dextrose
	$1 \text{ ml} \cdot h^{-1} \equiv 1 \mu g \cdot kg^{-1} \cdot \min^{-1}$
	At a dose not exceeding $10 \mu g \cdot kg^{-1} \cdot \min^{-1}$ there is little α-adrenergic activity.
Salbutamol	2.5–5 mg in 100 ml of 5% dextrose; 3–5 microdrops as an initial dose

Drugs used in cardiopulmonary resuscitation

Adrenaline (1:10 000)	$0.1 \text{ ml} \cdot kg^{-1}$	into central vein
Atropine	$0.03 \text{ mg} \cdot kg^{-1}$	i.v.
Calcium chloride (10%)	$0.25 \text{ ml} \cdot kg^{-1}$	into central vein
Dexamethasone	$0.25 \text{ mg} \cdot kg^{-1}$	i.v. 6-hourly
Diazepam	$0.2 \text{ mg} \cdot kg^{-1}$	i.v.
Sodium bicarbonate (8.4%)	$1 \text{ ml} \cdot kg^{-1}$	i.v.; then perform blood gas analysis

Appendix III
Normal physiological values in the neonate and adult

	Neonate	**Adult**
Hb	$18–25\,g\cdot dl^{-1}$	$15\,g\cdot dl^{-1}$
Haematocrit (PCV)	50–60 per cent	45 per cent
Blood volume	$70–125\,ml\cdot kg^{-1}$	$70\,ml\cdot kg^{-1}$
Extracellular fluid (percentage of body weight)	35 per cent	20 per cent
Water turnover per 24 hours (percentage of body weight)	15 per cent	9 per cent
Serum K^+	$5–8\,mmol\cdot l^{-1}$	$3–5\,mmol\cdot l^{-1}$
Na^+	$136–143\,mmol\cdot l^{-1}$	$135–148\,mmol\cdot l^{-1}$
Cl^-	$96–107\,mmol\cdot l^{-1}$	$98–106\,mmol\cdot l^{-1}$
HCO	$20\,mmol\cdot l^{-1}$	$24\,mmol\cdot l^{-1}$
Blood urea nitrogen	$1.3–3.3\,mmol\cdot l^{-1}$	$6.6–8.6\,mmol\cdot l^{-1}$
pH	7.35	7.40
Pa_{CO_2}	$4.7\,kPa$ $(35\,mmHg)$	$4.7–6.0\,kPa$ $(35–45\,mmHg)$
Pa_{O_2}	$8.7–10.7\,kPa$ $(65–80\,mmHg)$	$10.7–12.7\,kPa$ $(80–95\,mmHg)$
Base excess	−5	0
Total bilirubin	$100\,\mu mol\cdot l^{-1}$	$2–14\,\mu mol\cdot l^{-1}$
Total Ca^{2+}	$1.48–2.68\,mmol\cdot l^{-1}$	$2.13–2.6\,mmol\cdot l^{-1}$
Mg^{2+}	$0.7–1.1\,mmol\cdot l^{-1}$	$0.6–1.0\,mmol\cdot^{-1}$
Phosphate	$1.15–2.8\,mmol\cdot l^{-1}$	$1.0–1.4\,mmol\cdot l^{-1}$
Glucose	$2.7–3.3\,mmol\cdot l^{-1}$	$2.4–5.3\,mmol\cdot l^{-1}$
Total proteins	$46–74\,g\cdot l^{-1}$	$60–80\,g\cdot l^{-1}$
Albumin	$36–54\,g\cdot l^{-1}$	$35–47\,g\cdot l^{-1}$
Serum osmolality	$270–285\,mmol\cdot l^{-1}$	$270–285\,mmol\cdot l^{-1}$
Urine osmolality	$50–600\,mmol\cdot l^{-1}$	$50–1400\,mmol\cdot l^{-1}$
Na^+	$50\,mmol\cdot l^{-1}$	$30\,mmol\cdot l^{-1}$
Specific gravity	1005–1020	1005–1035

Index